Sarah Litvinoff has .... relationships for 15 years. Working closely with sex therapists and relationship counsellors she wrote three major guides for Relate, the British counselling and sex therapy service. These self-help guides have become standard reference works for professionals, and have been translated into a number of languages. In conjunction with a counsellor, she writes a monthly column, *Couples Counsel*, for *She* magazine, and was a former problem-page editor. She has also acted as consultant editor on a number of projects, including *Enjoy Satisfying Relationships* (published by Time Life). She is regularly invited to contribute to television and radio programmes on relationship issues.

Over the years she has become aware that although differences in sexual tastes are mentioned anecdotally by practitioners and in sexual literature, they have not been looked at systematically. She believes that for the majority of sexually well-functioning people, who are otherwise compatible, a clash of Sexual Styles is the single greatest cause of potential sexual problems.

Also by Sarah Litvinoff

Working Mother: A practical handbook for the 90s, co-author with Marianne Velmans (Simon & Schuster, 1993)
The Relate Guide to Better Relationships (Vermilion, 1991)
The Relate Guide to Sex in Loving Relationships (Vermilion, 1992)
The Relate Guide to Starting Again (Vermilion, 1993)

What's Your Sexual Style?

Solve the mysteries of attraction, love and sex by identifying your sexual personality

Sarah Litvinoff

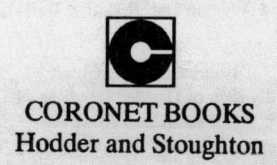

CORONET BOOKS
Hodder and Stoughton

Copyright © 1996 by Sarah Litvinoff

The right of Sarah Litvinoff to be identified as the Author of
the Work has been asserted by her in accordance with the
Copyright, Designs and Patents Act 1988.

First published in Great Britain in 1996 by Hodder & Stoughton
A division of Hodder Headline PLC

A Coronet paperback

10 9 8 7 6 5 4 3 2 1

All rights reserved. No part of this publication may be
reproduced, stored in a retrieval system, or transmitted,
in any form or by any means without the prior written
permission of the publisher, nor be otherwise circulated
in any form of binding or cover other than that in which
it is published and without a similar condition being
imposed on the subsequent purchaser.

A CIP catalogue record for this title is available from
the British Library

ISBN 0 340 68177 2

Printed and bound in Great Britain by
Cox & Wyman Ltd, Reading, Berkshire

Hodder and Stoughton
A division of Hodder Headline PLC
338 Euston Road
London NW1 3BH

For my Romantic, Sensual, Imaginative and Emotional loved ones, family and friends. You know who you are.

Acknowledgements

I would like to thank all the counsellors and sex therapists who have given me the benefit of their experience and told me case histories. Special thanks to Zelda West-Meads, who encouraged me when this book was just an idea, and throughout the writing of it. I would also like to thank all the friends and acquaintances I have talked to about their relationships over the years, whose real stories have helped me consolidate the theories and add missing bits to the jigsaw.

I have had great help and moral support from a number of people close to me: Lisa Eveleigh, more a friend than an agent, who makes me feel that what I write matters; my great friends, Lynn Picknett, who first commissioned me to write about relationships, and Jane Lyle, who gave me examples from her encyclopaedic knowledge of movies for this book; my mother, Cherry, who, as ever, read every word in progress, and whose comments are always relevant; my sister, Vida, whose love, enthusiasm and concern supported me through the good and bad times during writing; my daughter Jemilah, who understood the theory better than anyone, and helped me through our discussions and her own insights.

Contents

Discovering Your Sexual Style — 1

The Romantic Woman — 23
'This time I know it's the real thing.'

The Romantic Man — 49
'Desire dies because every touch consumes the myth ...'

The Romantic Combinations — 75

The Sensual Woman — 93
'Some creatures simply *die* if unmated.'

The Sensual Man — 121
'Those who restrain Desire, do so because theirs is weak enough to be restrained.'

The Sensual Combinations — 147

The Imaginative Woman — 167
'The brain is clearly the central erogenous zone for me, and he's got a big one.'

The Imaginative Man — 193
'The sensation of having "arrived" has never been a comfortable thing for me. Flirting with a woman has always been more exciting than *being* with a woman.'

The Imaginative Combinations — 219

The Emotional Woman — 237
'Anger and jealousy can no more bear to lose sight of their objects than love.'

Contents

The Emotional Man — 265
'I hate and love. You may ask why I do so. I do not know, but I feel it and am in torment.'

The Emotional Combinations — 293

Sexual Styles in Relationships — 311

The Romantic Man and Woman — 315
'I knew it was love, and I felt it was glory.'

The Sensual Man and Woman — 335
'The deep, deep peace of the double-bed after the hurly-burly of the chaise-longue.'

The Imaginative Man and Woman — 355
'There's a cool web of language winds us in,/Retreat from too much joy or too much fear.'

The Emotional Man and Woman — 375
'Love alters not with his brief hours and weeks,/But bears it out even to the edge of doom.'

The Romantic and The Sensual — 395
'I slept and dreamed that life was beauty/I woke and found that life was duty.'

The Emotional and The Imaginative — 415
'It has been well said, that heart speaks to heart, whereas language only speaks to the ears.'

The Imaginative and The Romantic — 437
'Come live with me, and be my love,/And we will some new pleasures prove/Of golden sands, and crystal brooks,/With silken lines, and silver hooks.'

The Emotional and The Sensual — 459
'Dumb swans, not chattering pies, do lovers prove;/They love indeed who quake to say they love.'

The Imaginative and The Sensual — 479
'For God's sake hold your tongue, and let me love.'

The Emotional and The Romantic — 499
'Now laughing friends deride tears I cannot hide.'

Discovering Your Sexual Style

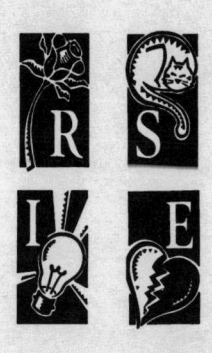

relationship with someone who has a different world view, different values, different pleasure principles, a different attitude to things that cause pain, then the result can be anguish and misunderstanding. Carl Jung, the psychologist, said that we tend to make judgements and assessments of other people based on our own perceptions and 'rules'. He says, 'People are profoundly astonished, or even horrified, when this rule quite obviously does not fit — when they discover that another person really is different from themselves. Generally speaking, they do not feel these psychic differences as in any way curious, let alone attractive, but as disagreeable failings that are hard to bear, or as unendurable faults that have to be condemned.' In other words a problem can arise when both people are quite 'normal' and consistent, but different.

So many people measure the health of their sexuality by the sexual behaviour of others. How often? With whom? Where? In what way? Never has so much sexual information and advice been so freely available, nor sex so graphically represented in the media. But there has not been a corresponding increase in sexual happiness and satisfaction. People still doubt or disregard their own feelings in favour of what 'everyone else' thinks, does — or says they do.

Sexual Style is not just individual. There is a prevailing sexual climate that influences the thinking and actions of people in society. Recently, in the West, this has been the do-anything-with-anyone-try-everything-once Style that I classify as Imaginative. Its hallmark, apart from variety and experimentation, is that sex is above all fun — and, so long as there is no coercion, sex need have no emotional significance, either in creating pain or love. If your Sexual Style is mainly Imaginative, you feel normal, healthy, and in tune. But what if it's not? There are many walking wounded who embraced the idea of 'free love' and found that, for them, it had a heavy emotional price.

When society's message is so strong it can cause insecurity

in the most unexpected people. I once interviewed a respected sex therapist who was nearing the end of a long and successful career. There was nothing she did not know about sexuality in theory or in practice. She had helped hundreds of individuals and couples improve their sex lives. She had had a long and happy marriage herself, which was clearly still sexually alive and satisfying. She had, as a young woman in more sexually reserved times, even had love affairs when sex before marriage was frowned on. Yet, she told me, in the late Sixties and Seventies, when the sexual revolution reached the pages of women's magazines, she wondered whether there was something wrong with her. Nothing she read shocked her, but she realised that there were many things she had never done sexually, and never wanted to do. Was she missing out? She didn't want three in a bed, an open marriage, a lesbian lover. Did it mean she was repressed?

I knew what she meant. I had been a teenager during those years, and even more painfully haunted by those questions. I was the last of my friends to lose my virginity – did it mean I was frigid? I read the magazines and the books, saw the movies, and knew every sexual possibility and permutation before I'd even kissed a boy. I was too embarrassed to admit to being a virgin when I first made love and was in a state of anxiety that I might betray my inexperience. Later, I realised with great relief that I was 'normal'. When I felt desire and love everything fell into place sexually. Even so, doubts lingered. 'Everyone' said that 'everyone was bisexual to a degree'. As it happens, I'd never felt sexually attracted to a woman. Was it, perhaps, fear or repression? It took me many years through my work writing about sexuality and relationships to accept that what 'everyone' said and did was irrelevant to me – to anyone. My own feelings, impulses and sensations were what counted.

I think the sexual climate is changing – the change heralded by the advent of AIDS. But whatever changes occur, they are going to make some people feel odd or left out. It will be the turn of the Imaginatives to question their own impulses and wonder if there is something 'wrong' with them.

In Victorian times sensuality was considered base. A woman with a natural liking for sex was thought to be abnormal. It was conceded that men had urgent drives, but self-control was judged the mark of a more civilised and honourable person. People whose Sexual Style was more Sensual than anything else felt ashamed and, sometimes, evil. In *The Making of Victorian Sexual Attitudes*, Michael Mason describes a climate I would classify as Emotional. He argues that Victorian high-mindedness was based on a belief that sex should be 'holy', an expression of all that was noble and ethical.

The pure Sensual culture is rarer but, as *Marie Claire* magazine described it in 1995, the island of Tonga is representative of the Style as I define it. Convention and stability combine with an earthy enjoyment of the range of sensual pleasures. The Tongan attitude to relationships is down-to-earth: 'I have asked them what a boy looks for in a girl,' reported a Tongan sociologist. 'The answer is someone who stays home, who behaves properly and has a nice face and personality. Likewise if you ask the girls what they look for in a boy, they want one who goes to church, who behaves properly.' This is not inconsistent with a love of pleasure. In 1995 there was a government-sponsored national competition to encourage Tongans to lose weight. They love their food, and both sexes prefer generously proportioned partners with abundant flesh. Pastimes are frankly lazy – sleeping is listed as a favourite activity.

The Romantics have held sway too, most notably in the Middle Ages. In Andrew the Clerk's *De Arte Honest Amandi*, written around 1170, he sets out 31 rules of love that reflect the atmosphere of the times: 'Nobody can have two simultaneous attachments; The ease with which one obtains physical solaces diminishes their value, whereas difficulties and obstacles serve to increase it; Once true love decreases, it soon ends: it rarely recovers its lost strength; When lovers marry love is violently put to flight,' and so on. Yet in other times and other places these 'rules' were considered ridiculous. I once watched a documentary about a tribe that had no concept of romantic love. One poor man, a classic Romantic, had conceived an intense romantic passion for a young girl and he became an object of ridicule and disdain.

That's why I wanted to write this book. If you can understand and respect your own Sexual Style you are less likely to feel odd in a society that presents another Sexual Style as the norm. What your friend does need no longer cause soul-searching when it conflicts with your own feelings and behaviour. If your lover's Sexual Style is different you can begin to work creatively with the differences, rather than think that one of you is wrong, or should change.

Of course, the variety of Sexual Styles is infinite. So complex are the ingredients that go to make up each person's sexual tastes that there are as many Styles as there are individuals. So, is it causing more problems than it solves to identify only four main Sexual Styles? I don't think so. Within this rich diversity of tastes there are basic characteristics – determining factors that establish where fundamental sexual pleasure is to be found, and where the seeds of potential problems lie.

This division by four is not a new concept. In 5th century BC Greece the theory was advanced that everything (animate and inanimate, including human temperament) is made up of the four elements: fire, earth, air and water. This influenced much thinking, including medical, for many centuries thereafter. Most people are aware of it in astrology, where the 12 signs are grouped into these elements: Aries, Leo and Sagittarius are fire signs; Taurus, Virgo and Capricorn are earth signs; Gemini, Libra and Aquarius are air signs; and Pisces, Cancer and Scorpio are water signs.

But this elemental division had more mainstream proponents. Doctors would treat people according to their mixture of

Melancholic (water), Phlegmatic (earth), Sanguine (air), and Choleric (fire). In more recent times, Jung looked freshly at these categories in his book *Psychological Types*. He redefined them as Thinking (air), Feeling (water), Sensation (earth) and Intuition (fire). Sexual Styles, as I define them, are also fairly close to the elements, although there are differences: Romantic (fire), Emotional (water), Sensual (earth) and Imaginative (air).

What I am saying is probably closest to Stendhal, the 19th century novelist, who proposed four categories of love: Passionate (water), Friendly (air), Vain (fire) and Physical (earth). This is because I am not necessarily talking about the whole person, but concentrating on *Sexual* Style. In other words, that part of your personality that affects your sexuality and your attitude to love. There are, of course, some 'pure' types, for whom every aspect of their behaviour, personality and sexuality are consistent – and I have looked at these Sexual Styles in detail. But many people are a mixture, with a bit of this and a bit of that, in differing quantities and combinations. It's a little like the mix of genes. Two children from the same parents can turn out very differently – one has her mother's looks and her father's brains, the other has it the other way round. One person may be a mix of Romantic and Sensual, but it is expressed somewhat differently from his friend who also has the same combination.

In your relationships it is your Sexual Style that matters – the way you approach sex, what love means to you, how you function in long-term relationships. For instance, you might have the Sensual's earthy attitude to food and the need for stability, the questing restlessness of the Imaginative in your career, but if your Sexual Style is Romantic you will always feel the need for your relationships to be magical, out-of-the-ordinary and intense. Sometimes Sexual Style 'breaks through', such as in your attitude to food and drink, or the clothes you wear, or how you like to spend your leisure time. That's why it can be possible to pick up clues to another person's Sexual Style, even when you know nothing about his or her love life.

People often turn to popular astrology books to tell them in what way they are different from others. But these books can disappoint. Suppose you were born with the sun in Cancer. You look yourself up and find that some of it fits, but much of it doesn't. That is because astrology is far more complex than these books are able to show. Yes, you might be a watery Cancerean, but a closer look at your chart reveals many key planets in earth or fire, or planets in 'airy' houses. Some of your personality reflects your watery sun, but what affects your emotions and your sexuality can be quite different. Serious astrologers despair when astrology is dismissed as nonsense by people who only know about it through astrological columns in newspapers or sun-sign books. I'm interested in astrology, and have often been able to see why a person born in the fiery sign of Leo, say, has a love-life which is much more like an earthy Taurean. But not always. There are so many other things to consider: the angles planets make with each other, for instance. And people 'live' their charts differently. Two people with very similar charts can express one part of it more than another, and so end up appearing quite unalike. In the final analysis, only you know what you feel, how you behave, your likes and dislikes, and so on.

That's why this book asks *you* to decide which Sexual Style you are, based on your knowledge of yourself. The questionnaire that follows can help you decide which Style is most like your own. There is no substitute, however, for reading the sections on the individual Sexual Styles to see the examples of famous, fictional, and ordinary people, and how they feel and operate in relationships. It helps in knowing which Style you are if you have had some years of experience of loving and living with others. Sometimes your fantasies of what you think you want in a relationship, how you will behave, and what you will put up with, turn out to be very different from the reality. In

Discovering Your Sexual Style

a way, your Sexual Style becomes most apparent when the going gets tough. Most people want it all when it comes to relationships – the excitement of romance, the physical rewards of satisfying sex, a relationship that is emotionally compelling and intellectually satisfying. And when you are first in love you put up with a lot, and dismiss nagging doubts.

But there is a bottom-line tendency which is often easier to see in a relationship that has settled down, or is going wrong: what makes you finally snap? The Romantic finds it hard when a relationship loses its quality of magical specialness. The Sensual can put up with this so long as life is comfortable and there is regular physical contact. The Emotional finds this hollow unless there is a continuing strong emotional bond – not necessarily a happy one. The Imaginative finds routine unbearable, but lack of verbal communication even worse. These are broad generalisations, and the more subtle manifestations are explored further within each section.

What sexual style are you?

Look at the following statements and select the one that comes *nearest* to your own feelings. It is best to complete the questionnaire when you are alone – you can be affected by what another person answers, or what you think that person would like you to say. You may prefer to note down your answers on a separate sheet of paper, rather than in the book.

1 The most important ingredient in love is: ✓
a An exciting meeting of minds: you find each other fascinating. ☐
b High passion: thrilling and compelling. ☐
c Complete identification with each other, deeper than words. ☐

Sexual Styles

d   Profound contentment generally and specifically sexually. ☐

2 Long lasting love needs: ✓
a   To be based on more than sex: ideas, interests in common, shared experiences. ☐
b   Continuing romantic feelings: never taking each other for granted. ☐
c   An enduring emotional connection that goes beyond feelings of contentment. ☐
d   Sexual satisfaction and a feeling of well-being when you are together. ☐

3 Love at first sight is: ✓
a   A mixture of lust and infatuation that has little to do with real love. ☐
b   Essential: without an instant attraction real love won't develop. ☐
c   A recognition of a deeper emotional connection. ☐ ☐
d   Sexual attraction – it can last if you turn out to be sexually suited. ☐

4 If a relationship has a lot of emotional turmoil you feel: ✓
a   Exasperated and unloving – it is uncivilised and gets you nowhere. ☐
b   Threatened – but as long as you also show you love each other you put up with it. ☐
c   It shows the depth of your feelings for each other. ☐
d   You don't like it – too much is a sign of incompatibility. ☐

5 A relationship that is predictable and settled makes you feel: ✓
a   Bored and restless, possibly trapped. ☐

Discovering Your Sexual Style

b Uneasy; unhappy if the romance has gone as well. ☐
c Secure – you feel you have truly merged. ☐
d Content and in control. ☐

6 When you are totally delighted with each other and can think of no one else you feel: ✓

a It's a wonderful stage, but it will soon pass and may even die. ☐
b This is the best it gets – you hope it will last. ☐
c Love should be like this, but deeper love is different. ☐
d It's exciting but unsettling, love will feel more real when it becomes less intense. ☐

7 Talking about problems in the relationship is: ✓

a The only way to deal with them – it brings you closer. ☐
b Possibly a help, but problems are a sign that love is on the way out. ☐
c Difficult – it doesn't touch the feelings involved. ☐
d Irritating – a good cuddle or good sex is more healing. ☐

8 Sex with someone new is: ✓

a Intensely exciting and erotic, whoever it is. ☐
b Intoxicating when you have fallen in love. ☐
c A big step. ☐
d A try-out for the future. ☐

9 If you are a woman and sex with someone you like turns out to be a one-night-stand you feel: ✓

a It was very exciting anyway. It would have been nice to see him again, but you don't feel too disturbed. ☐
b Humiliated. Your confidence takes a knock. Weren't you good or attractive enough? ☐
c Upset and betrayed. Sex is so intimate that you feel your whole self was rejected, not just your body. ☐

Sexual Styles

d Disappointed. One-off sex can never be as satisfying as when you get to know each other's bodies. ☐

10 If you are a man and you have a one-night-stand you feel: ✓

a It was very exciting, whether the sex was good or not. It couldn't have been bettered by seeing her again. ☐
b You enjoyed it for what it was, but it would have been more exciting if you had felt more for her. ☐
c The sex was fine, but you feel vaguely disgusted with her or yourself. ☐
d Having sex made you feel great, but the experience could be spoilt if the sex wasn't especially good. ☐

11 Trying new positions and new ways to make love is: ✓

a Essential if sex is to remain erotic. ☐
b Good to a degree, but only if it is spontaneous and not contrived. ☐
c Irrelevant – it's what you feel for each other that makes sex satisfying. ☐
d Good for finding out what you like, but not beyond that. ☐

12 In a relationship that lasts many years, the sex: ✓

a Is bound to become boring. ☐
b Must be kept exciting with mystery and romance. ☐
c Might become less frequent, but will remain good so long as you feel deeply. ☐
d Matures like fine wine, becoming even *better* if your sexual tastes are similar. ☐

13 To keep sex good you must: ✓

a Be prepared to talk about it and not slip into a routine. ☐

Discovering Your Sexual Style

b   Show how much you love each other all the time. ☐
c   Continue to feel profoundly connected emotionally. ☐
d   Make love often, and take your time. ☐

14 As a woman, you are more likely to be attracted to a man who is not good-looking if: ✓
a   You find him fascinating to talk to. ☐
b   You admire him. ☐
c   You feel that you 'know' him, even if you've just met. ☐
d   There's a sexual chemistry between you and you desire him. ☐

15 As a man, you are more likely to be attracted to a woman who is not good-looking if: ✓
a   She is a good conversationalist or witty. ☐
b   She has style. ☐
c   You are emotionally touched by her. ☐
d   Something about her physically turns you on. ☐

16 Sexually, a good body and good looks are: ✓
a   An initial attraction, but fail to be noticeable after a while. ☐
b   Enhancing to the experience. Both of you should continue to look good. ☐
c   Irrelevant compared to your emotional interaction. ☐
d   Attractive, but not necessary. How you make each other feel sexually counts more. ☐

17 What is your reaction to the statement 'you can learn to love someone you weren't attracted to at the outset'? ✓
a   It's possible when you spark each other off mentally and have mutual interests. ☐
b   It won't be a great love without that initial passion. ☐

Sexual Styles

c It can be even more enduring when you get to know the 'real' person first. ☐
d If you discover you are sexually suited love can grow. ☐

18 Sex without love: ✓
a Is just as good, and sometimes more exciting. ☐
b Is less thrilling. ☐
c Cheapens relationships. ☐
d Can be just as good – but when it is, love may follow. ☐

19 Love without sex: ✓
a There's no essential connection – love is sometimes more intense without it. ☐
b Is perfectly possible, but somewhat worrying. ☐
c Is perfectly possible, and doesn't affect the quality of the love. ☐
d Diminishes over time. ☐

20 A relationship thrives when: ✓
a You can operate independently, and interest each other. ☐
b You continue to make each other feel special. ☐
c You feel so bonded you can't imagine life apart. ☐
d You feel physically satisfied and comfortable together. ☐

21 When you no longer feel a pressing need to talk to each other you feel: ✓
a Bored and unhappy. ☐
b Neglected. ☐
c It doesn't matter, the important feelings don't need words. ☐
d Content, as long as there is no hostility. ☐

22 Sexual fantasies are: ✓
a A great turn-on, especially when shared. ☐

Discovering Your Sexual Style

b Enjoyable when they are yours, less so when they are your lover's. ☐
c Powerful and sometimes disturbing. ☐
d Usually rooted in experiences you have had. ☐

23 Talking about sex: ✓
a Can occasionally be more erotic than love-making. ☐
b Takes away the spontaneity. ☐
c Is difficult – the feelings are beyond words. ☐
d Is a poor substitute for doing it. ☐

24 If you are not in the mood for sex, you can be turned on by: ✓
a A thrilling, stimulating conversation, or an unusual sexual approach. ☐
b Being treated in a romantic way. ☐
c Feeling intensely moved by your partner. ☐
d Being cuddled, and caressed in ways that you like best. ☐

25 Intimacy is: ✓
a Constant conversation and sharing ideas. ☐
b Constant displays of love and affection. ☐
c Feeling needed and possessed. ☐
d Satisfying love-making, and physical closeness. ☐

Your sexual style rating

The **a** answers are Imaginative, **b** answers Romantic, **c** answers Emotional and **d** answers Sensual.

If you have most in one category – more than half, say – then you can be fairly sure that this is your dominant Sexual Style. If two categories run close, then you are likely to be one version of that combination. For instance, you might have nine Sensual answers and eight Emotional answers. You may well be a SENSUAL-Emotional, but if you often hesitated between the two, you could be an EMOTIONAL-Sensual – the elements are the same, but are expressed differently according to whichever is the stronger. Reading both of these categories will give you a better idea which one you are.

If your answers were evenly distributed through the four Sexual Styles, then you might be a combination, but one will predominate even though this wasn't made obvious by answering the questions. You will have a better idea which is most like you when you read the chapters devoted to each Sexual Style. Looking at the combinations at the end of each chapter will give you further insights into how these combinations might be expressed in your relationships.

But questionnaires are never completely reliable. Sometimes you can't help answering in the way you think you should, or as you would prefer to answer. Answers can also be unreliable because, sometimes, we don't know ourselves as well as we think we do – and how we behave in a situation is very different from our imaginings beforehand. By their very nature, questionnaires are simplistic: in real life the choices aren't so stark or exclusive – how you behave can depend on your mood, and so can how you answer.

For all these reasons, regard your results as a rough guide. It can't be emphasised enough that the most reliable way to check out your Sexual Style is to read them all, to see which one corresponds most closely to your own experience.

The Sexual Styles in brief

The following explanations give the main characteristics of each style, sexually and emotionally. The individual chapters explain more fully the subtleties, and how they are expressed in relationships.

Discovering Your Sexual Style

The Romantic

The essence of romance is that you feel special, and are convinced of the specialness of your partner. For the Romantic this is essential to release the catch on sexuality. While many Romantics love the traditional romantic hallmarks of flowers and candlelight, particularly Romantic women, none of these matter so much as the certain knowledge of being all-important, or of feeling that the partner is uniquely wonderful. Romantics can adore the physical side of sex, can be highly sexed and sexually expert, but none of this is satisfying in itself. The Romantic woman will feel 'cheap' when sex is casual, the Romantic man will despise casual sexual partners. Being 'in love' is the greatest aphrodisiac for Romantics, as it is for many people. But, unlike the other Sexual Styles, the Romantic doesn't usually find more 'ordinary' love a turn-on — nor does quiet compatibility substitute for heady rapture. Sexual variety, once the romance has gone, won't revive flagging sexual interest.

Emotionally, Romantics are volatile and dramatic, and show their feelings easily. To love, they need to adore or be adored, preferably both. They are great flirts, but are very jealous — they need to know they are the best loved of all, and are the best in bed. Love for them doesn't depend on 'liking', but it does need to feel compelling and important. Too much domestic intimacy destroys their illusions, and the magic. When these go, so does love — and the Romantic yearns to rediscover the wonder with someone else.

The Sensual

For this Sexual Style the bodily sensations are all-important. The feel of skin, the texture of flesh, the nature of the caresses, the preferred sexual positions and acts, the intensity of orgasm — these are the essential characteristics. While all of this is important to every sexual being, for the Sensual these elements are paramount. When they are right nothing else matters: not love, atmosphere, compatibility nor occasion. What does it *feel* like? That's what counts. They often give their hearts to a partner who suits them profoundly on a sexual level. The Sensual man or woman is not necessarily more sexy, more sexually active, or better at sex than the other Sexual Styles, but the physical sensations are more important than anything else. This can make them quite selfish and demanding sexually, though they can learn to enjoy long, slow love-making that is mutually satisfying. The Sensual type can be quite promiscuous when young – 'if it feels good, do it' – but they prefer to find a compatible partner and settle down together for life.

Emotionally, Sensuals are realists. The here and now is what matters: if it is pleasant and satisfying they are supremely content. If it is not, they can be quite stoical, but may feel depressed. Sensuals like to feel secure, so stability in relationships is important to them. They are not emotionally demonstrative or demanding, and prefer a calm emotional atmosphere. Warmth, comfort and tolerance are more important to them in a relationship than excitement or romance.

The Imaginative

It is said that the mind is the main sexual organ, and this is particularly true for the Imaginative. On one level this means that sex has most meaning for them when there is a true meeting of minds – when shared intellectual concerns or interests are strong. The excitement of stimulating conversation is the most potent aphrodisiac. Another expression of this is that many find boredom hard to tolerate. After some time, they find it difficult to remain sexually interested in their partners, even when they love them very much. They often need their interest to be piqued and sustained by sexual variety – either by changing partners or by experimenting sexually. This is the Sexual Style most likely to enjoy a complicated but uncomfortable sexual position because the novelty makes the experience so erotic. Sex engages their interest more than their emotions, which means they can take casual sex lightly, being neither moved nor hurt by it. While Imaginatives are not necessarily more or less intelligent than any of the other Sexual Styles, if their interest or their mind is not engaged then sex itself seems mundane and pointless.

Emotionally, the Imaginative is happiest when emotions are not intrusive. They respect what they think more than what they feel. Strong emotions seem irrational to them, and are therefore somewhat frightening. They find emotionally demanding partners suffocating. They operate best in relationships where there is some separateness and independence, and they love longest someone who can interest and surprise them.

The Emotional

For this Sexual Style the intensity of the sexual experience is directly related to the depth of the emotions. Sex without a strong emotional connection is insipid and unsatisfying. While the other Sexual Styles can be just as emotional, and it can be a factor in their sexuality, it does not have the same power to affect the fundamental quality of sex. Depending on the life experience of the Emotional type, the underlying feelings that need to be activated to give sex its significance can be positive or negative — in some hate or fear can be a force as erotic as love, and for most they are preferable to indifference. While Emotional men and women can have high sex-drives which lead them to play the field, they rarely feel good about it, and can find casual sex deeply disturbing. Sex can seem over-rated to them until they find partners who affect them deeply. Then, the mechanics of what they do in bed are secondary, transformed by what is happening in their hearts.

Emotionally, Emotionals never take anything lightly. They are driven by their feeling-nature in every aspect of their lives.

Sexual Styles

Even when highly intelligent, they trust their instincts and their gut reactions above logic or reason. In love, they are intense and possessive. They can make life-long relationships of passionate and obsessive commitment with the soulmate who touches deep emotional chords in them. These relationships can even be difficult or unhappy without affecting their commitment.

The Romantic Woman

'This time I know it's the real thing.'
Jane Seymour, actress, on her fourth marriage

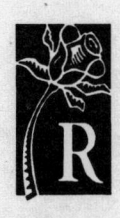

The Romantic Woman

Every woman is the Romantic in some corner of her being. It's a rare woman who has never been ecstatically infatuated with what she thinks is the world's most wonderful man. Almost every woman revels in being treated like the most beautiful and desirable woman on earth. But for the other Sexual Styles love has more to offer than this. And the Romantic woman's attitude to love is only one of the ingredients in her emotional make-up.

The uncritical eye that she tends to turn on her new love is often echoed by an eager, uncynical attitude to life itself. She *wants* things to be perfect, lovely and happy. It takes a lot of disappointment or many hard experiences to turn her into a moaner who looks on the dark side. Indeed, she can be very good at dismissing or forgetting past difficulties, and can have a touching faith that everything will be all right *now*. This makes her sound foolish and gullible, but that's not so. It's the product of optimism. And there's something about an optimistic attitude that seems to draw good experiences, just as pessimists seem to have a knack of attracting the bad. But it's more than a sunny disposition. Ms Romantic refuses to allow life's vicissitudes to get her down. Or rather, problems might bring her down, but they rarely *keep* her down. There is something childlike in this which attracts other people — men and women — who find her fun to be around. It can also make for an electrifying or disconcerting person when it is joined, as it can be, to a sharp intellect or a formidable business brain.

Unlike the Romantic man, Ms Romantic almost invariably needs to have love in her life. *His* nature can be expressed almost exclusively in his work or lifestyle without compromising his image of himself. She, on the other hand, needs her femininity to be acknowledged. She likes to know she is desired and admired as a woman throughout her life. Without this her triumphs can seem hollow. Even when she operates on equal terms out in the world; even if she can think like a man and be just as ruthless in business, there is a part of her that yearns to be the little woman at home. She wants a man to adore her, cherish her. Inside the Romantic feminist lurks a traditionalist who needs a big, strong worshipping male — or a man that she can look up to and admire.

There is something in her that needs applause and admiration for herself, not her achievements. In the absence of a man she will look to friends or others for this. She doesn't especially want to be told that she has done something wonderful, but that *she* is wonderful. This is because, like her male counterpart, she is always somewhat insecure, even when she seems most bouncy and out-going. She's actually quite easily crushed by people who show they don't like her, even if she conceals it by acting haughty. Fortunately, it is in her nature to uncrumple just as quickly when exposed to the warmth of approving attention. Indeed, this is her area of gullibility. A feature of insecurity is that it often alternates with a sense of superiority. They go together because the superior feelings she harbours are difficult to live up to. There are moments when she feels no one could be better than herself. When this is disrupted she judges herself harshly and her confidence plummets. When a man tells her she's the ideal woman he activates her sense of superiority, and she doesn't question it. The same with the most perfunctory praise. She believes it all.

A good example of the Romantic woman is the actress Debbie Reynolds, whose screen stardom was built on the portrayal of the sunny, wholesome girl next door, in movies such as *Singing in the Rain.* Other keynote roles were as Tammy and the Singing Nun, and in films such as *The Unsinkable Molly Brown.* Acting draws Romantic women like a magnet. Apart from anything else it brings with it attention, admiration, and a chance to craft their own image. As Carrie Fisher, the actress and writer who is Debbie Reynolds' daughter, says: 'She is an extraordinary woman who was able to create herself. She invented herself and she is constantly changing herself.'

Debbie Reynolds' three marriages show most clearly her Romantic nature. She was married first to Eddie Fisher, who left her for Elizabeth Taylor; then to the shoe magnate Harry Karl, who ran through his fortune and hers in quick time; and lastly to Richard Hamlett, whom she married in 1987 when she was 55, and whom she left in 1992. In an interview with *Vanity Fair* she said: 'I fall for the wrong people. We all do it. We fall for the romantic side of life. We're all looking for the white knight on a horse.'

She's right – but only about Romantic women. Why should a rich, successful, and powerful woman need a white knight? It's that insecurity. She explains: 'I looked for fathers all the time. I thought Eddie was the sweetest thing but he never loved me. Harry Karl adored me, worshipped me, but he destroyed me in the end financially. My present husband loved me, but the going got too tough. I want them to take care of me. I want them to handle everything.'

It's not unusual for Romantic women to reverse roles with their children in later life. In the same interview Carrie Fisher and Debbie's son Todd spoke of her as if they were concerned parents. Carrie's perceptions were acute: 'My mother's way of loving people is to endow them with great gifts in her mind. They therefore become worthy of her great devotion. She likes to give up her power to men. My mother is always constructing palaces. I think she thinks she's a queen, and so when she picks someone he must be a king.'

Romantics dream grand dreams. Since 1992, Debbie's has

been to create 'The Debbie Reynolds Hotel/Casino' in Las Vegas. She bought the derelict premises cheaply, but the restoration work has cost millions, subsidised by her children. She couldn't see the problems, only her vision. Carrie Fisher said: 'I wept when I first went into the lobby. She would be waving at these black caverns of space and saying, "This is going to be Bogart's Bar!"' Debbie wants it to house her enormous collection of Hollywood memorabilia – costumes, furniture, props and posters. It is quite in keeping for Romantics to collect obsessively, and Debbie protected her collection even when she was down and out. Todd says: 'She's married to 200 rooms, a showroom, a museum and a couple of restaurants. That's her husband. It's probably the best husband she's had. She's frantic, but I think she's happier now than I've ever seen her.'

But Debbie's view of what her 'husband' is differs, and is more shrewd. She says of her adoring audiences: 'This is my love. This is my kiss. This is my husband. Look at the love they give me. That may sound corny, but I'm corny. My life has been corny. All I can say is that my dreams are being fulfilled.'

Debbie Reynolds has all the elements of the Romantic woman: the blindness in love; the beautiful vision; the desire to be looked after however successful; the ability to bounce back from difficulties; and the craving for admiration, from wherever it is to be found.

Ms Romantic can retain a zest and girlishness throughout her life. She never loses her femininity, however long she lives. She is never too old to flirt. In later life she often relates better to younger people than those of her own age, and can play with children at their own level – even to the extent of getting upset when she's beaten at Snap by a five-year-old. Indeed, the state of her emotions can be quite obvious to others. She cries when she's sad and she laughs when she's happy – and she looks mortally offended when she's crossed. This can lead others, and even herself, to believe that she is Ms Emotional. But unlike women of this other Sexual Style, once she has experienced the emotions they can pass away without leaving a deep wound or marking a personality change. Even when she is very sad there is something in her that urges her towards happiness. In fact, when she feels unhappy it is an offence against her nature. She doesn't like it. It's not fair. She won't stand for it. Indeed she finds it difficult to understand people who become depressed for long or who, as she sees it, wallow in misery or can't 'pull themselves together'.

To see her at her most typical she must be in love. But even when she's not, she is usually fairly recognisable in a crowd.

Identifying Ms Romantic

Ms Romantic cares about her image. Some Romantic women fit the stereotype neatly by wearing floaty, frilly, flowery, pastel clothes, but by no means all of them do. It's feminine to be fashion-conscious, and she often is — which means that if it's all hard edges and silver and blue, that's what she'll be wearing this season. The less secure she is the more likely she will be to rely on fashion to dictate her wardrobe.

The more confident Romantic woman — or at least, the one who is most sure about the image she wants to project — will be less attuned to the trends and more to her own style. She might dress exclusively in pink. Or black. She might always go for the same shapes and cut that enhance her best features and minimise her worst. Of course, many women aim to do this, but she will be more dedicated than most. She's also prepared to put up with a fair bit of discomfort to achieve the look she's after. Even when her style is very individual she will often be aware of fashion. If she goes for the classic look her skirts will always be the current length, her lapels the 'in' shape, her jacket the latest cut, and the touch of colour she chooses will be this season's hot favourite.

The exception to these rules is the Romantic woman with a more theatrical self-image. She might see herself as the urchin, the gypsy, the diva or the vamp, and dress accordingly. She might, indeed, change her image regularly, and act and dress according to the latest role.

On the whole, she prefers long hair, if it suits her at all. And if it does, she'll never consider herself too old to wear it long. Even if it doesn't suit her, or her image demands a shorter style, she will take great care of her hair. She knows it is a distinguishingly feminine feature, and a 'crowning glory'. She will usually take care of her skin too – if not when she's young, certainly as soon as she notices any signs of age. She'll rarely leave the house without make-up, even if it's to put the rubbish out, although it may be so discreetly applied as to be almost invisible.

All this is on the surface, but it doesn't stop there. Ms Romantic's underwear is not only spotless, but usually distinctive, sexy or luxurious – even if no one will see it but herself. A Romantic friend of mine once told me that the extent of her depression during a bad time could be measured by the fact that she hadn't bought any pretty underwear *all year*. It's the same with the clothes Ms Romantic wears to do the housework or the gardening. There'll be a chicness about them, the colours will suit her, the cut will be good. She doesn't feel right in something merely comfortable, and will be disturbed in anything too shabby. In bed, even alone, she'll wear something glamorous or sexy, and if she wears nothing at all she'll certainly be smelling sweet or sultry. Part of her is always standing back to survey the effect she's creating, whether there is an onlooker or not.

She prefers to live somewhere up-market. She'll often prefer a poky apartment to a large house, if the area is better. If she can't have her first choice, she'll tell you that where she lives is up and coming, or remarkable in some way. She needs her living space to look very nice. So do many women, and lots of men, but in her case it is as much to do with the fact that it is an extension of her image as anything else. Part of her is aware that it is not

The Romantic Woman

just home, but a means for people to judge her – and she wants to be sure that they come to the right conclusion.

Ms Romantic thrives in company. She's usually outgoing and wants to have fun. She likes the whole business of dressing up and can enjoy spending hours at it. She rarely looks less than her best when she's going to a party, or even if she's just seeing a friend. She's a great flirt – especially, of course, with men. It's delicious for her to gain a man's attention, know that the female in her has caused the male in him to respond. That's usually all there is to it. She'll flirt with your grandfather or your 11-year-old son, or the unattractive bore who everyone else avoids. Oddly, she sometimes finds it hardest to flirt with the man she really fancies. That insecure side of her can be frightened of not provoking the right reaction when it really matters. Even a shy Romantic woman will flirt. She never wants to fade into the background, as other shy women do. She'll look up through her eyelashes and smile tremulously. She makes men feel wonderful. She might not be the most beautiful woman in the room or have the best figure, but she's the one who attracts the most men.

Other women often misunderstand her. They stand icily tapping a foot and gripping a wine glass as she appears to be making a dead-set at their man. She can be genuinely bewildered at their hostility. Don't they know she's not interested, that it's only a fun, sociable game? Men can misunderstand her too. She often comes across as extremely sexy, in the shortest, lowest-cut, tightest number in the room. She might be very sensual and love sex, but equally she might not. Looking sexy means being womanly to her, it's not an invitation. She can be irritated when she can't shake a persistent man off, and outraged when he makes a pass, or besieges her with phone calls after a meeting. When she dances at a gathering she's very aware of the effect she's creating. She has usually practised in front of the mirror. She'll rarely go red, sweat or look ridiculous. She is *displaying* as much as responding to the music.

She flirts with women too. Not in a sexy way, but to make sure she's liked. She'll be vivacious, pay compliments, tell amusing anecdotes. She might not take her turn at listening much. She's more concerned about making a good impression than she is about forging a connection. To this end she'll bend the truth if it makes her story better — even bend the truth about herself to enhance her image. It's not that she's *lying*, more that she's caught up in her own fantasy of how she would like life to be.

She usually has some women friends of whom she is very fond. Equally, she needs close male friends as well. She's not at her best in all female gatherings, as the presence of a man — any man — lights her up. Sometimes, however, she prefers the company of women. This tends to be when she sees men in the abstract, as conquests rather than human beings. Sometimes this makes her disdainful of men — she's so good at manipulating them that she finds it hard to respect them. She can be more herself when she doesn't have to concentrate on the effect she's creating on them. On the other hand, some Romantic women see all other women as competition. This kind of Romantic is very insecure and when she is not being desired or flattered by male attention she feels only half there. In her case women are for seeing when there's nothing better to do. She will stand up her best friend if a date with a man comes along — even if she is only slightly interested in him.

She can be a jolly friend. She is often infectiously enthusiastic. Deeper intimacy can be harder for her. If her friend is miserable she wants her to cheer up, and can be exasperated at having to listen to tales of woe. And if she is upset she often hides it. She sees it as a failure, and she doesn't like people feeling sorry for her. She wants to be admired, not pitied. This pride can make her hard to help. Help seems patronising. She often finds it easier to look to male friends for support. Exposing vulnerability to a man, after all, is feminine. When she is as happy as she wants to be and life is looking good, she can be generosity personified. There's a touch of *noblesse oblige* about her attitude — she's the loving princess, sharing her largesse. When things are going badly for her, in contrast, she can be uncharacteristically crabby or spiteful, and envious of others who have what she wants. She hates herself for being like this, which is why she is always motivated to look for the silver lining, restore her confidence, and regain her rightful, regal position in the world.

She likes to feel her friends have something special to offer. When she has the chance she can be a bit of a name-dropper. When they are not famous she'll tell you what they are good at, or how much money they have. She doesn't like her friends to be ordinary, and is proud if they are attractive, so long as they don't cast her in the shade. When she's especially lacking in confidence she might choose a plain friend to go around with, but often she enjoys the effect created by stepping out with someone who looks as good as she does.

She can care more for her figure than she does for food. When she does like eating she can sometimes worry that it looks unfeminine to tuck in hungrily. In these cases she might eat in private before she does so in public, so that she can toy gracefully with her meal. She prefers food that is elegant and well-presented. She can be rather a food snob, and follow fashions in ingredients as closely as she follows styles in clothes. She is often a good cook, or knowledgeable about food — she sees this as an essential feminine characteristic. When her Romantic nature has a strong undertone of the Sensual she can be one of the best cooks you know, as she combines a good sense of flavour with beautiful presentation and skill.

She may well know her wines, too. Whatever she drinks has a touch of elegance to it — even if it's beer it's likely to be the best! Her relationship with alcohol can be more complicated than this, however. In the autobiographical *Postcards from the Edge*, Carrie Fisher portrays her mother Debbie Reynolds as an alcoholic. Whether this is so or not, it is certainly true that some

Romantic women drink too much as a way of blurring the edges of reality and keeping their dreams intact.

When she works she is drawn to anything with a touch of glamour in it. If she must work in a factory, then she at least needs to feel that it makes the best products. She will often use her femininity at work, too. She doesn't know how to switch it off — and if you've got it, flaunt it. Sometimes she's unaware that she is doing so. This can cause difficulties with colleagues, men as well as women.

On the whole, she likes going out and having a good time. She has quite a lot of energy that needs using up. Sometimes she doesn't even recognise when she *has* used it up. When she's excited and involved she doesn't notice the signs of fatigue. Sitting at home doing nothing has a limited appeal — unless she is doing it with an interesting man. She does, however, like to be transported to another world. If this can't be an exotic trip, then she will read or watch movies — preferably things with a lot of passion and fire, or that are escapist, such as thrillers or soaps. She likes dramatic music that can make her cry or feel excited. She often has a creative streak, and may draw or write for pleasure if not for profit. She can also be intensely interested in the esoteric and unknown. Unlike the Romantic man she doesn't feel the same need to fight mystery with logic. She likes to be thrilled and chilled — to feel the world is a dramatic and magic place, with many hidden wonders.

The unattached Romantic woman

Little Ms Romantic threw herself into imaginative play. She liked dressing up and organising other children to act out her fantasies. The quieter child was probably a bookworm, intensely living the parts of the characters in her storybooks. Although other children like these activities too, in her case they indulge an essential part of her nature, which continues to be important in her adult life. The fact is that real-life experiences and real people are often not quite perfect enough, and she has a tendency to superimpose her own wishes and fantasies on to them. This can be particularly marked if her childhood was not very happy. While this will lead little Ms Emotional to expect unhappiness in later life, and the Sensual little girl to develop a dogged attitude to difficulties, it propels the Romantic child into her own world, and increases her determination to make sure that her future will be better, brighter and pain free. She will be attracted to people who seem to promise this. The little boy with the angel's face will gain her devotion. He fits the part, and her imagination supplies the rest.

She continues to have an eye for a good-looking man throughout her life. Looks are always important to her and she is easily led to believe that beauty of face and form signals an inner beauty. It's special. As her ideas gain in sophistication, however, so does her interpretation of what makes a person special. She might then be drawn to talented, brilliant, successful or rich men – people marked out as being above the ordinary. In these cases she will forego good looks, although she would prefer the two to go together. She believes her choice of man enhances who she is. She likes to be envied for her catch. When she adores and admires him she will put up with a certain amount of bad behaviour in the interests of keeping him.

The part of her that wants to be cared for will also be drawn to powerful men – not because power itself is an aphrodisiac, as it can be for the Emotional woman, but because she believes they will look after her. She has a preference for tall, masculine men that she can look up to, and older men – big daddy types – although she will go for smaller, slighter, younger men if they have other outstanding characteristics. Sometimes she likes the idea of big, sweaty, physical men because they seem so masterful and masculine. Usually the reality puts her off however, and if she becomes involved with such a man she'll try to groom him into something more sophisticated and less animal.

All adolescent girls have crushes on unobtainable people, but hers will often be more intense and long-lasting. She invests the adored target with all the elements that most appeal to her, and the boys she knows look poor value in contrast. She will flirt with them however – that starts young – and she can be the object of the devoted attention that she always craves.

It doesn't suit her to embark on an early sex life. The romance gives way too soon to a concentration on the physical. She prefers a tantalising, long-drawn-out courtship, and if he is maddened and rendered devoted by unconsummated lust, then it's all the better as far as she is concerned.

Later, of course, when she discovers her sexuality, she will want to make love with the man she loves. But she will always cherish the build up to sex, and will rarely feel happy going to bed with someone soon after they meet. She will only allow it if she can feel that it was love at first sight and they were swept away by grand passion. Indeed, promiscuity doesn't suit her. A one-night-stand makes her feel cheap. If he doesn't want to see her again she is devastated. Her belief in her powers and her femininity takes a knock and her self-confidence suffers. Actually, she needs to feel that he wants her forever and has never loved anyone so much. And she is quite easily convinced that this is so by a smooth talker. Some Romantic women are flattered into a series of short and unsatisfactory sexual encounters because they want to believe what the men say, but this is always harmful for them.

The exception is the Romantic girl who becomes a groupie – hanging around famous singers or actors and offering sexual favours. The glamour of the encounter can outweigh the brutality of the sex, as she feels she is borrowing some of the star's specialness. She can also believe it shows the world that she is highly desirable – he has picked her out from the adoring crowd. Ultimately, however, she becomes disgusted, or her self-esteem suffers. Really she was hoping he would fall in love with her.

Although most Romantic women want to be married and live happily ever after, they need heightened romantic intensity more. This leads some Romantic women to have a series of passionate attachments, none of them lasting more than a couple of years. Once the high-voltage feelings go they feel that love has gone, and they need to find a new man to love. Actually, although she is never happier than when she is in love, she has a streak of emotional independence which allows her to be choosy about the quality of her love affairs. When ecstasy evaporates she prefers to be free to find someone else rather than to be shackled.

Surprisingly, this can lead some Romantic women to prefer the role of the mistress. The enforced separations, the dramatic, ardent meetings, the way they focus on each other exclusively when they are together can be exquisitely satisfying. Being parted from him can make her unhappy, but secretly she enjoys the star-crossed situation. She is centre stage in a poignant tragedy. She might even be oblivious to what makes it so powerfully compelling for her. Sometimes, indeed, when he leaves his wife the lessening of the intensity can mark the end of her love for him.

Throughout her life she is susceptible to a man who says the right thing. The plainest Romantic woman will believe the man who tells her that she has an unusual beauty. She is always a young girl inside, and the man who treats her as such, whatever her age, will never be mocked. An example is the women who visit The Gambia, West Africa, known as the 'Gigolo Coast'. It is famous for its 'bumsters' – young men, and even teenage boys, who sell their bodies to visiting women, most of them well into middle and old age. Most of the women want uncomplicated, cheap sex with a vigorous young man. Some, though, want more. There is a rising incidence of women who accept the gigolo chat-up line as the real thing. Some of these marry their suitors, often after knowing them for two weeks or less. They have been taken in by protestations of love. One 57-year-old

British woman married a 34-year-old Gambian she met on a short holiday. She sold everything to go to The Gambia to live with him. Six months later she was back home with nothing. There are many like her. The local registrar tells of refusing to marry a 70-year-old to a 14-year-old Gambian boy!

These are the tragedies, but the Romantic woman's ability to re-experience the wonder of love anew can also be glorious. She sees romance everywhere. A brief encounter with longing sultry looks can be the real thing as far as she is concerned, even if they barely exchanged a word and never touched. Being in love is the best feeling she knows. 'It is the ultimate ecstasy,' says an 80-year-old woman in Linda Sonntag's *Inside Marriage* — the words of a Romantic. 'It makes me feel worthwhile as a person,' says another, betraying the insecurity of a Romantic. But love, as far as the Romantic woman is concerned, is what other people would call infatuation. It's not about real, fallible people, but about a dream. Of course, Ms Romantic can feel the deeper reaches of love and genuine concern for another, but this is not as satisfying for her as the intensely exciting period when he seems perfect and so does she. She can see his faults, but they don't seem to matter: they're part of his charm. Those same faults, when they lose their charm, can be precisely what makes her feel most disillusioned. She can wilfully invest him with all sorts of characteristics that he doesn't have. Love is often truly blind for the Romantic woman when it comes to the inner man.

She also needs him to adore every little bit about her. A more prosaic acceptance of her shortcomings can seem upsettingly offensive and the reverse of true love.

Sex and Ms Romantic

The Romantic woman often has a sexy aura about her. She might indeed like sex very much and have a keen sexual appetite. But even if she doesn't, she still comes across as if she does. Some Romantic women are more glacial. They have a queenly presence. Even so, the obvious femininity of these women leads men to believe that once they get them between the sheets they will be deliciously yielding.

The best sex, as far as she is concerned, is when she is madly in love. Everything about being in love is delightful. She looks at her best, for a start. Her skin and eyes glow and her vitality is insuppressible. Her mind is filled with thoughts of him, even when she should be working. Life seems sweeter; problems don't matter any more. When they are together no one else exists. They can't keep their hands off each other. That's one of the reasons the sex is so good. It is so connected to the loving feelings that it has a special quality. It's not just sex, it's making love. The erotic atmosphere that envelops a new and exciting love affair also means that she is very easily turned on. She's more ready for sex than she ever will be, and because of this every touch is sensually pleasing. He seems to be the perfect lover with an instinctive knowledge of what her body wants.

Every woman experiences this when she falls head over heels in love. The Romantic woman, however, finds it harder than most when these feelings run their natural course and turn into something less ardent. Sex, particularly, can seem disappointing when it becomes more routine. Sometimes this is because now that she is less easily turned on she realises that he is not such a wonderful lover after all. The caress on her hair, which used to send electric shivers through her entire body, now just makes her feel her hairstyle is being messed up. When they are making love he doesn't actually touch her in quite the right way. If her sex drive is not high she can lose much of her interest in sex at this stage, and be irritated by his continuing sexual demands.

But even if her sex drive is high, and even if he is a consummate lover, she still finds it hard to adjust to the fading of the romantic intensity of infatuation. Sex becomes less meaningful and exciting because there is no longer that passionate need to be in each other's arms all the time. She can't help realising that sometimes it *is* as much about sexual satisfaction for itself as it is about making love, and that can be sad for her.

Sex will never transport her in quite the same way again – at least with her current man. The right lover, however, will know how to make it nearly as good. She needs to be wooed and courted. Unlike the Romantic male, all the trappings of romance are very important to her. She likes flowers, presents, love notes, valentine cards (preferably more than once a year) thoughtful gestures – and particularly sweet-talking. She needs to be told that she is loved, beautiful, mesmerising. The words 'I love you' never sound hollow or perfunctory to her, and she can't hear them enough. The man who remembers all this knows how to put her in the mood for love-making.

She needs the circumstances to be right to give herself fully to enjoying sex. It's only in the early days that she can feel right making love in the lobby the moment he comes through the door. Normally her passion builds more slowly. She needs soft lighting, soft music, a loving atmosphere. She prefers to be feeling desirous already before they start touching intimately. Kissing is important. She will be put off if he grabs her breasts first. She also needs to feel that she is looking her best. If she thinks she's having an 'ugly day', or her hair is unwashed, or she's feeling fat, almost nothing will turn her on, even if he finds her perfectly desirable just as she is. Similarly she can be turned off by love-making positions that expose what she sees as her faults. She won't like rear-entry positions if she thinks her bottom is too big, or to be on top if she thinks the angle is unflattering to her breasts. She feels self-conscious, and her desire wanes. Because of this she sometimes finds it difficult to 'lose' herself in love-making, which can make it hard for her to reach orgasm. When she is mentally standing outside herself to focus on the effect she is creating she won't be concentrating on her physical sensations. Indeed, she needs to feel very trusting to let herself go, which is one of the reasons that casual sex can be so unsatisfying for her.

She might prefer not to make love first thing in the morning. There's no build up, and she worries that her breath is smelling. Or she is put off by the fact that his breath smells. She likes a man to take care of himself too. Usually she likes him to be well turned out, with a hint of aftershave. Taking her to dinner in a smart restaurant can be excellent foreplay for a number of reasons. She feels spoilt and cherished. Their attention is wholly concentrated on each other. She has made herself look her best, and so has he. She often finds men in a suit, especially a dinner jacket, or a sharp uniform, most attractive. If he comes in sweaty and dirty from a game of squash, raring to make love, she can be very put off. This is not the woman who can fancy a man who wears his socks in bed, doesn't care about his personal hygiene, or picks his nose or his toenails in front of her. She always makes an effort, and she doesn't see why he shouldn't as well.

The modern Romantic woman is likely to feel that she should be an artist when it comes to making love. Like her sisters in history, she can privately prefer the man to take charge during sex: it makes her feel very feminine. Nowadays, however, she may feel that an almost oriental attention to making the experience good for him is equally feminine. She will rarely make the very first move, though. Feeling that he wants her often marks the first stage of arousal for her. What she is prepared to do, however, is always limited by her preference for remaining feminine at all times. Sex acts that seem brutal or dirty are usually not in her line. She rarely wants to make love during menstruation, even if she has erotic feelings at that time. She might find giving oral sex humiliating or distasteful. She can be equally uncomfortable receiving it, particularly if she is worried about her intimate smell. Some Romantic women find genitals – hers and his – ridiculous or ugly. Typically, she often likes dressing up for sex, even if it's only a satin negligee. The actress in her can also enjoy more theatrical costuming –

stockings and suspenders, or a sexy French maid number, or a demure schoolgirl or nun's outfit. Equally, she can become adept at the striptease, enjoying the feelings she arouses in herself as well as the desire she sees in his eyes.

She usually finds his desire for her erotic, particularly when connected to adoration. If he makes her jealous by his admiration for other women, the result can be a temporary ferment of heightened sexuality on her part as she tries to compete, often followed by a complete loss of sexual interest. In the same way, she can be furious and offended if he has an interest in pornography. She doesn't want to be the recipient of sexual attentions inspired by someone else. It is in her nature, however, to want to excite his jealousy from time to time. She'll flirt with other men even when she adores her partner. Apart from anything, when he becomes jealous she feels that he still loves her and wants her. If he's not good at reassuring her in other ways she will use this weapon more frequently. Indeed, a man who forgets to let her know he loves her will often drive her to provoke a reaction from him in any way she can. She might throw scenes, start rows – anything that centres his focus on her and their relationship.

Her idea of a good sex life doesn't include having to guide her man to give her sexual satisfaction. That seems mechanical and the opposite of erotic. Even if she is an experienced woman who knows what she likes, she believes that a good lover should know what to do. She is prepared to go in for a certain amount of hinting, manoeuvring and leading, but she stops short of telling him outright. If she is compelled to, something good disappears for her. She might know consciously that it is silly, but it doesn't change the fact that she wants him to touch her in exactly the right ways because that's how he *wants* to touch her – not because he has to in order to satisfy her. On the other hand, she responds to him taking the initiative to learn. When he asks whether she likes this or that, and proceeds accordingly, she feels he is being wonderfully caring and masterful.

The Romantic woman and marriage

She is the marrying kind. When Ms Romantic is in love she wants to spend her life with the man. She's not interested in practical details of compatibility or long-term considerations. She is swept up in the miracle of the heady feelings she is experiencing, and she can't imagine them not lasting forever. Inevitably, sometimes the feelings fade before she does marry him, or she may marry in haste and her marriage can be a mistake. She is the woman most likely to make a series of marriages, convinced each time that she has got it right. She trusts implicitly her romantic feelings, and her optimism leads her to believe that, with the right man, the magic of infatuation can endure. Only when she has had many disappointments does this optimism fade. Then, as a point of pride, she might vow never to marry at all.

On the other hand, the Romantic woman can often choose well. When her idea of specialness includes wealth and success, she will fall in love with a man who has these attributes and her marriage can have ingredients that give it a staying power. When he provides the means to give her freedom to indulge in the things that are important to her, such as making a beautiful home, spending time and money on the way she looks, creating a lifestyle that is glamorous and enviable, indulging her children, and so on, she has enough to keep her happy even after the first flush of romance has faded. When she is successful in her own right, however, she is likely to demand more from him in terms of love and devotion.

Despite the fact that she needs the excitement of romantic love to be truly happy, she is more committed to seeing her marriage through the natural disappointments than is her male counterpart. This is because more of her self-image is invested in her role of wife and home-maker, than the Romantic man's is in being a steady partner. Her femininity requires her to do it well; superbly. Mr Romantic is likely to believe his wife is to blame when the romance goes, whereas she will often take the blame on herself. Her basic insecurity can lead her to believe that she is doing something wrong, and she will often make every effort to put it right. Similarly, she can see her children as extensions of herself. While the Romantic man needs to shine himself, she can be just as happy working towards giving her children the opportunity to fulfil her dreams. Sometimes this makes her over-indulgent, or conversely a pushy, or 'stage' mother. When the school complains about them, she'll take their side. She tends to see them as she wishes them to be – which is often extraordinary, talented, even perfect.

The Romantic woman who needs to adore more than she is adored can put up with a badly behaved man so long as her image of him remains intact. If she admired him as a poet, for instance, she can be prepared to struggle in a garret for years while she believes in his talent. If she admires his power, strength and success she will tolerate him putting most of his time and energy into his work. But if she is disillusioned her patience can run out. The big daddy who needs support when his own confidence goes can find her icily withdrawn. The artist whose talent is exposed as negligible will attract her scorn eventually. She might soldier on in such a marriage if there is no alternative, but her heart isn't in it. Indeed, her romantic, optimistic heart will be ready to embrace someone more admirable. The search is on, even if she is unaware of it. She will only play mummy to her children. It does not suit her to have to do it for her man.

The Romantic woman who prefers to be adored and desired herself can make a lasting match with a devoted partner. Indeed she is often adept at making him continue to see her as the gorgeous girl he fell in love with, even after decades together. She will retain her flirtatiousness, play up her helplessness, continue to make sure she looks as good as she possibly can. Sometimes she remains in a time-warp, unable to learn more mature strategies. If he tires of this behaviour she may redouble it, because she doesn't know what else to do. On the other hand if she tires of it herself, and is looking for more adult interaction she might find his devotion lessens. Either way, she loses the adoration that nourishes her, and her marriage feels empty. Concern for her children will sometimes keep her in a marriage she sees as loveless. But her resolve will waver if a white knight on a horse should cross her horizon.

On the other hand, some couples are good at retaining romance within their relationship, long after it usually expires. It requires some privacy, some respect, and a lot of outward displays of love while never taking each other for granted. If she constructs a marriage like this, Ms Romantic can often live quite happily without sex, if her husband is equally happy. Sometimes, indeed, she sees sex as having a purpose: to bond them in the first place, and then to create children. After this it can appear quite natural for it to fade away.

When Ms Romantic will stray

She doesn't want to be unfaithful. When she is in love it wouldn't cross her mind. But if she believes she has fallen in love with someone else it can seem like the right thing to do. She'll sometimes throw away everything when she is in a passionate haze, even leave her children. When the mist clears she may realise that she has lost something valuable.

She might be acting on impulse if she has an affair, but she never does it lightly. She is usually swept up in something that seems inevitable. It won't usually be sexual reasons that drive her into the arms of another man, though if she has been sexually disappointed the awakening of her erotic nature can be infatuating. If she wants to make love with someone else, however, it is usually because she feels that something has irretrievably died in her marriage. Even if the affair remains secret, or is very short-lived, it exposes a lack of the quality she feels is essential.

She is always vulnerable to a man who lays siege to her and tells her how much he desires and loves her. This will give her great pleasure, but it only becomes dangerous when she feels her own partner is taking her for granted. If things are merely comfortable and gently loving at home she can miss the intensity of more passionate courtship. Then the right man (or often the wrong one) can beguile her into believing she is in love.

She rarely intends to have 'just an affair'. It might turn out that way if that is all the man is looking for, but generally she commits sexually where she places her heart. She is usually ready to leave for him. Only occasionally does a Romantic woman want someone on the side, as the Romantic male can do, to compensate for missing dramatic thrills. She is more whole-hearted than he is in her relationships. Sometimes, though, she does take a lover in this way. Usually it is because she has a strong sensual or practical streak and doesn't want to jeopardise her lifestyle, particularly if she has made it as beautiful and glamorous as she could wish. Then she will dally with a good-looking man for excitement alone. Her romantic heart has been given to something more reliable than a man.

Ms Romantic and sexual problems

As sex is most thrilling when she feels herself to be passionately in love, and loved and desired in return, she misses the intensity when it passes. Unless her natural sex drive is high, sex that is merely companionable and affectionate can seem a waste of time. When she is married with children and the natural constraints of a busy life mean that sex is relegated to the last thing at night on the same day every week, she can find it hard to respond. A man who expects sex as his due, and doesn't feel that he should have to woo her beforehand, will excite only distaste, not lust. Sometimes it takes only small adjustments to bring back her desire. A single flower, or a phone call telling her that she is loved can touch her heart, and make her more responsive. When the relationship has good things going for it, her partner will find that their sex life improves when he shows her loving attention, is flattering, kind and generous. She also needs time with him on her own – either for an evening or preferably a holiday – so that she can feel like his woman, rather than his housekeeper or mother to his children.

Anything that makes her feel better about herself is likely to have a knock-on effect on her sexuality. Because she needs to feel good, and to feel she looks good, if her confidence is low then so will be her interest in sex. She's not being difficult when she worries about getting fat or growing older. Her attractiveness and her femininity are central to her feelings about herself, and she needs to have them reaffirmed or she will feel too vulnerable to want to make love.

She will also find it difficult to desire a man who is a slob in his personal habits. Neither will she take kindly to him using the lavatory while she is having a bath. She can't see him as a sexual being if she's had to endure him farting in front of her. There's such a thing as being too natural, as far as she is concerned. A man who wants his Romantic woman to enjoy making love with him, rather than tolerate it, needs to bear these things in mind.

A more profound problem arises when time shows that the sex life they have constructed doesn't really move her. After the first flush of new love has passed she is rarely motivated to do anything about it, other than withdraw sexually. What's the point, she wonders, when the great feelings have gone? Sometimes, indeed, she may have been faking orgasm from the early days, in the interests of making him feel good, or because she believes it means she's not good in bed if she doesn't climax. She may never mention it, but suffer her disappointment in silence.

Sometimes a couple like this go for sex therapy, because he is angry or bewildered, and she can't explain. Therapy that concentrates solely on the physical mechanics of what they do is unlikely to work for her. She needs to feel desire first, before her body switches on. Without this even the most sensitive love-making can leave her cold. When the loving feelings are rekindled she will be receptive to gentle sensual exploration to awaken her responses. If she can't find it in her heart to adore or admire him again, however, or she feels that he cares more for sex than he does about her, she is unlikely to allow herself to feel the necessary pleasure.

The Romantic man can use fantasy to stoke his passion. Sometimes she, too, finds it helps to replace his image with someone she considers more ideal. Some Romantic women, indeed, keep their marriages and their sex lives going by indulging in a rich fantasy life, and can continue to have crushes on unobtainable men, as they did when they were adolescents. She'll rarely want to share her partner's fantasies, though. The exception is if he gives her a starring role as the desirable, eternally beautiful icon that she yearns to be.

The Romantic Man

'Desire dies because every touch consumes the myth...'

W B Yeats

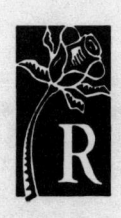

The Romantic Man

There's a misconception about the Romantic Man. *SHE* magazine once awarded six men the 'most romantic' title. Tim flew his girlfriend to Paris for a surprise only a week after they met. Kevin left love notes under the pillow. Crispin had an antique table delivered to the restaurant where he was taking Catherine for her birthday. It was covered with a tablecloth while they ate, and whipped off afterwards to reveal the surprise. These are wonderful romantic gestures, but it has to be said that although there are millions of Romantic men out there, it would not cross the minds of most of them to act like this. Indeed, thinking up special treats and surprises can seem too much like hard work for the man who thinks love should be grand and passionate, but also effortless.

Mr Romantic loves being loved. He loves falling in love, and no one is more likely to do so at first sight. It's what comes afterwards that sometimes proves more difficult. Among the dictionary definitions of a romantic is someone 'given to thoughts and feelings of love, especially idealised or sentimental love'. Another one is 'impractical visionary'.

At his most extreme, the modern Mr Romantic has much in common with his ancestors, the troubadours of the 12th century. They glorified unconsummated passion for a married woman, a 'courtly love' that expressed itself in romantic songs and devoted attention. The point is that they never got close enough to know the real woman and could love with hopeless passion a vision of perfection, who was, to a great extent, a figment of their imaginations. Nowadays, Mr Romantic would have to be very shy or very young only to love at a distance, but this intensity of feeling, which can include the delighted, wondrous belief that the woman is flawless, is one of his trademarks.

Most men have experienced this heady feeling. So have most women. It is characteristic of falling in love. When you are 'in love' all your normal critical faculties are suspended. You don't or can't see imperfections in your lover, or even faults seem adorable. It is incredibly exciting, too. Some crazy mechanic has tuned up your body: it shows in your eyes and your skin, your speeded-up responses. When you are with your lover your body is one gigantic erogenous zone. Even a touch on the elbow is exquisitely erotic.

Mr Sensual and Mr Imaginative are well aware of the part lust plays in the process — in fact they might put it all down to hormones and sexual chemistry. Mr Emotional is less cynical, but knows there are deeper emotional depths to plumb. They are all prepared to listen to the expert's view that falling in love is an altered state that cannot last, and is comparable to a euphoric drug-high or an anaesthetised alcoholic fog.

Mr Romantic, instead, dismisses these ideas. This, he knows, is love. This is *real* love. It doesn't matter how many times it has happened to him before, this time it is even better, this time it will last.

It is when he is in love that sex is most fulfilling for Mr Romantic. He is not alone. Virtually everyone remembers the early days of a relationship as a sexually intense and thrilling time. You are so easily turned on by each other that technique hardly matters. There is no sense of duty about it. You want to touch constantly whether you are making love or not, so the idea of 'foreplay' is irrelevant — and lazing together afterwards, continuing to stroke and talk lovingly is no hardship. Sex, when this phase has passed, is never quite the same, but for Mr Sensual and Mr Emotional at least, it can be rewarding in a different way. Not so for the Romantic man.

It's not just because sex is so passionate and easy in these circumstances that Mr Romantic is hooked on it. The sexual passion is directly related to the intoxicating atmosphere of the romantic partnership. In the rapture of early love only the two lovers exist. She's wonderful, special. And she thinks he is, too.

This is one key to understanding the Romantic man. He knows he's special, but the world conspires to put him down from time to time. He hasn't reached manhood without noticing that not everyone shares his evaluation of himself. Whether he has learnt to come across with a certain self-effacing modesty, or whether he seems overbearingly self-confident, there is often a dented ego lurking somewhere. When a woman is madly in love with him he feels he has come into his birthright. Her adoring attention restores his sense of specialness. This increases his feelings of power and potency, particularly sexually. When the romantically intense phase passes, and the woman he loves starts to appraise him more critically, Mr Romantic takes it hard. He doesn't see it as 'realistic', but as a betrayal. Never mind that she still loves him, or insists she loves him even more, or that she wants to spend her life with him. That's not what he calls love. She doesn't think he's perfect, and it hurts.

On the other hand, there is also the Romantic man for whom idealising his partner is enough. If it suits him to feel that he has made the catch of the century, then it can even feed his romantic fantasy to see himself as unworthy of his prize. Owning her proves he is special. I once worked on a magazine with a woman I shall call Angela. She was a great flirt. More than that, she gave the impression that she was seriously sexually attracted to – even in love with – many men she met. She wasn't especially attractive, but the men felt they were on to a good thing. They often propositioned her and pursued her, but she held them at bay. I knew she had lived with Ben for many years, and assumed that she was unhappy with him. She once invited me to dinner, and I realised I couldn't be more wrong. Much of the evening was spent telling Ben about the latest 'unwelcome' attentions from her admirers. Ben glowed with pride, and wanted every detail. Clearly their long relationship was nourished by this strange game. As a typical Romantic man it suited him to see her as a wildly desirable woman who sent other men insane with lust.

Ideally the Romantic man would like both of them to be madly in love with each other forever. What usually happens is that he settles for either being the lover or the loved. Whatever the case, there must be something special and out-of-the-ordinary about this relationship for it to hold his attention, especially his sexual attention. Mr Romantic thrives on drama, and being at the centre of it — if their personal drama can't be Romeo and Juliet, he will settle for the bitter jealousy of Othello.

A classic Romantic is F. Scott Fitzgerald, the writer who used himself and his life in all his work. The way he described Anson Hunter in the short story *The Rich Boy* is telling: 'I don't think he was ever happy unless someone was in love with him, responding to him like filings to a magnet, helping him to explain himself, promising him something.'

Scott Fitzgerald maintained he first fell seriously in love at the age of nine. He kept the valentine he received when he was 11 for most of his life. As a child he fantasised he was the son of 'a king who ruled the whole world'. He fell in love with the wild and beautiful Zelda when he was 21 and she was 19. They had a tempestuous two-year courtship before marrying, and he only won her when his first novel was published to great acclaim. Like all Romantic men he loved glamour and excitement. Zelda personified this, and it was said of them as a couple: 'There was a golden innocence about them and they were both so hopelessly good-looking.' When they had money they lived grandly and ostentatiously, with wild parties, servants and endless expenditure.

Scott Fitzgerald said of his relationship with Zelda after some years together: 'We're still enormously in love and about the only truly happily married people I know.' For many people this happiness seemed like hell: 'Zelda and I sometimes indulge in terrible four-day rows that always start with a drinking party.' They tortured each other by flirting with other people and flinging destructive and unforgivable accusations at each other during arguments, then making up extravagantly. Sex was not so important to Scott Fitzgerald, who worried about his penis size and of whom his friend, the critic Ernest Boyd, said: 'Where so many are conscious only of sex, he is conscious of the soul.' It was most important to him to live life on the edge, to live with drama and heightened feelings, good or bad, realistic or not. The theme of *The Great Gatsby*, he said, was: 'The loss of those illusions that give such colour to the world so that you don't care whether things are true or false as long as they partake of the magical glory.'

For some Romantic men the need for the highs of love and for one or both of them to be on a pedestal is frustrated. They respond by withdrawing. Sometimes they hate women for being such a disappointment up close. Their need for romance is projected outwards into their work and life generally. There is a streak of emotional independence in all Romantics that makes life on their own tolerable, if not so much fun as when they are in love. Indeed many Romantic men, even those who settle down, or continue to have affairs, find that love does not provide all the romance they require. It defines their sexuality but it is not exclusively linked to it. This is why it is possible to spot Mr Romantic as he goes about his daily life.

Sexual Styles

Identifying Mr Romantic

If you ask many men to shut their eyes and tell you what they are wearing they would be hard put to say which sweater or suit they had on, or the colour of their tie or shirt. Not so Mr Romantic, who dresses with the care that complements his sense of being a special human being. What he wears, however, will then be affected by his personality, age, constraints of his job, and so on. A Romantic adolescent might slavishly copy his current hero — another boy he knows, a rock star or sporting personality. A conservative businessman will co-ordinate his colours with care and buy the best quality. Labels are often important to him, as if the glory of the established name is reflected on himself. On the other hand, if he fancies himself as a poet he might dress entirely from thrift shops, favouring period clothes from a more romantic decade. Mr Romantic usually has a strong sense of the image he wishes to project, and clothes are the best way of doing so. Whatever he wears, he will usually be privately delighted if you notice it, and will be happy to tell you where and why he bought it.

Liking 'the best', in whatever way he personally defines it, is another clue to his essential nature. If he has money this will be shown by the restaurants he goes to, the holidays he takes and the area in which he lives. He prefers the top of the range, whatever the depth of his pocket: if he can't afford the best car, he would prefer the best motorbike or, failing that, the best skateboard. What he drives tells you more about him than he might be aware. There's usually a touch of flash to it. The retiring Romantic man who dresses exclusively in shades of grey often favours the brightest red car. If not, it'll be very sleek, very fast, a classic, or equipped with the latest in modern technology. This liking for 'things' often turns him into a collector. Again, how much he has to spend determines what he collects. Whether it's Old Masters or old watches, collecting feeds his Romantic soul. On one level this is because the child in Mr Romantic needs to play, and collecting is a legitimate, adult way of playing. And while some collectors are driven by obsession — a need to order and catalogue something — Mr Romantic is in pursuit of a magical perfection. Perfection is the completed collection, which will always remain tantalisingly out of reach, and thus can never be a disappointment to him.

Mr Romantic is easily beguiled by the extraordinary, the out-of-this-world, the magical — anything that is not mundane and which suggests that we don't know all there is to know. The more outwardly conventional he is the more he struggles to hide it. He might loudly rubbish astrology, for instance, but watch his face at a party when he meets an astrologer who proceeds to tell him about himself. For a moment you'll see a yearning to believe. He'll tell you why there aren't such things as UFOs, or give you the physiological explanation for near-death experiences, or the reality behind a ghostly manifestation. The difference between him and other sceptics, however, is that he has bothered to read up on what he dismisses so contemptuously. Indeed, his irritation often masks a secret disappointment. Part of him longs for it to be true. There is something attractively childlike in his enthusiasms, and even in his irritated rejection of them when they let him down.

Confusingly, the most obviously Romantic man might not signal his Sexual Style in these ways. That is because these are, to a degree, methods of sublimating his romantic nature. The more he expresses it in his love life or in his way of living, the less likely he is to need to find other outlets. There is nothing distinguishingly romantic about Marcus, for instance, unless you know about his life. On retiring from the army he settled down with a wealthy, beautiful, loving wife and had several children. Then some years into the marriage he suddenly ran off with another woman. She was wild, unsuitable, and not half so nice or good-looking as his wife. But he was madly in love. This was the 'real thing', for which he was prepared to give up everything. Marcus went from affluence to poverty almost at once, and a short time later this great love evaporated. He was without home or money, and necessity drove him back to the only thing he knew — soldiering. He became a mercenary, travelling the world. For the last few years he has alternated fighting away with loving at home. He has had a series of relationships, each one the 'true and only' great love, all of which last no longer than two years. He has never been happier.

For the warrior, like Marcus, is a classic Romantic. He could be a campaigner, a trade union activist, a politician. *What* he is fighting for matters less than the battle itself. Whether he is literally fighting for his life or fighting for his beliefs, what he thrives on is the intoxicating rush of adrenalin that makes him feel alive and vital. Love narrows his focus onto one woman and the rapture of the moment. There is a different excitement in fighting but it has its own drama, and the similar effect of increasing the significance of *now* — this crucial moment of engagement. The optimist in him can't conceive that he might be the one to be killed or hurt, which can lead to glorious acts of bravery. He's always capable of pushing himself well beyond his physical limits — partly because he doesn't know what they are. His image of himself can continue to be of a vigorous young man, even when the reality is somewhat different.

Some Romantic men gain the excitement they need by living on a precipice — lurching from one love affair to another, perhaps deeply in debt. They find something poetically gratifying in having nothing — in fact they often have a grand, if undefined, sense that the world owes them a living, and that by doing unsatisfying work they are compromising themselves. Alternatively they have a childlike belief that a miracle will happen and all that they need will be magically provided. Sometimes they look to women to provide that miracle. Even the most down and out Romantic will have a vision of how wonderful his life could be — indeed *will* be. Unlike the more focused Emotional or Imaginative man, however, he often doesn't like the hard work involved in making his dream a reality. This is one of the elements that attracts him to gambling. The act of gambling is exciting in itself, and there is always the possibility that the next win will be the big one. He rarely contemplates losing, even if he has lost more often than won.

Many artists, actors and other performers are Romantics. The glamorous professions enhance the Romantic man's view of himself as chosen and special. He can express his romantic nature and get paid for it. Anything creative gives him the opportunity to rework life and substitute his own vision. As Scott Fitzgerald noted, writing was 'a back door way out of facing reality'. Most Romantic men, of course, don't have these kinds of careers, but a proportion secretly wish that they did. Some undervalue their work if it is considered boring or unglamorous. Then they might aim for success, money, or becoming the boss – as tangible proof that they stand out from the crowd.

The Romantic man usually likes to feel that there is something special about his friends, as well. He subscribes to the view that you can tell what a man is like by the company he keeps. Consequently he likes people around him to be admirable in some way – or rich, famous or influential. There is often an element of hero-worship. Scott Fitzgerald said: 'When I like women I want to own them, to dominate them, to have them admire me.' His feelings about men were different: 'When I like men I want to be like them – I want to lose the outer qualities that give me my individuality and ... absorb into myself all the qualities that make them attractive.' On the other hand, the Romantic man doesn't like to be overshadowed, and needs the opportunity to shine. He is often gregarious and enjoys large gatherings and parties. When he is out-going, he is easy to spot. He works the room, charming men as well as women: he likes to be liked, and each conquest raises his self-esteem a notch.

However nondescript he might appear, he has an enviable success rate with women. He'll whisk the most beautiful woman in the party away from more obviously sexy men. It's something to do with the intensity with which he pays court to them. It's also because his belief that he is a prince among men (albeit sometimes in disguise) casts its own spell. He is capable of great acts of generosity. When he's delighted by a woman he will tell her so with immense flattery and charm – and will be willing to spend everything he has (or hasn't) got on her.

The shyer Romantic man still manages to draw attention to himself, often by looking soulful and brooding or aloof. While Mr Emotional broods for real, Mr Romantic is usually playing at it. His substitute for being unable to hold court is to give out an unspoken message that he is above all this. He's a contradictory creature, really: either brash and confident on the outside, concealing much self-doubt, or with a quiet and unassuming exterior hiding a fierce and proud sense of superiority.

The pure Mr Romantic might eat heartily, but his basic attitude to food is that it is a necessary evil. Unless he is a food snob, endowing food with glamour, he sees it as something to be got out of the way. His attitude to alcohol is less simple. He likes altered states of mind, and for this reason might experiment with drugs as well. Usually it is just a social pleasure, but some Romantic men drop more seriously into alcohol or drug abuse. A heavy drinking Romantic is trying to blur the edges of real life and soften the harshness. Too much that he sees and experiences is far from ideal, excitement is rare, and perfection so often disintegrates that he can find reality hard to take. The less confident he is inside, the more likely he is to turn to alcohol to drown these uncomfortable feelings. Scott Fitzgerald was a hard drinker who became an alcoholic. One friend from his youth said: 'I felt that he was one of those people who could never be satisfied with life. He seemed to feel there must be something more that he hadn't gotten and could never get.'

Some Romantics find falling in love works better than alcohol. That's why this is the Sexual Style most likely to be a love-junkie. Infatuation cocoons him from the world and allows him to indulge grandiose ideas about himself, life, and his love. Any man who is tattooed with a woman's name is a Romantic. It wouldn't occur to him that he would ever feel differently or want to change it.

The unattached Romantic man

He has been falling in love ever since he can remember. He might even be able to tell you the exact pink of the dress of the little girl in the park who won his heart at the age of three. Puberty confused him, however. The purity of the love he had been used to feeling was sullied by a torrent of hormones that sent his head spinning with all sorts of lascivious thoughts and kept his body in a permanent state of sexual excitement. There are two main ways Romantic Junior is likely to respond to this. One is to reserve a special place in his heart for an exquisite and untouchable princess of his acquaintance and expend his 'dirty' thoughts and deeds on girls he considers more ordinary. The other way is to believe that he has fallen in love every time he is swamped by lust. To a degree, the way he deals with these adolescent attempts to reconcile lust and love will set a pattern for his romantic and sexual dealings in adult life.

Some Romantic men marry very young. They believe that the first great passion over the age of majority is 'it', and they commit themselves in a very short time. The Romantic man who has taken to placing women on pedestals is most likely to do this. If he has fallen in love with every woman he desires, however, he is less likely to marry in haste – some of his 'loves', after all, have not survived the night. And, of course, some Romantic men never marry. These men usually start off with high ideals, looking for the perfect woman, but then a procession of disappointments disillusion them. Often this kind of Romantic man has a better than average understanding of his own Sexual Style. He recognises that he needs to be in the intensely exciting first phase of love for sex to be good and for the relationship to be worth it, but he knows, too, that it doesn't last. Rather than marry, therefore, he prefers to find new loves as and when he can – until he either can't or he isn't bothered any more.

That is not to say that Mr Romantic is necessarily promiscuous. Once past the sexually indiscriminate youthful phase he usually doesn't derive maximum enjoyment from sex unless he's in love with the woman. It can seem tacky. A Romantic man I know was once plied with drink and seduced by a woman. It was a sordid memory for him; he said he'd felt 'raped'. Some Romantic men separate their romantic feelings from their sexuality and become enthralled by women that they wouldn't dream of touching sexually. Nevertheless, Mr Romantic is likely to change sexual partners more often than anyone apart from Mr Imaginative, because when love dies he is impelled to rediscover the wonder of it with someone else. Whether he has many lovers or not depends on how quickly he learns to distinguish between pure sexual fascination and an attraction that has more to it. It also depends on how fastidious he is – in other words, how quickly the reality of the woman punctures his romantic dream. It has to be said that some Romantic men require an impossible degree of perfection in women – his love without make-up, or with garlic on her breath, or not understanding his jokes, can finish it for him. Fortunately most Romantic men do allow their women to be human beings as well. Whether his love lasts five days or five years depends on these and other aspects of his personality. If he is a classic Romantic, however, while he is in love he will be intense, focused and faithful.

This is both the joy and the danger of the Romantic man. When he tells you that he loves you, that he thinks you are extraordinary, beautiful, the most sexy woman he has ever seen, and that he has never felt like this before – no one could be more sincere. Other men will say similar things in a cynical attempt to talk you into bed – but an experienced woman knows the difference. You believe Mr Romantic, and you are right to — because he means every word. You should just watch that bit about it lasting forever, or wanting to marry you, or even merely wanting to see you again. He means all that, as well: *today*. Tomorrow, or three weeks' time is another matter. A Romantic man's passion can suddenly flare up — and just as suddenly die down. When this happens, the woman feels used, bruised and furious. Strangely enough, so does he. The Romantic man, particularly one who is not strong on self-awareness, believes it must be the woman's fault. His feelings were genuine, so she must have misled him in some way. My friend Lynn was unlucky enough to excite the undying love of a Romantic to whom she was strongly attracted. He was an intelligent man in his fifties, who said he'd never felt like that before. He begged Lynn to marry him: it was a mere detail that he was already married. His undying love, unfortunately, died soon after his proposal and was replaced by an outraged conviction that she had bewitched him — that she was a wicked woman with evil powers who had tempted him off the straight and narrow.

Many Romantic men are more moderate in their reactions than this. Nevertheless, Romantics are attracted to emotional extremes — if they're not flooded with excited feelings, they are not quite sure whether they are feeling at all.

Mr Romantic likes beautiful women. What man doesn't? However, in his case it's not just because they appeal to him aesthetically or sexually, but because they appeal to other men as well. He likes a woman to be desired and sought after — it gives her glamour, and winning her proves that he is the better man. If he prides himself on his sophisticated taste the woman he goes for might be less obviously attractive, but has, he believes, a connoisseur's value. Romantic men who look for more from women than their appearance like their partners to be outstanding in some way — clever, witty, successful, unusual. Whatever she looks like, however, he usually wants her to dress as well and carefully as he does, and might have strong ideas about what suits her. He is the man most likely to nag if she puts on weight or 'lets herself go'. Sometimes what she looks like is all he is concerned about. He is the man most likely to fall for and marry a foreign woman with whom he can barely exchange a word. He can indulge himself by inventing an entire personality and intellect for her. When they can communicate he might discover that it was all a fantasy.

The Romantic man is happiest as a hunter. He'll be flattered by a woman who makes a bee-line for him, shows she wants him, calls him for a date — he might even pass the time with her until his new great love shows up. With few exceptions, however, he's unlikely to fall in love with a woman who makes the running. He'll wonder if it's because nobody else wants her. He'll worry that there's something wrong with her. Deep down, just as Groucho Marx said he wouldn't want to join a club that would have him as a member, Mr Romantic has a similar feeling about women who take the initiative. It's another sign of his fragile ego. Once she's his he wants her to adore and idealise him, but he needs to win her first. While men of other Sexual Styles can also share this preference for being the chooser rather than the chosen, for the Romantic it touches that deeper need for dramatic excitement. It's the hunter in him, for instance, that often draws him to wild, unpredictable women. There's not much skill involved in taming a rabbit, he would say, but a tiger is something else. Difficult, wayward women also hold his romantic attention for longer. When his woman is capricious he can continue to see her as special and to a degree unattainable. Even if he is sometimes driven mad by her, or made very unhappy, he often prefers this turbulence to homey contentment. At his most perverse, he will ardently pursue a woman, sometimes for years, who does not return his feelings. But in some cases when he finally wins her his love dwindles in a very short time.

This is Mr Romantic at his most desperate, however. It is how he generates drama in the absence of rapture. For the need for drama is what defines the Romantic man and powers his love-life. This is different from the excitement required by Mr Imaginative, for whom novelty and variety are essential. For Mr Romantic, to be adored is exciting; to worship is exciting. It is the excitement generated by bliss – that light-headed transformation of perception that comes with being in love. When his life is without drama he feels flat – or worse: restless.

Sex and Mr Romantic

The Romantic man can be a very good lover, if he wants to be. The actor in him likes to put on a good performance, and to a degree he will be watching himself and taking pride in how he does, sometimes at the expense of his own physical sensations. Not all Romantic men are good lovers, however. Sometimes this is simply because technique has never been an issue during their highly charged passionate encounters – or because they perceive the magic to have gone once they are required to think about how to turn a woman on or satisfy her. Other Romantic men see sex as low priority, or find the sheer animality sullying. Even when sex is more important to him he can sometimes be put off by a woman who frankly revels in sexual contact. When she becomes sweaty, her hair sticks up, she is mottled by a sexual flush, or makes unfeminine noises, he finds it disturbing. If the rictus of orgasm spoils her prettiness it can mar his pleasure. When a woman tells him what she does or doesn't like sexually it destroys the passionate inevitability for him, or he feels it is a criticism of his prowess. In some cases he is more excited by a woman who accepts his love-making with gracious indifference, so long as she is not disgusted. A woman who wants more sex than he does will profoundly irritate him – sex for its own sake seems brutal; it is unerotic for him if it is not connected to an emotional outrush of love or even anger. Remember, love, as far as he is concerned, is sentimental, rose-tinted – not the quieter, deeper, unselfish concern that moves without drama. As his sex drive diminishes he is the man most likely to be prudish about sex.

Most Romantic men like a touch of Hollywood at bedtime. Freshly-pressed silk or satin nightwear, freshly brushed hair and teeth, a face that doesn't look made-up, but is not heavily creamed or too well scrubbed either. He doesn't subscribe to the view that a man's shirt or pyjamas look better on a woman, nor will he be turned on by her wearing an old winceyette nightgown, or a baggy tee-shirt. A woman coming to him naked can be very exciting in the early days, but nudity *per se* is not especially erotic to him over time, particularly if she is not physically flawless. He likes her to 'smell nice', but that usually means perfume, not soap or her natural smell. He's not comfortable being reminded that his princess has normal bodily functions. This is not a man who will be happy watching his woman shave her legs, or accepting that she too suffers from wind.

The Romantic is beguiled by the right atmosphere. Creative lighting, moody music, and anything that evokes the thrilling and the mysterious is desirable. He is less likely to be aroused when surrounded by casual untidiness, and can only be turned on in sordid or uncomfortable surroundings when in an illicit, complicated relationship which leaves few options. Then this, too, will seem romantic.

As far as sexual technique and preferences go, Romantic men are highly variable, but there are some distinguishing characteristics. Unless they are concerned to prove that they are good lovers and that they have read the right books, foreplay as such holds little interest for them. From their own point of view, they usually want to make love when gripped by powerful feelings, and then they need no readying themselves. Consequently, the idea of having to coax a woman into readiness dampens the fire of their passion. Unless their Romantic nature is strongly underpinned by sensuality, caresses might arouse their groins, but little else. The best foreplay from their point of view is non-physical — the drama of a row, reconciliation, sentimental love-talk or admiration — him for her, or vice versa. Non-sexual massage, however, is different. Mr Sensual might bask in the physical sensations, but Mr Romantic is moved by the love, concern and care his partner shows by wanting to ease his muscle tensions and relax his body. The woman who understands her Romantic partner well knows that if he is not in the mood for love-making, offering him a back-rub is more likely to result in sex than a more openly seductive approach.

Because Mr Romantic prefers to make love in the heat of passion, he finds the 'quickie' — when both are overtaken by desire, which flares up suddenly and is consummated quickly — most satisfying. Many men enjoy a brief and lustful coupling from time to time, but for this man the best part of it is the feeling of being carried away by something too powerful to resist. If it was just for sexual relief he would end up feeling disgusted with himself, his partner, or both. On the other hand, when he is feeling deeply delighted by his partner, spending hours lazing together in bed, punctuated by bouts of love-making is also bliss for him. What he doesn't like is extended love-making for the sake of it.

When he is in love, sex has a meaning for Mr Romantic which transcends the physical. He is the man least likely to enjoy sex as sport. While his sex drive is high, and in between great loves, he may go to bed casually with someone who means little to him, and might use the experience to hone his technique, as well as to get some relief. Although this is very much second best as far as he is concerned, he might, paradoxically, be a better lover with someone that he doesn't love — when he is not transported with ecstasy he is more able to concentrate on what he is doing. But if his vanity requires him to be an expert lover, he might well be fairly adventurous and experimental, even with his adored partner. Orchestrating a complicated sexual routine can make him feel talented and smug. Sex for show, however, creates a certain distance and is ultimately low on intimate contact. Bluntly, the heady, inflamed feelings he labels as love are not the same as truly intimate love, which requires a depth of openness, acceptance of reality, and mutual tolerance which he finds off-putting.

Sex is a serious matter for the Romantic man. He tends to leave his wit and sense of humour outside the bedroom door. Laughing during, or at, sex, like laughing in church, undermines the significance for him. He can sometimes be laughed *into* bed — when his partner's wit and humour are part of her charm for him, but she must then remember where she is. Sex, at its best, is a hallowed, religious experience for him.

During adolescence Mr Romantic might have a scientific interest in pornography, but it is rarely the sort of turn-on he likes in later life. The exception is the Romantic man who keeps his woman on a non-sexual pedestal. In the well-known madonna/whore split he will cherish her tenderly and believe she is above sex, while venting his sexual feelings on less worthy women. He might then use pornography and even prefer dirty, degrading sex as an antithesis to his pure feelings for her.

Safe sex and condoms are anti-romance. Mr Romantic hates to have to talk about these things — it's so calculating, he feels. He's capable of lying, if it suits him, but with a woman he loves he feels more fated about it. The past means nothing to him when he is newly in love — he can't believe that it could rise up and cause disease. We are in love, he explains. Nothing will happen to us.

The Romantic man and marriage

Some Romantic men marry early, others never do. Most are in between. Whichever he chooses, the institution of marriage is difficult for the Romantic, whose preferred emotional state is somewhat divorced from reality. It's hard to idealise the person you see every day over breakfast, or to be admired by someone with intimate knowledge of your quirks and failings.

In some ways, the Romantic man who marries for pragmatic reasons has the best chance of marital stability. If the relationship has never seemed intoxicating or powerfully fated it is easier for him to keep in view his reasons for marrying in the first place. When he marries on a high, however, he will eventually have to battle with his disappointment when the intensity of excitement passes.

The Romantic man who has managed to separate his sexual urges from his romantic feelings can make a marriage that endures for a long time, or quickly goes wrong. He has often pursued his woman ardently and relentlessly, but once she is his wife he doesn't want to make love to her. Sometimes it is abrupt – within weeks of marrying, and occasionally accompanied by distaste for sex with her. A sex therapist told me about a man who went off on a month's holiday and came back married to a woman he had met while abroad. He stopped wanting sex with her after two weeks, and when six months had passed she began to despair. She tentatively suggested one morning that he see a doctor about his lack of libido. Instead he stayed away for 24 hours, and when he eventually returned home he handed her a prostitute's calling card, on which the woman had scrawled 'your husband's a very good fuck'. As the sex therapist said, he had behaved cruelly because he had been wounded by what he saw as his wife's criticism. But: 'He didn't see it as a problem: it was in his nature to put loved women on a pedestal. Previously this position had been reserved for his mother, now he expected his wife to occupy it, and she shouldn't be thinking about sex on her pedestal – that activity was for naughty girls.'

Sometimes he only goes off sex after his wife has had a child, when by turning into a mother she breaks his image of her as girl-woman. The Romantic man who loves his wife because she adores him is the man most likely to resent having to share her love and attention with children. If she is similarly unconcerned about sex this is workable – indeed the lack of physical closeness, when it suits them both, can allow the distance necessary for mystery to be maintained. If sex is more important to her, however – either physically or symbolically – unbearable tensions can build up between them.

Nevertheless, Romantic men can and do make lasting marriages that are happy and continue to have an undercurrent of excitement in them. Scott Fitzgerald and Zelda achieved this by battling and infuriating each other. They eventually divorced, but the breakdown was more to do with his alcoholism and failing success as a writer, and her increasing mental instability, than it was with the way they chose to interact.

Not that this extreme of behaviour is the only way to hold the attention of the Romantic husband. His liking for enigma and his preference for distance over intimacy has its positive side. He can often tolerate better than other men his wife having an identity of her own – he sometimes loves her more as a wife when he continues to see her as an individual. A vital, busy, popular woman is a constant reminder of how lucky he is to have won her. It is important to this kind of man that his wife continues to be attractive – when she is no longer young he likes her to be chic. He can also be excited by other men's admiration of her, so long as there is no danger of her reciprocating their attentions. As one Romantic man said petulantly to his beautiful wife: 'Why don't you ever flirt with other men, or make me feel in danger of losing you?'

Danger it is, however, if he is the more jealous Romantic who needs to be adored more than he needs to adore. These men have the most fragile egos, and a constant need for reassurance. They don't take kindly to criticism or less than unwavering admiration. They are men it is hard to get close to, because they don't want their outward image penetrated. This kind of man can remain faithful and attached to a wife who is dedicated to shoring up his ego, or who, for her own reasons, is not keen to get close enough to see his flaws.

On a day-to-day level marriage to the Romantic man works best when a respectful distance is maintained. The couple should use the bathroom separately, even dress alone, and be as private and careful in their personal habits as they would with strangers. He likes her to look nice for *him*, not just when they are going out. She's mistaken if she thinks that after some years he will just take her as he finds her. When space allows, it even works for them to have separate bedrooms. He doesn't enjoy being reminded that the face he loves owes much to the pots on the dressing table, or to be confronted with her discarded underwear. For the undiluted Romantic man, snuggling up together every night is not as rewarding as the freedom of choice to sleep together or have sex when it feels right. Indeed, the Romantic man often remains most passionately committed to a relationship with enforced separations — when he has to travel for work, or even if circumstances place them in different countries with only occasional meetings. Time apart restores the magic, allows the little irritations to fade, and heightens his desire. In some cases, the Romantic man's attention can be held forever if she refuses to marry him, even if they live together. Knowing that he can't own her enhances his commitment: she is close enough, but tantalisingly out of reach.

Ultimately, the Romantic man can tolerate a relationship without sex, but there needs to be an enduring sense of specialness about the union, a feeling that no other woman could make him feel like this.

When Mr Romantic will stray

Of all the Sexual Styles, Mr Romantic is the most likely to give up everything when a new love explodes into his life. If he is a pure Romantic, he can leave wife, family, home, job — and consider it all well lost, even if he has spent years building a lifestyle that suited him. Fortunately for the partners of Romantic men, most of them have a leavening of the other Styles and are less likely to be so devil-may-care.

Nevertheless, Romantic men find it hard to resist temptation when intoxicated by a new love. If his sexuality is well integrated into his nature he will only stray when his feelings are engaged, and is less likely to be unfaithful purely out of lust. This, however, makes his liaisons more unsettling and potentially fatal to his marriage. He'll never leave his wife because sex is better elsewhere, but because he is compelled by something that seems greater than himself. If he feels more strongly for his mistress than his wife it can damage his commitment to his wife forever. On the other hand, the Romantic who finds it difficult to be sexual with women he truly loves might be unfaithful more often to 'get the sex out of his system', but he will be casual and contemptuous of the women he sleeps with. He might even prefer prostitutes.

The Romantic who has recognised that he is a love-junkie – and that all his loves evaporate over time – can indulge in a series of affairs as a way of protecting his marriage. He needs the fix for excitement, but doesn't want to jeopardise his home life. He is less in danger of leaving his wife because he recognises that the highs he seeks are inevitably followed by lows.

On the whole, the Romantic man is less likely than most men to be remotely interested in sex with someone else while his central relationship continues to obsess him. While he is focused on one woman he barely notices others, except to compare them unfavourably with her.

Mr Romantic and sexual problems

As the best sex is linked to heightened feelings of excitement for Mr Romantic, it follows that when these are absent he is less interested. If his natural sex drive is high then this might not be immediately apparent: his need for regular sex obscures the fact that it is a second-rate experience for him. If his need for sex is low, or as it wanes, he can go for long periods without feeling desirous. If his partner feels differently, then a problem emerges. It is his nature, in these circumstances, not to perceive it as a problem, or else he places the blame elsewhere — he is fully functioning, after all, so it must be because the relationship or his partner is at fault.

In these circumstances sex will not improve unless the relationship is regalvanised. Sometimes a measured dose of jealousy acts like a shot in the arm, but this should be approached with caution. Some emotional fireworks — as long as they are not too threatening — can also lead to satisfactory making up. Often, drawing back from too much cosy domesticity, and injecting a bit of mystery and glamour works best. The much-mocked women's magazine advice to women to make an effort with their appearance, dress alluringly, make him feel special and so on, is tailored to the Romantic man. The other Sexual Styles are less likely to be influenced by these tactics alone, but unless there are deeper problems in the relationship Mr Romantic responds as the magazines say he will. The Romantic with this kind of problem is most resistant to sex therapy that seeks to uncover the source of the trouble. Anything that lays bare his faults, or his partner's dissatisfaction will make him truculently resistant to the process. If he's disappointed by sex or has gone off it, he believes, it's because the wonderful feelings between us have gone, and tinkering with the mechanics or talking about it won't put it right.

The Romantic man who has only ever had sexual encounters in a blaze of passion can find that in a settled relationship his technique is limited. When he is low on sensuality and all his sensations are concentrated in his heart and his penis, the erogenous potential of the whole body can be lost on him. While appealing to his senses might not work in this situation, an appeal to his vanity has more chance of success. Don't criticise. He needs you to think he's a wonderful lover. Then a tactful but tactical programme to introduce him to new ideas through films, perhaps, or books, can arouse his competitive instincts to show that he can do as well or better. It helps his ego to think that it is his idea, rather than yours.

A more intractable kind of problem is faced by the Romantic man who has successfully managed to separate his sexual feelings from the romantic. He can function sexually, but rarely with the women he cares most for. Putting the two together, indeed, can kill his finer feelings: women are to be adored, not used, and when they become sexual beings they fall from grace. As has been said already, this can work well when the woman colludes and she too can live harmoniously without sex. When this makes her unhappy, however, the beautiful relationship is set to fail. Therapy, sexual or otherwise, can sometimes help to increase the man's understanding of why he has split in this way, and if he is motivated to change progress can be made. But it is unlikely that he will be able fully to integrate the two facets of his nature without some loss: and the most likely casualty is his romantic dream. The most successful marriages made by this kind of Romantic man are those that are based on an unromantic realism, boosted by his sexless crushes on unavailable women. It's not ideal, but his tolerant wife is prepared to put up with his occasional yearnings for someone else in the knowledge that he is unlikely to be unfaithful.

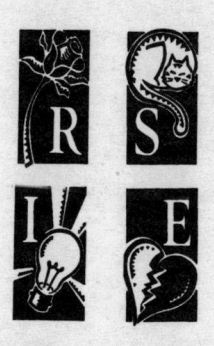

The Romantic Combinations

The Romantic Combinations

This section looks at Romantics who have a strong subsidiary Sexual Style. It should be read in conjunction with the main Romantic chapter, and you should also look at the sections on sex and love for the secondary Style, or Styles. Each person will manifest their sexual combination in a unique way but, if you have identified your Sexual Style correctly, the broad themes will apply.

The ROMANTIC-Sensual (R-S)

A Sensual element in the Romantic personality has the effect of keeping the Romantic's feet on the ground. This combination is much easier to contain than it is when the balance is reversed (the SENSUAL-Romantic). A more Sensual person is made uncomfortable by the Romantic need for extra drama, whereas a Romantic finds the practical extension of a down-to-earth Sensual streak can help make dreams come true. Less often, however, Romantics find that a Sensual element manifests as a carping inner voice of convention or over-caution ('You *can't* do *that*'), so that their Romantic yearnings remain unrealised.

The R-S woman has a special allure for men. Her extreme femininity and the attractive way she presents herself has follow-through. The Romantic woman *wants* to be sexually responsive and sexually pleasing; she *wants* to be a good cook and home-maker: it's feminine. With a strong dose of Sensual in her nature she does more than wish: she delivers. This is the woman who flirts and means it, although she is still unlikely to let her earthy, lustful nature lead her into a sexual embrace for the sake of it. Like other Romantic women, she needs to feel that she is in love to make sex meaningful and so as not to feel cheap. Unlike the thoroughgoing Romantic, however, a sexual attraction can lead her to believe she is in love – and even if it lasts only for that night or a week it won't shake her conviction that it was real while it lasted.

The Romantic male has this tendency anyway. Love makes him feel lustful, and vice versa. The difference when Sensual combines in his temperament is that he derives more pleasure from sex itself. What this means is that he is less likely to need air-brushed perfection from his woman in bed, and sexual compatibility intensifies his romantic satisfaction. He is unlikely to be dazzled by the sexless icon who can be very compelling to other Romantics, or to go in for intense unrequited passions beyond adolescence. He is drawn to genuinely sexy women – so long as they look good to him – and finds it difficult to retain an infatuation for a woman who is not attracted to him or who does not enjoy sex. Other Romantic men can sometimes find these sexual obstacles strangely thrilling, increasing their desire to win and conquer. The R-S, on the other hand, loses interest.

It is similar with R-S women. They are usually attracted to overtly sexy men. They respond to the words of Tennyson: 'He is all fault who hath no fault at all:/For who loves me must have a touch of earth.' Actually, their dominant Romantic side rarely allows them to act on these attractions unless the men have more to offer, and they could find it embarrassing to be partnered by them, but they need more than other Romantics to have the romance in their relationships validated by an active sex life.

Grace Kelly was a good example of this Style. Alfred Hitchcock, who directed her when she was an actress, compared her to a snow-covered volcano — a reference to the sexuality that smouldered beneath her beautiful, virginal exterior. Becoming a princess, by her marriage to Prince Rainier of Monaco, was the ultimate Romantic dream, and the riches and stability this offered were important to her Sensual nature. Nevertheless, the Romantic in her was disappointed. 'I have come to feel very sad in this marriage,' she told Gwen Robyns. 'He's not really interested in me.' A Romantic needs to feel special and vital to her man, and, as Robyns said: 'She operated on adulation.' Her Sensual side gave her the grit to stay in her marriage despite disappointment, and the Sensual in her also loved food and drink. It was rumoured she had affairs with good-looking younger men: 'What she wanted was eternal glamour, and those young men supplied it.'

Aristotle Onassis epitomised the male R-S. He caught his own version of the princess: Jackie Kennedy, widow of the US president, who was as beautiful, glamorous, famous and charismatic as his Romantic nature demanded. She was not interested in him sexually, however, and sex was very important to him. He returned for comfort to his former mistress, Maria Callas, the opera singer. Nevertheless, he remained married to Jackie because, as a Romantic first, it suited him to flaunt such a prize even if there was no substance to the relationship. If Sensual had been dominant in his nature, Maria Callas, who adored him, probably would have been his choice of wife. But his Romantic craving for the right image won in the end.

Usually the Sensual component in the R-S character makes for more stability in relationships. The R-S woman in particular settles down to married life prepared to make it work — a concept difficult for many other Romantics. Their passionate involvement is extended in a relationship that includes satisfying love-making, and they find the business of daily life and home-making more rewarding than is usual for a Romantic. But they need to bring glamour and excitement to the mundane, unlike the Sensuals, or even SENSUAL-Romantics. Cooking becomes an art, as does decorating, gardening and child-rearing.

Romantic men are often the least likely to stick in relationships that have lost intensity, and their tendency to risk all for love can can turn them into much-married serial monogamists. But when Sensual forms part of their make-up they tend to weigh the consequences with care, and their commitment is fuelled by security at home and the pleasures of an enduring sex life.

Nevertheless, they are Romantics. Commitment can feel like an endless austerity when the special intensity of romance goes, or when they stop admiring their partners or feel over-looked themselves. Sensual compensations then lose their power. Indeed, an R-S woman, while retaining a need and desire for sex, can find she is unmoved by her partner's attentions if she feels taken for granted or she no longer finds him admirable. An R-S man is more easily beguiled into believing that love is present while sex is frequent, but he will lose his desire for a woman who ceases to look attractive to him. For R-S men and women the Sensual might then be expressed as a timidity about leaving the relationship unless a concrete and safe alternative has been set up. On the other hand, when the relationship retains its special quality of mutual admiration, or is a show-case for happy family life and a refined lifestyle, the R-S ultimately feels that sex is not an essential element. It's a bonus, but there are other rewards.

The ROMANTIC-Imaginative (R-I)

These Romantics are usually top of everyone's party list. When Romantic combines with Imaginative you have an electric personality: the kind of person who is fun, interesting and gregarious, who makes every social occasion memorable. Inevitably there's a drawback. They won't necessarily turn up to *your* party if a better, more exciting offer comes along. Indeed, they often accept a number of invitations for the same night, and then see what they feel like when the time comes. These emotional butterflies are charm personified, but they're not prepared to make concessions to convention, and having to take other people's feelings into account is boring, not to say irritating. This is often reflected in their love relationships as well. Being mainly Romantic, there is nothing they like better than the heady thrill of being madly in love, heightened, for their Imaginative side, by the fact that it is all so new and uncharted. But when, over time, this exciting phase passes, they find it hard to think of a good reason for hanging on to the relationship. Of course, they *can* feel deeper love, but if their interest is not profoundly engaged, or sex has become routine, and the dynamic interaction between them and their partners has slid into a gentle acceptance, something in their temperament makes staying together seem illogical.

Talking of sex, some R-Is are highly sexed, but sexual contentment alone is not enough to bind them to one other person. Variety is too important to them and that includes variety of partners. Their dominant Romantic nature makes them more sexually constant than the reverse combination, the IMAGINATIVE-Romantic (I-R) — certainly for as long as they continue to feel there is something magically special about their partners. But should this admiration go, or they feel taken for granted, they re-experience the Imaginative itch for something new. Some R-Is, indeed, have much less interest in, or need for, sex. They can be thrilled by a relationship that is intensely engaging intellectually — wondrous, pure mutual admiration — and virtually sexless. This kind of interaction is exemplified in the film *Brief Encounter*, which starred Trevor Howard and Celia Johnson. Their absorbing, fated passion with its snatched meetings could never come to anything because of their commitments elsewhere. The hero departing for Africa made a perfect ending – a romantic encounter that could never be sullied by domestic detail.

A real-life R-I is Janine, who conducted a 25-year relationship with a man she rarely saw. Richard travelled the world for work. They corresponded, telephoned, and had occasional, passionate months together. For the sake of this relationship she was prepared to forego marriage, children, and a partner who was there for her emotionally and sexually. All Romantics have a soft spot for a relationship in which excitement is kept on the boil by distance, but with a strong leavening of Emotional or Sensual in their make-up a relationship such as this would ultimately disturb them.

Emotions are disturbing anyway to the R-I. Not that they don't have them, but they are frightened by their illogical power, and connect best to emotions that Romantics understand – passionate infatuation and the jealousy and rows that can result. They are uncomfortable with anything gloomy, and have a good repertoire of evasive tactics – filling their lives with fun and adventure so as not to be trapped by emotional turmoil. When they do suffer they have a talent for turning it into a story to amuse or rivet their friends.

A good example of the R-I male is Gay Kindersley, the Anglo-Irish aristocratic millionaire and amateur champion jockey. Interviewed by the London *Evening Standard* at the age of 64, he described his constant sexual adventuring while expressing devotion to his second wife, the beautiful and much younger Phillipa, 'who understands me completely', and to whom he had been married for nearly 20 years. Like all R-Is he is renowned for his charm and openness: his autobiography chronicles his three great passions – drinking, horses and falling in love. Like many Romantics, he wears his heart on his sleeve, 'I still burst into tears frequently', but he seems untroubled by deeper emotional considerations. Phillipa knew all about his infidelities – when he was interviewed he was having an open affair with the local barmaid — and she tolerated his frequent sex holidays to Thailand, only cautioning him to ration himself to sleeping with five girls. It wouldn't occur to him as an R-I that she might be harbouring more troubled feelings. R-Is say what they think, and anything unsaid does not seem real to them. Kindersley's Imaginative streak is strong: 'I've got this infidelity thing, I've always had to be chasing.' But the Romantic overlay means that he doesn't see it as pure sex. 'If I'm going to a party I long to be drawn next to a pretty girl. I have a great capacity for falling in love.'

If a relationship is going to have any lasting power, an R-I needs to feel important, while being beguiled by an intellectual or sexually inventive partner. Their relationships last longest when there is genuine, undimmed admiration — preferably on both sides, but at least one way. It is the dominating Romantic in their sexual personalities that needs to feel that they are with someone conspicuously special, with good looks, wealth, status or talent — best of all when they are combined. Alternatively they need to feel constantly adored — their susceptible egos return admiration with grateful love, and won't take kindly to criticism. If this element is missing, however, the relationship will lose its power for them — whatever the brain-power or the sexual sophistication of their partners. They find it fairly easy to be casual in sexual adventures, particularly male R-Is, so long as there is a compelling central romance in their lives. But if casualness, coolness, or sometimes even cosy affection, should become the keynote of this primary relationship they will feel the heart has been wrenched out of it. In this case, the quest will be on for someone new.

Fundamentally R-Is are happiest when they are in love. But the Romantic's streak of emotional independence is fortified by the Imaginative ability to find comfort as well as fascination in new experiences and adventures. R-Is won't sulk or pine when there is no one special in their lives. They will be out and about doing interesting things and having fun. This *joie de vivre* inevitably makes them attractive to others, and they rarely have to wait too long before the next romantic opportunity presents itself.

The ROMANTIC-Emotional (R-E)

When a Romantic's Séxual Style is tempered by Emotional the result is a complex character with the capacity to make enduring relationships, albeit often tempestuous and difficult. The R-E has all the allure of the traditional Romantic, but is far less straightforward than he or she may seem. In a way, the R-E is like the spider in the nursery rhyme: '"Will you walk into my parlour?" said a spider to a fly;/"Tis the prettiest little parlour that ever you did spy."' He or she is attractive, winning and fun, but the 'pretty parlour' conceals a person with a need to feel intensely bonded to another, sometimes in misery. The R-E can be much more deeply hurt than the pure Romantic, and hasn't the same capacity to recover when a promising romantic relationship fails. An extreme example is Dickens' tragic, fictional Miss Havisham in *Great Expectations*, who was jilted on her wedding day. To the end of her long embittered life she sat amidst the ruins of her cobwebby wedding feast, wearing her tattered bridal gown. Romantically fixated on her erstwhile suitor, the dark, Emotional side of her nature gained comfort from wreaking revenge on all men, and blighting the love-life of her apparent protégé, Pip.

More usually, R-Es are attracted — as Romantics tend to be — by people they perceive as stunningly good-looking or special. Long-lasting unions are created when these people touch a deeper and more mysterious emotional need.

Lucille Ball, the mega-successful comedienne most well-known for the Fifties' television series *I Love Lucy*, was a typical R-E. This was most apparent in her marriage to Desi Arnaz, alongside whom she starred, and to whom she was married for 20 years. It was love at first sight. He was dazzlingly handsome and somewhat younger than Lucy. Theirs was a passionate, jealous and tempestuous relationship from the start. 'My friends gave the marriage six months,' Lucy said later. 'I gave it six weeks.' Their relationship continued to be stormy – some would say destructive – throughout their marriage. Four years after they married Lucy was filing for divorce because of Desi's chronic infidelity, but she soon dropped the case. They fought constantly, but continued to work and live together. A power struggle was central to their interaction, as is often the case with people who have an Emotional element in their characters: Lucy held the professional power, while Desi's vengeance was expressed in heavy drinking, womanising and, finally, violence. She divorced him for real in 1959 for extreme cruelty and causing grievous mental suffering. Only a woman with a strong Emotional streak would have put up with it; even enjoyed it. Lucy was the richer and more successful partner: she certainly did not have to stay with him for reasons other than choice. As with all R-Es, it was precisely the torment and difficulties between them that fed the excitement and romance from her point of view. For this Sexual Style emotional fireworks are usually preferable to placid contentment, or 'quiet' love. A pure Emotional might have stayed the course, even with an increasingly violent and alcoholic husband. Where Romantic is more dominant, however, as in Lucy's case, ultimately self-preservation wins. Neither is the Romantic impressed by the physical ravages caused by alcoholism. Romantics, even R-Es, have to bear their own physical decline, but it's not necessary for them to have to endure it in a partner. Love is rarely blind to the physical for the mainly Romantic person.

Some R-Es are also sexually passionate people. But what happens in bed is far less important for this Sexual Style than the sense that a relationship is life-changing in its intensity and its quality of significance. It needs to touch deep and possibly unconscious emotional chords. This lights the love-flame which all Romantics need to feel that nothing else matters so much as the two of them.

An example of the male R-E, for whom sex was only a minor consideration, was King Edward VIII. He made the ultimate Romantic gesture by giving up the throne of England in 1937 to marry his great love, Wallis Simpson, an American divorcée, who, in those days, could not be accepted as Queen. Wallis was 38 when their relationship began, and she had never been a beauty. The Prince of Wales, as he then was, found her fascinating. He was enraptured by her chic, her style, and her informal American manners, which he thought daring and glamorous. As it happens, she was his Romantic ideal. But to give up being King for her, to accept the lesser title of Duke of Windsor? To remain passionately dazzled by her until the day he died? People wanted to know what her secret was. It was said by some that it was refined sexual technique, picked up during the time she had spent in China being taught, it was rumoured, the secrets of high-class prostitutes. But the Duke of Windsor had little interest in or desire for sex, as earlier mistresses testified. Instead, Wallis appealed to the Emotional in his nature. His parents had been cold and his childhood was unhappy. Wallis became a mother to him – domineering but loving. She fostered his Romantic attachment by bolstering his ego. She also recognised that the man who was born to rule had a deep need to serve. She made him fear her as much as he loved her and, while flattering him, also treated him as a lackey. Sex played a small part in their relationship, and what there was apparently continued this power play. One close friend believed that they indulged in elaborate sex games – nanny and child scenes, where she was dominant, and he was happily submissive.

There are, of course, R-Es with more conventional, happier

Emotional requirements. The long-term relationships they make are not so perplexing to outsiders. Certainly, when deeper needs are met it often invests their partner with the aura of specialness that they, as Romantics, need to feel satisfied with life.

But although R-Es take relationship breakdowns hard, and might stay in a partnership longer for fear of being alone, their stronger Romantic qualities will give them the impetus to leave a relationship that disappoints. Their Romantic propensity for feeling wounded when no longer highly regarded by their partners, or if they lose respect for an erstwhile loved one, is intensified by their secondary Emotional sensitivity. This outweighs any fears about loneliness. The Romantic urge to merge in a delightful way, fuelled by the more primitive Emotional need to bond will force them out on the hunt again. On the other hand, even R-Es will put up with the loss of profounder feelings in a relationship in the interests of a partnership that has what they deem to be the right ingredients. The 'perfect' partner who can be shown off, the good lifestyle – these elements might seem to others to have only superficial glamour, but for the R-E there is something emotionally satisfying in them as well.

Combinations of three or four

It is rare to have a genuinely equal balance of Sexual Styles. One will be dominant – in these cases Romantic – and the remaining two or three are also unlikely to be found in equal measure. In most cases one of them will combine most strongly with the main Romantic Style (in the ways described above) and the third and possibly fourth will add colour and subtlety, but little more. Most usually, aspects of the weaker Styles will be noticeable in other aspects of your personality – your attitude to clothes, career, loved ones other than partners, and so on. The following descriptions are therefore only broad guidelines to the possible ways the Styles can coexist.

The ROMANTIC-Sensual-Imaginative (R-S-I)

This Romantic knows what feels good — and it feels even better with a partner who stimulates more than the erogenous zones — but only when this is heightened by the essential ingredient of feeling this relationship is special, intoxicating even. Or, to put it another way, the R-S-I falls in love with someone who is interesting and with whom he or she is sexually compatible. Adding Sensual to the Romantic and Imaginative cocktail earths the volatile nature of this combination. This person has more need for a relationship with staying power.

When the Sensual component is stronger than the Imaginative, the R-S-I has a greater capacity for loyalty in an exclusive relationship. The Imaginative requirement in this case is usually confined to needing a partner who is interesting and mentally stimulating. When the proportions are reversed and Imaginative dominates, the R-S-I is likely to have a more roving eye, and the Sensual need for stability is less obvious than the Sensual precondition that sex be truly satisfying as much as it is experimental.

As Romantic defines this person's nature, however, the Sensual and Imaginative elements only contribute to an ideal package. Even good sex and a lively mental interaction are not enough unless R-S-Is are made to feel special and important, or feel great and enduring admiration for their partners. With Romantic as the main ingredient in this Sexual Style, what the world thinks is also important. While the facade remains intact, much is bearable. When there is mutual — or even one-way — admiration, the rest seems less important.

In the end, this Sexual Style can tolerate life without good sex or intellectual stimulation, but is likely to look round for a substitute if the relationship has become mundane, or when too much disillusion has crept in.

The ROMANTIC-Sensual-Emotional (R-S-E)

Deep currents of feeling run through this Romantic's relationships, and there is a strong tactile element. This is the steadiest of all Romantics, as both the Sensual and Emotional contribute in their different ways to a profounder need for stability and deep bonds in a relationship.

When Sensual is dominant, there is a stress on certainty and security, as well as the physical elements of comfort and sexual satisfaction. This will often open the channels to the deeper feelings that the Emotional demands. If the Emotional side has a higher priority, then this Romantic has a greater need for profound and sometimes more difficult emotional needs to be met. This then paves the way for good sex, but does not depend on it so strongly.

The R-S-E is the least carefree kind of Romantic, and the most cautious about entering into relationships. Fear of being hurt, and wanting to know that there is a guarantee of stability before being able to commit makes for an uncharacteristic defensiveness. In some cases, especially when he or she has been hurt and disappointed, this creates such a mistrust of relationships that the R-S-E retreats into a self-protective Romantic position of loving from afar. These Romantics then yearn for physical and emotional closeness but choose impossible love-objects who do not return their feelings.

More frequently, however, they will cling on to their partners for longer than Romantics usually do. They can forego the profounder satisfaction of emotional and sexual connections if the relationship still bears the hallmark of specialness that Romantics require. But if the R-S-E begins to feel that there is nothing inherently special between them in the Romantic sense then the relationship won't feel worthwhile. Parting will cause great anguish, but this pain is ultimately more tolerable than remaining in a relationship that seems, from a Romantic point of view, empty.

The ROMANTIC-Imaginative-Emotional (R-I-E)

Sex, however good, is never ultimately an essential factor for this Style, whose representatives need intellectual stimulation and an emotional connection with strong reverberations much more.

In this case the Romantic's deeper emotions are likely to be activated by a sparky, intelligent and interesting partner, and sexual variety gives more of a kick than sexual security and compatibility.

But, to a degree, Imaginative and Emotional elements tend to war in any temperament. One wants to bond and merge, and the other needs more unpredictability. The Emotional component strengthens the Romantic need for eternal love, and the Imaginative enhances the Romantic demand for excitement and drama. This can be an uncomfortable pairing, unless the R-I-E's Emotional side thrives on fear, or when abandonment or rejection is an underlying theme in this person's life. In this case, the R-I-E of either sex is the greatest potential drama queen — secretly thriving on turmoil, uncertainty and difficulties that can seem insupportable to others.

The R-I-E with less destructive emotional impulses is happiest in a relationship that continues to feel romantic, and also has a creative intellectual element with some variety of experience, as well as deeper emotional roots. But the Romantic needs to feel special, adoring, or in an enviable situation even more than he or she needs the less tangible-seeming pleasures that motivate the Imaginative and the Emotional. Without this dramatic quality, the other elements seem less satisfying, and eventually the R-I-E will look elsewhere — or at least wish for an alternative.

The ROMANTIC-Sensual-Emotional-Imaginative (R-S-E-I)

Of all Sexual Styles, Romantics are the most likely to have impossibly high ideals about relationships. In their hearts they want only the very best: the most brilliant and attractive partners; a sexual relationship that is enduringly good and special; an emotional attachment so profoundly right that it is like meeting a soulmate. No one would turn down such a prize, but while the other Sexual Styles are more likely to see it as a wonderful vision which is ultimately fantasy, Romantics tend to feel that this person exists out there somewhere — and can be found if they look hard enough.

Most Romantics, indeed, will believe that they are R-S-E-Is, for precisely this reason. In reality, however, when they are making their relationships, they will find that one or perhaps two of the other Sexual Styles is more dominant in their nature. They cease to mind the missing element, or elements, in a relationship that otherwise meets their requirements.

It is a rare relationship, anyway, that manages to keep all these elements in perfect balance all the time. Relationships change, have their ups and downs, disappoint at times, however good and strong they are. The Romantic who continues to feel the need for this delicate balance of perfection is more likely than most to feel that low points in a relationship are truly unbearable. In the quest for the ideal, therefore, this Romantic has the propensity to leave relationships that other people would deem good enough — or even better than good enough. Compromise of any sort can seem a betrayal of the Romantic dream. Indeed, this demanding Romantic is likely to chase the mirage for so long that he or she ultimately ends up alone.

Nevertheless, Romantics also have an ability to see what they want to see. Their essential requirement is for a unique and exclusive attachment, which relegates all other relationships to second place or lower. The Romantic who has this can invest it with all the qualities that he or she desires: perfect sex, lively interaction and potent emotional bonds. Until the glamour fades, that is.

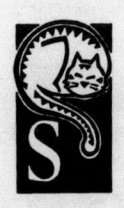

The Sensual Woman

'Some creatures simply *die* if unmated.'

Marie Stopes, pioneer in birth control, in
'Married Love' (1918)

The Sensual Woman

When Marie Stopes first published her books *Married Love* and *Wise Parenthood*, in which she wrote of women's sexuality and the need for contraception, she almost single-handedly gave respectability to the Sensual woman. For a long time previously the Sensual woman was thought to be an aberration. A contemporary gynaecological text expressed the accepted view: 'In the normal woman, especially of the higher social classes, the sexual instinct is acquired, not inborn; when it is inborn, or awakens of itself, there is *abnormality*. Since women do not know this instinct before marriage, they do not miss it when they have no occasion in life to learn it.' Sensual women had to conceal their natures with care. Since then, of course, much has changed — nowadays many women who enjoy sex would be quite happy to categorise themselves as 'Sensuals'. Not all of them are right.

Yes, as Marie Stopes was one of the first in modern times to state, every normal healthy woman experiences the desire for sex, the ability to enjoy it and to have an orgasm. But for the Sensual woman the pleasures of the body go far beyond this — and define not only her sexuality but every aspect of her life.

Ms Sensual's approach to sex is very basic. It is food and drink to her — and this cliché expresses a fundamental truth in her case, because food and drink are very important too. She responds strongly to what she experiences through the five senses, although touch, taste and smell give her most satisfaction.

The Sensual woman thrives on being touched, not just sexually. She likes to be patted, stroked, hugged, her hand held – and to do the same to others. She likes to have close contact with everyone she cares for – women friends, relatives, children. When she takes a baby on her lap – any baby – she revels in every aspect of the experience: the warm pressure on her body, the smell and texture of the fine baby hair, the exquisite softness of the skin on the baby's arms. She's the woman least likely to give the bundle back to its mother when there are ominous sounds from down below, or he possets a little sour milk. To her, these natural smells combine into a heady cocktail with the scent of soap and clean baby flesh.

Not surprisingly, she's like this with a man too. She might be attracted by his looks or his character initially, but what she wants to do is touch him. This is not pure lust. Indeed, she gets as much enjoyment from investigating the textures of his body hair – softer on the head, the bristles on his chin, the coarseness of pubic hair, and the different feel of the hair under his arms and on his chest. She is delighted by the contrast between the calloused skin on his hands and the smoother skin on his back. She likes to explore with her mouth: the extra sensitivity of her lips can detect even more subtle variations than her fingertips, and the sensation is enhanced by what she can smell – the traces of soap or aftershave giving way to the more earthy scent of an aroused male. And she glories in being touched in return. Like a cat, she gives herself up to the sensations, getting almost as much pleasure in a different way from a finger tracing the line of her eyebrow as she does from purposeful stimulation of her clitoris. Indeed, when she is very aroused she will want to be penetrated, and will enjoy vigorous sexual intercourse, but she can be just as content with less specifically sexual contact, revelling in warm flesh on flesh or a fully-clothed prolonged cuddle as an end in itself.

She has always been like this – ask her mother. When she played with modelling clay she enjoyed the squish of it through her fingers as much as what she was creating. She liked to smell it, nibble it – long after most children had passed through the stage of putting everything in their mouths, she was still taking surreptitious licks and bites at non-edibles. She can continue this right into adult life, sometimes waging a constant battle against an addiction to cigarettes or nail-biting. The more dainty little Ms Sensual and her refined adult counterpart might be more fastidious and controlled altogether. There may be more tastes and general sensations that she doesn't like – but she will still be acutely sensitive to those she does, and gain great pleasure from them. In a way, things only become real to her when she experiences them through her senses – when she can touch, hold, taste and smell them. She might develop into an intellectual, but classifying through theory or learning from others is never enough for her. She must experience in her own body and through practical experience to be able to absorb and verify.

Dolly Parton, the award-winning singer, songwriter and actress, is mainly a Sensual woman, as she reveals in her autobiography, *Dolly: My Life and Other Unfinished Business*. Sex is important to her: 'I have always loved sex. I've never had a bad experience with it ... It was never dirty to me. After all, God gave us the equipment and the opportunity. There's that old saying If God meant for us to fly, he'd have given us wings. Well, look at what he *did* give us.' Her sensual approach goes beyond the sexual. As she says of her husband: 'I love to smell Carl's clothes ... especially if he's not around.' Almost equal in importance is food. She says: 'Men are my weakness. Men and food.' As a child, she promised herself that when she was a star she would eat all the things she enjoyed: 'One need only look at the width of my butt in *The Best Little Whorehouse in Texas* to know that I kept that promise to myself.' Indeed, at one point when her weight threatened to escalate out of control, she devised the 'Dolly diet'. This involved eating whatever she fancied — but in minute quantities, sometimes it simply involved *chewing* what she wanted and spitting it out. She is quite clear that it is the taste of food that matters, not the emotional comfort from eating: 'I do not overeat because my mother slapped me when I was five. I overeat because I'm a damned hog.' She loves cooking rich and fattening food — and always makes lots of extra, which she packages up to give to friends and family, and the homeless.

The most telling example of Dolly's Sensual nature, however, is her attitude to her husband, Carl Dean. They married in 1964 when she was 18, and have been together ever since. Sensuals need to be in long-term committed relationships. She says there is no jealousy between them: 'That's just what comes from being sure of each other and our relationship. We trust the strength of the foundation we have.' She hints that she might have had affairs, but will not enlarge on it: 'That's for me to know and you and Carl Dean to find out.' Indeed, she has the usual Sensual reluctance to go into sexual details. Sensuals would always rather do it than talk about it, yet she believes that everyone, like herself, is very focused on sex: 'Sex is a much bigger part of what we want than most of us will admit.'

Dolly definitely has a strong streak of Romantic — most evident in her obsession with her appearance, and her admitted numerous submissions to the cosmetic surgeon's knife, but this is all superficial: 'Although I look like a drag queen's Christmas tree on the outside, I am at heart a simple country woman.' She only wears sexy nightwear on special occasions. When it's cold: 'I'll sleep in a flannel gown or one of Carl's flannel shirts.' She tolerates the fact that Carl is completely unromantic: 'He's cheap. He's the kind who'll go to a drugstore on Valentine's Day and get two boxes of candy. He'll give one to me without a card and say, well, here. The other he'll put in the freezer for next year, just in case he might forget.' She *knows* he loves her, in the instinctive Sensual way, and because he's always *there*. The only thing that bothers her is that: 'He's not a big cuddler like me.' She deals with it in the typical Sensual way: 'I force him to let me baby him and I make him baby me.' Dolly can't bear to sleep alone, and when there's not a man around, she'll often share a bed with her childhood friend and companion, Judy. It amuses her that people assume that it means she's bisexual: 'We have always slept together since we were kids ... We sit up in bed, watch TV, read. We lie in the darkness and talk just like an old couple would. Why scream across the room when you don't have to?'

Like most Sensuals, Dolly is emotionally robust, and tougher than she looks. As she says: 'A southern woman who looks soft and pretty on the outside but is as strong as forged metal on the inside is called a steel magnolia. I am proud if people think of me as one.'

The French writer Colette is another example of the Sensual woman. Her first novel was published in 1900 when she was 27. Like all her work, it bursts with sensuality — more acceptable in France, at that time, than it was in Britain or America, where the view that an inherently sexual woman was abnormal still prevailed. The critic Raymond Mortimer, writing an introduction to the volume containing *Cheri* and *The Last of Cheri* in the Fifties, said: 'She is not so much a novelist who has written memoirs, as an autobiographer who has disguised some of her experiences more or less transparently as fiction.'

Colette's writing was not exclusively about sex: she expressed her rounded sensuality through her work. Mortimer explains: 'Her subject matter is carefully limited to the life of the senses ... How odd to treat cookery as an exacting art; and, worse still, to elevate love-making into an erudite, almost religious ritual! ... She accepts the validity of any sensuous pleasure, however abnormal, provided that it does not give pain to others ... She avoids ideas, never discusses religion or politics, and seldom refers to literature or any of the arts except the theatre ... Her work is devoted to the visible, tangible, audible, tasteable, and smellable world ... So intense is her love of life, so responsive are all her senses, that she envelops every experience in poetry.'

The Sensual woman cannot love for long at a distance, nor is she able to tolerate a relationship with a man for whom physical contact of any sort is rationed. Something in her shrivels and dies when she is left too long untouched, and when she is required to control her sexuality her feelings of love fade. On the other hand, Ms Sensual is capable of great constancy and loyalty when she is physically satisfied and comfortable. Comfortable is, in fact, a key word. Creature comforts are crucial to her happiness, and the less sexual Sensual woman places greatest emphasis on being well-fed, cosy and healthy. While many women share these needs, for the Sensual woman, whose sense of self is grounded almost exclusively in her bodily functions, a lack of any of these elements makes it hard for her to be at ease. In other words, she can put up with a lot that others find hard to tolerate – the absence of romantic, emotional or intellectual contact, for instance – so long as there is harmony within her bodily needs. This includes a demand for solidity – bricks and mortar, or at least a home that is a long-term base. She thrives on familiarity, preferring the unchanging view from her window to more exotic locations.

Sometimes she tends to depression. She finds it hard to look beyond her day-to-day existence for comfort. If life isn't treating her well she doesn't have a natural capacity to rise above it. She is hemmed in by what she is experiencing now. Mind you, she is stoical. She can soldier on through bad times with a grim determination. If she had a difficult or unhappy childhood she develops stalwart coping abilities. She often learnt that little treats helped her endure bad times. Whether it was cuddling teddy, eating sweets or burying herself in warm, soft bedclothes, she has ways of hanging on until the misery passes. She will usually find adult substitutes for these coping techniques as she grows older.

This no-nonsense attitude determines her ability to stick at relationships that others might deem inadequate. Compatible, even boring, comfortable day-to-day interaction counts for a lot. Ideally, there will also be much smooching, tactility, and sweaty sex, but if she is less highly sexed she will even forego love-making so long as they still feel happy snuggling up together at night.

Identifying Ms Sensual

Despite her usual earthy appreciation of sex, Ms Sensual is unlikely to be a smouldering, walking sex bomb. She is too taken up with her own sensations to think much about the image she projects. Although some Sensual women come across very sexily, on the whole they find it hard to be interested in the trappings of sexual signalling: the revealing clothes and the game of flirtation are not especially appealing. When she wants sex, she wants it with the urgency of hunger, and all that game-playing seems like delaying tactics. On the other hand, when she is not sexually hungry she can't be bothered to act as if she is: she's more interested in whatever other sense is currently being delighted. For instance, at a party she will throw herself into a dance for the sheer thrill of feeling her body working, and won't even think about what it's doing to her hair or make-up or the effect she's creating. As a type, therefore, she's less likely to be a Marilyn Monroe, than the nondescript librarian, who turns out to be a tiger in the bedroom. Indeed, she might often seem quite prudish. She likes sex, but she sees it as a private matter.

Not that she is any easier to typecast than other women. A more telling distinguishing characteristic is her relationship with food. Ms Sensual eats and drinks with gusto. When she's hungry she can't think of anything else. If she drinks to excess it's often because she likes the taste, or she enjoys the sensations of being drunk – not usually because she wants to escape from reality. About the only time she loses her appetite is when she is newly in love, and all her senses are yearning towards physical contact with the beloved.

She loves everything to do with food: handling the ingredients while she cooks, the smells released by cutting and heating, the taste and texture in her mouth, and the feeling of well-being that spreads through her when hunger is assuaged. She is usually a good cook, expert at imagining flavour combinations. She doesn't resent time spent in the kitchen devising meals. But she can derive as much pleasure from a perfectly boiled egg as she can from more exotic fare. Not surprisingly, she might fight a tendency to plumpness. Some Sensual women are frankly fat – often because denying themselves is very difficult, but more usually because they have turned to the pleasures of food in the absence of satisfying physical contact. Ms Emotional, too, can be prone to putting on an unhealthy amount of weight, but in her case she is usually eating to fill an emotional void, often joylessly. Ms Sensual, on the other hand, relishes every mouthful.

It doesn't, in fact, suit a Sensual woman to be fat – not just because she worries about whether it is attractive or not, but because she needs to feel good in her body, and the heaviness and discomfort of obesity is disturbing to her. Indeed, a health-conscious Sensual woman finds it easier to be moderate in her intake because she is more comfortable when she is in sleek condition than when she is indulging herself.

You can spot Ms Sensual by her relationship to her body. Unless she has had damaging experiences in the past or is shy, she is at ease in her skin. She walks well and freely. When she sits down, she burrows herself into the most comfortable position. When she is not touching someone else, she is usually touching *something*: feeling the texture of silk and brocade on a cushion, stroking the smoothness of wood, playing with her table napkin or her glass. She is confusing to the body language experts: they maintain that a woman who strokes the stem of her glass is covertly signalling sexual interest, whereas she is just enjoying the contrasting sensations of the slippery facets and the sharp edges. According to the rules of body language, a woman who touches her face and hair, or smoothes the fabric on her thighs, really yearns to be touching the man she is with. This could be so in Ms Sensual's case, but not necessarily. She likes the feel, and in a way she is checking that she is really there. A woman I know used to slip her hand inside her blouse and hold her breast in public – until it was pointed out to her that it excited or alarmed onlookers. It was a habitual, unconscious gesture with no sexual overtone which just felt cosy and nice to her.

The feel of things also determines her style in clothes. At one end of the range she likes to wear all the natural fabrics that feel good: silk, satin, cashmere, the softest cottons. At the other end she likes clothes that have become old friends – shabby, moulding to her body, impregnated with her natural smell. Whether she is fashion-conscious or not, the comfort of her garments is most important. She'll very rarely suffer to be beautiful or fashionable. Usually she will adapt the current fashion to make it easy to wear. Unless she is very young and still into slavishly copying the latest trend, she also baulks at being the wrong temperature. She wants to be warm in winter and cool in summer. If she doesn't mind what she looks like she'll even wear something warm and woolly under her blouse – or will nod to current convention and make it a sexy silk number.

Whatever she wears when she's out and about, it's a rare Ms Sensual who doesn't favour some old clothes for slopping about in at home. Apart from the comfort, she becomes attached to what's familiar. If she wears anything at all in bed it's likely to be something like this, although she might keep a more glamorous article for when her lover calls. Quite apart from anything else she ceases to be objective about things and people she loves. She can be genuinely surprised to have it pointed out to her that her favourite tee-shirt has gone a funny colour with repeated washing, or that her cherished jumper has lost its shape and gone into holes. Even when she notices, it's part of the charm. I once forcibly had to separate a Sensual friend of mine from her bag, when she was going to an interview for a job. She looked immaculately well-presented, but the bag looked as if it had been rescued from a dump. 'But it's *beautiful*,' she wailed, as I substituted a more respectable one.

Her home is almost invariably comfortable too. For some Sensual women this is more important than beauty. This type will hang on to the aesthetically unappealing armchair with its tatty upholstery because it is heaven to snuggle into. Her house might be untidy, but it is always warm and welcoming. You know it won't matter too much if you spill wine on her carpet. Another kind of Sensual woman needs more refinement in her comfort. Her need for solidity and security is often expressed through acquiring good quality objects and furniture, so that she can look around with satisfaction knowing that it all belongs to her. She will be less happy about friends dropping cigarette ash on her priceless carpet. Nevertheless, that antique sofa she bought is not only worth something, it feels good to sit on. Comfort is always as important as looks to her.

Feeling comfortable extends to her relationship with friends. She enjoys the companionable pleasure of eating well together and then settling down cosily in front of the television. It doesn't matter if they scarcely exchange an interesting word. If other aspects of her personality and intellect demand lively interaction she will also have more stimulating encounters and friendships, but none will be so satisfying to her as time spent with an old friend with whom she can just *be*. This is partly because she tends to be conscientious and reliable in her working life, sometimes denying her own needs in the process. Getting back in touch with herself, therefore, is more important than more obvious ways of having fun. Sophia Loren, the actress, is a Sensual woman like this. She works very hard, but she does not enjoy the glamorous social life of a star. She prefers being at home with her husband and children, cooking and doing domestic and ordinary things.

For these and other reasons Ms Sensual is often quite conservative in her pursuit of pleasure, including sexually. She enjoys sex, but it doesn't have to be anything extraordinary, so long as it is physically satisfying. She likes what are often called the simple pleasures: she prefers a walk in the countryside to time spent in an art gallery. Walking gives her the wind and warmth on her face, the sounds and smells of nature, the feeling of her muscles and lungs working and benefiting from the experience. She enjoys gardening, too, and often has green fingers. The rhythm of the seasons makes sense to her. If she hasn't got any land, she will compensate with indoor plants and window-boxes. If there's no man or children in her life (and often when there is) she needs to have an animal – preferably a furry one that is good natured enough to put up with endless stroking and cuddling.

The Sensual woman who glories in the working of her body also likes exercise of various kinds. It's not so much that she is pursuing a future physical perfection, but that she enjoys the activity of the moment. She is unlikely to 'go for the burn' – indeed, the burn tells her that she has done too much. Lazier Sensual women (and there are many of these) prefer putting their feet up by a roaring fire: basking in the heat, the scent of woodsmoke, the pictures in the embers, and the shifting, snapping noises of the coals and wood. When she finds something she likes doing, then she wants to do it over and over again: while it's satisfying she won't be bored. She prefers her excitement in measured doses, and usually becomes attached to her routines. Spur of the moment invitations can alarm rather than excite her.

Bathing is one of Ms Sensual's pleasures, and not just for the purpose of becoming clean. The feel of soft warm water on her skin is what she likes. Psychologists talk about returning to the womb, and perhaps there is this element in it. At her most basic, Ms Sensual will enjoy just as much the water that someone else has bathed in, so long as the temperature is right. Indeed, the most earthy Sensual woman is not too keen on over-scrupulous hygiene. It's not that she's unclean, but she actually relishes the natural smells of the body — her own and others. Overlaying these with artificial scents of perfumes or aftershaves can sometimes be more offensive to her. She's bewildered that some people think 'good clean sweat' is dirty.

The more 'ladylike' Sensual woman has a more conventional attitude to these matters. She feels better squeaky clean, and is less uninhibited about her natural secretions. She'll shower rather than bathe for freshness. When she does take to her bath, however, it is likely to be a sybaritic experience: lit by candlelight and perfumed with aromatic oils. The Sensual woman who likes perfume on herself and others, however, does so because she genuinely enjoys the smell, not because she wants to mask what is underneath.

Ms Sensual is happiest when she finds her own style, understands her own body, and allows herself to follow her own instincts about what suits her best. While this is a universal recipe for contentment, the Sensual woman who denies the importance of her physical surroundings and bodily comforts cannot be consoled or elevated by spiritual, intellectual or emotional considerations. Other women can rise above physical restrictions, or even be inspired by them, but the genuinely Sensual woman feels depressed.

The unattached Sensual woman

Sensual women tend to mature early, either physically or emotionally. It's not surprising, therefore, that some Sensual girls start being sexually active young. In a way, she's the original girl 'who can't say no' — not because she wants to please or is very biddable, but when she is sexually excited she can't even remember the word. Depending on her upbringing and the social climate she might be full of regrets afterwards, but in the heat of the moment she did just what she wanted to do. However, sex with an inexperienced boy can come as a nasty shock, or at least a disappointment. All that touching and kissing felt so wonderful that she thought the sex itself would be even better. If it was hasty and clumsy she can feel very let down. Sometimes it puts her off for a long time.

On the other hand, some Sensual girls wait for years after puberty before getting close to a boy. They want to touch a person for whom they have strong, positive feelings, and they won't want even to kiss or hold hands with a boy unless they feel very attracted to him. This goes back to childhood. The little Miss Sensual who threw herself into grandpa's arms, couldn't even be coaxed to peck the cheek of her disliked Aunt Sadie. At the time when her best friend was quite happily indulging in heavy petting with any boy who would do, she held herself aloof, not allowing even the most chaste and tentative explorations. She, and others, might think it's because she's a Romantic, but what happens next reveals her true nature. When she is seriously struck by lust, the first kiss can very soon lead to full sex.

Lust is always important to her when she is looking for a partner. She confuses it with being in love, indeed she can't fall in love without it. When in lust she is quite blind to the unsuitability of the boy or man in question. Her body reacts first and most intensely, and she is good at ignoring any warnings from her heart and mind. She always finds it hard not to give her body what it clamours for, be it food, sleep or sex. If physical contact feels 'wrong' with him, however, or she doesn't like his attitude to sex, or his love-making is perfunctory, lust dies and so do the feelings of being in love. This is where she differs most from Ms Romantic and Ms Emotional. They too might be motivated by lust at the start, but to fall in love requires much more for them –

and it takes more than disappointment with sex to spoil the romance.

Often, Ms Sensual will stay with her first boyfriend for a long time, especially if their sexual investigations are satisfying and fun. She just won't be as interested as other girls in playing the field if she feels physically fulfilled. They can be a pair of teenagers who behave like an old married couple. On the whole, she's happier in long-term relationships anyway, and is able to accept the ups and downs with an equanimity that is less easy for her sisters from other Sexual Styles. An unawakened Sensual woman, who has no idea of her own potential, will even settle for a comfortable relationship in which sex hardly figures.

A smaller number of Sensual women change partners more frequently. These are the ones for whom sex itself is the most urgent of their sensual needs. They are looking for the ultimate sexual partner and aren't prepared to put up with love-making that is only adequate. Not every Sensual woman is as aware of her sexual needs as these women are. Indeed, some Sensual women are conscious of sexual disappointment without realising that anything can be done about it.

The Sensual woman who shops around for better sex is often demanding. Knowing her body so well can mean that she is quick to give orders about what she likes, sometimes with scant regard for tact. She usually gives as good as she gets sexually, however, although the more selfish Sensual woman is primarily concerned with her own satisfaction. When she lies back immobile she is paralysed by the intense pleasure she is receiving. It can be so good that she doesn't want to have to move, or do anything to him because changing her focus might diminish her sensations.

Sometimes a man can be a good and generous lover but 'something' puts her off. She can be hard put to explain it – he doesn't 'feel right' or 'smell right'. It is an instinctive animal reaction, below the level of her conscious, rational mind, although she may come up with some plausible explanation.

Then she's off. She can't see any point in sticking with him when her body has rejected him. Unlike Ms Imaginative, who finds one-night-stands erotically appealing even when the sex is poor, Ms Sensual needs more time. A lover is not going to learn her body in one night together. Ms Imaginative is concerned to investigate pastures new however good the sex, but the sexually adventurous kind of Sensual woman will linger longer when the sex is good.

When he feels right, smells right, and she feels very comfortable with him, this often outweighs other considerations such as what he looks like, or what he does. Looks, indeed, are less important to her than that indefinable something that a man 'gives off'. She can see objectively when a man is attractive, but even when he is her type she relies more on the reactions of her body to his physical presence than the evidence of her eyes or intellect.

Ms Sensual enjoys falling in love, of course, but there is something about this excited altered state that makes her anxious. She can be quite relieved when it settles down into something quieter. In her book *Inside Marriage*, Linda Sonntag quotes women who express this: 'It's exciting and worrying at the same time', 'the intensity can sometimes be overwhelming', 'I'm not too happy that it is an overpowering emotion which, for a time, makes one neglect other aspects of life'. I suspect these are the words of Sensual women. Falling in love is fine and can be wonderful, but it is more important for sex to be good, and for her to be sensually replete and comfortable. There is nothing comfortable about intense new love, but the sexual and sensual satisfaction can endure even when it passes. The more practical Sensual woman can even prefer sexual encounters without the complication of love, particularly when her sexual appetite is large and she is feeling deprived. For her, in fact, love and even liking often follow sexual satisfaction rather than preceding it.

Sex and Ms Sensual

The fully-fledged Sensual woman has the capacity to enjoy every aspect of sex with great intensity. This doesn't mean that she's a sexual athlete, or wants to try every possible sexual variation, though it can. Actually, she can be extremely unadventurous and find an unvarying sexual routine quite blissful when it feels good and exactly suits her requirements. As this is so, she can often be quite shocked when she hears what other people get up to, and rarely wants to talk about her own experiences. It feels good: that's about all she is able to say about it.

Ms Sensual is alert to the physical sensations of every touch and caress. She wants her nerve-endings to tingle, and to feel each part of her body awaken and respond. She won't be especially interested in trying new positions, unless the change intensifies or enhances her responses. Much more satisfying is a lover who is prepared to spend time exploring her body to find the unique combination of touch and pressure that excites her. The man who believes there is a standard way to arouse a woman can miss out on the fact that she is more turned on by warm, tickly breath on the nape of her neck, for instance, than she is by having her breasts touched. A virginal Sensual woman might be unable to manoeuvre him into doing what she likes, because she doesn't yet know what that is. The only solution is to try it all, and discover whether her earlobes or her feet are more sensitive, where she likes the scrape of nails or the lick of a tongue, when she prefers softness to hardness, and so on. The sexual game she most revels in is experimenting with different textures on her body: does she prefer the ostrich feather or the soft bristles on the inside of her thigh? Does she like to be stroked through silk or to make love on a rubber sheet or fur? It's a good game, but once she knows what she likes, she wants it again and again. Don't run out of ostrich feathers.

All women are similarly unique in their sexual preferences,

but for other Sexual Styles a certain amount of cack-handedness is tolerable, so long as other elements are right. The Sensual woman, in contrast, will be yours even if you forgot the flowers, were irritable two minutes ago, don't really love her, and so on – as long as you know the secrets of her body and how to vitalise it. Touching her with generous care and consideration, indeed, *is* love as far as she is concerned, and can generate an outpouring of love in return.

For the Sensual woman it all comes back to the physical. While Ms Romantic and Ms Emotional might get an erotic charge from being given a piece of jewellery, Ms Sensual is gratified but unmoved sexually. She might like being wooed, but she doesn't need it. Foreplay is wooing enough. Not that she really understands the concept of foreplay as a means to an end. Touching, caressing, and kissing are delightful in themselves, not part of an obligatory prelude to the 'real thing'. Even when she is very aroused she can enjoy delaying indefinitely the moment of penetration when love-making speeds to its conclusion. It's not just that she wants him to go on caressing her: she also needs to get her fill of him. When she loves his body she wants to experience all of it, checking out every crevice with her hands and mouth. Sometimes this is as arousing as being touched herself. After orgasm she enjoys lying close in a sweaty heap, liking the heat, heaviness and scent of him. Indeed, she wants the touching to go on and on. He needn't feel alarmed that she is not satisfied: it is just her nature to bask in contact of any kind. It's how she knows love is real. This woman will rarely want to leap into the shower to wash off the smell of sex, and she will be offended by the man who needs to do so. In fact, although she adores the feel of crisp, fresh sheets, she also loves bed linen that lingers with the scent of sex and her man ('nesty' is one Sensual woman's affectionate word for it).

She's not too concerned with other aspects of scene-setting. If it feels right she's just as happy under the glare of a single naked lightbulb as she is by candlelight. She won't necessarily hear the soft music, or be put off by the workmen clattering outside. On the whole, however, she prefers to be comfortable. Assuaging passion on the back-seat of a small car only suits her when she is in an agony of lust, and it won't be erotic to her otherwise. Similarly, she is less likely to be concerned to find new venues for love-making. She thinks the kitchen table is too hard and the floor too cold for all but the occasional high-voltage quickie. The bed will be fine, thank you. She prefers to take her time. Ms Imaginative can be excited by an encounter on the stairs, but Ms Sensual finds the carpet burn detracts from her pleasure and would prefer to relocate. On the other hand, when her sexual hunger is sharp, Ms Sensual is not opposed to the occasional short vigorous sexual encounter. When she's feeling very turned on it can be just what she wants, and unlike some other women she feels obliged to the man rather than short-changed by him.

Her attitude to love-making is essentially uncomplicated, driven solely by her responses. Her adventurousness is usually limited to differences in touch rather than variety of position and technique. The Sensual woman who is driven to experiment with different ways of having sex has usually not found what profoundly suits her. When she does, she is happy to settle for variations on a theme.

When it comes to ways to touch, however, there are usually few holds barred. The more oral she is, the more she feels she would just like to 'eat him up', and she savours the flavour of him. She will often enjoy giving oral sex as much as she likes receiving it. One Sensual woman was given some chocolate 'body paint' by her lover, but preferred to eat it with a spoon, saying that he spoilt the taste of it — and it spoilt the taste of him. Of course, the dictates of her palate are so important that if she happens not to like the taste of a man she will be turned off if oral sex is expected of her. Similarly she might need reassurance that she 'tastes nice' to allow her to relax when he is pleasuring her.

When nothing in her past has occurred to inhibit her sensuality, Ms Sensual tends to reach adulthood being very knowing about her body. She is likely to have masturbated, and understands what she needs to reach orgasm. Until she has experimented with a lover, however, she will be less knowledgeable about the rest of her body, or her response to his, but will approach the investigations with joy. For one reason or another some Sensual women are more inhibited. This can happen if they came from physically undemonstrative families, for instance, or they were sharply discouraged from touching themselves and others, or, indeed, their affectionate exuberance was misinterpreted as a sexual invitation from certain adults. These and other experiences can make a Sensual woman less comfortable with her own body, less able to trust her instincts and her senses, and more fearful about sex altogether. Some of the knots can be untied in a long-term loving relationship, but she might always be happier with close contact that is largely unsexual.

Indeed, there are some sexually well-adjusted Sensual women who do not have strong sex drives. They need physical affection, but only occasionally want it to develop into erotic love-making. They enjoy being physically fussed over, and fussing back — lots of hugging, hair-rumpling, stroking, kissing, and generally being close. While other women like this sort of attention as a sign that they are loved, many can do without it so long as there are other signs — such as loving pet names and sweet-talk, presents, love-notes and ardent phonecalls. She, on the other hand, enjoys the sensations as much as anything, and when she is patted and petted she feels loved in every fibre of her body. In fact, if anything is going to turn her on, this will. As the scent and the feel of him seeps into her senses her desire to touch more intimately can grow. The more sexual Sensual woman finds it nearly impossible to cuddle her man for long without her thoughts turning to sex.

The Sensual woman can also enjoy love-making that doesn't reach the heights of arousal — she doesn't necessarily have to be close to orgasm. Even the more highly-sexed Sensual woman sees this as part of the sexual experience. She can allow herself to be made love to when she knows she is not going to become aroused herself because it feels nice anyway. Orgasm is not better, only different. While some women feel used in these circumstances, she simply appreciates the low level of pleasure she is receiving. Some women of other Sexual Styles, in contrast, can't see the point in making love unless they want to, or are moving towards what they see as their goal: orgasm.

Sex can also be fun for the Sensual woman. She sees nothing wrong in having a good laugh if their bodies make strange noises, or they try something new that ends in failure. The more openly sexual she is the more she will see it as essential exercise — a sporty and uplifting way of giving her body a thorough work-out and a mode of releasing tension — leaving her feeling bonelessly relaxed and content. Sometimes it is the only exercise she is prepared to tolerate.

The Sensual woman and marriage

Because sex can be so important to her it is easy to assume that Ms Sensual will marry the best lover she can find. This is not necessarily so, however. The strong streak of conventionality that runs through her means that she never quite loses sight of long-term objectives. While Ms Romantic can be blinded by infatuation, and Ms Emotional can be led by deep wells of emotional response, the lust that drives Ms Sensual is not so all-encompassing as to leave her blind to practical considerations when it comes to something as serious as marriage. Ms Imaginative will run a mile or two before settling down, but Ms Sensual knows that it answers one of her deep needs — for security. It could be for this reason that Sophia Loren chose the older, less attractive Carlo Ponti, over the glamorous and romantic Cary Grant who was also desperate to marry her.

Ideally, Ms Sensual will marry a man who satisfies her physically, and who shares her need for comfort and tactility. When she finds such a man it takes a lot for her to let him go. She is often a natural home-maker. When she feels secure she is able to accept a degree of deprivation or imperfection that her more demanding sisters would never support. She knows that she chose him for qualities beyond the personal and physical, so she won't allow herself to be too disappointed if he doesn't come up to scratch. When she is predominantly a Sensual woman she has the grit to take disenchantment in her stride, even if she has strong elements of another Sexual Style and married her husband for romantic or other considerations.

What helps if she is dissatisfied — and even if she's not — is being able to construct a daily procedure that suits her well. A comfortable home, luxurious or not, makes a difference, as does a satisfying routine. The business of cooking and eating, which takes up a good slice of every day, is also a solace. A garden to potter in and an animal to pet is healing and sensually satisfying. Having children is best of all. Her urgent need to be physically involved with and close to loved ones can be satiated for many years while she has a growing family, even when she is let down in this by her husband. Her sexual side might have to be sublimated for a while, but her other senses can compensate.

In other words, all being well, she is an agreeable marriage partner. Her husband doesn't have to make too many adjustments for her to be happy. If he hugs and kisses her on leaving and returning, opens his arms for her at every opportunity, doesn't play too fast and loose with their money, and likes regular sex, she will accept a lot. With these undemanding ingredients she's unlikely to complain if he puts his feet up on the furniture without removing his shoes, isn't too scrupulous in his personal hygiene, or occasionally forgets her birthday or their anniversary. What she finds harder to tolerate is a man who is away too much, who punishes by withdrawing all affectionate contact, or who shows ostentatiously that he doesn't accept her natural self. When her married life suits her she can even be fairly tolerant of discovered infidelity, so long as it doesn't threaten the marriage. Lust itself isn't likely to tempt her away from her settled lifestyle, and so she is more likely to accept that it won't lure him away either.

The drawback in this easy-going attitude to marriage is that she can miss signs that her husband is more restless. Her own contentment makes it harder for her to understand a more demanding nature. Her ability to be phlegmatic in the face of depression means she can tolerate disillusionment when she is secure, and not notice if he is less resigned. Another potential difficulty is that her talent for routine can dig her into a rut. Years along the line she discovers to her surprise that she is bored, and she hasn't developed the skills to remedy this.

The Sensual woman can be a lusty, willing sexual partner throughout her married life, uncritical of her husband's changing physique or failing prowess, so long as they can find different ways of satisfying each other. If sex has been of paramount importance to her, however, then the loss of sexual contact can eventually propel her out of the marriage. On the other hand, most Sensual women are also prepared to look for non-sexual ways of gratifying their senses – and when blessed with a large and extended family they do not have to look far.

When Ms Sensual will stray

She doesn't make a habit of being unfaithful. Before she has committed herself she is more likely to leave one man for another than she is to cheat on him. On the whole, however, the Sensual wife cares more for stability than she does for satisfaction. The older she is, the more this is likely to be true. Most Sensual women will be able to resist temptation while their marriages are more good than bad. That doesn't mean she will never stray, however. If her relationship has become sexless, and sex is important to her, she often prefers to find a lover than to allow herself to become too discontented. She might, in this case, choose not to dally with men who will pose any threat to her primary relationship, but exercise an almost masculine regard for physical satisfaction alone. Because love tends to follow lust in her case, however, even these dalliances can be perilous.

The Sensual woman who is in more danger of jeopardising her marriage is the late flowerer. She went through adolescence, early adulthood and even marriage without discovering her sexual potential. Classically, she came into her own after hitting 30. If this is the case she is vulnerable to a man who shows her what she is capable of physically. This woman is most likely to be torn between what she knows and what she could become. Even then, the purely Sensual woman often chooses familiarity over excitement. But the more unaware she has been of her sensual nature the more likely she is to believe that these wondrous new lustful feelings are true love.

Her husband can believe their marriage is over if his wife strays. But if he understands her essential nature then it can be saved if he makes an appeal to her conventional side. He has an even better chance if he takes advantage of her newly awakened sexual responses to seduce and satisfy her himself.

Ms Sensual and sexual problems

Ms Sensual is less vulnerable than other women to sexual problems of an emotional nature, but that doesn't mean she is problem free. Her sexuality often acts as a relationship barometer. Sometimes she only knows she's unhappy with her man when her body tells her. If she inclines to depression she might not be aware for some time that her relationship is going wrong. She used to find his pre-brushed breath sweet in the morning, but now he smells wrong all the time, even when he is perfectly clean. She doesn't want to touch him, and doesn't want him to touch her. When she gets to this stage the relationship probably needs major surgery to survive.

Usually, however, if she goes off sex it is because it has never been quite right for her. In the early lustful days it all felt good, and only as their sex life settled down did it become clear that she wasn't being touched in the way that suits her best, and that she rarely comes close to orgasm. Or sex has always been – or has become – too quick for her. She hasn't had time to become aroused before it's all over. Sometimes politeness inhibits her from saying anything, although she's not much good at talking about sex at the best of times. She might try to signal her needs through movement, sound or taking the lead, but if he doesn't get the hint she has used up her tactics. When she knows her body less well she may not even know what's wrong. If dissatisfaction drives them to sex therapy at this point, she blossoms with the sensate-focus programme, in which the couple relearn their physical relationship from scratch. They take it in turns to find out how each other likes to be touched, non-sexually at first, moving in slow stages towards full sex. You don't need to be in sex therapy to try this remedy.

Ms Sensual can also develop problems with a man who believes physical contact should be reserved for sex, especially when it is infrequent. If they are not making love often then she craves to be fondled, cuddled and kissed anyway. When she is not, and she is discouraged from touching him, she shuts down physically. This is an automatic self-protection to stop herself longing for contact. She'll find it hard to reawaken to order when he's in the mood for sex. This can also happen when her sex drive is naturally higher than his. She can find it difficult to control her sexual thermostat, and in the process of trying to turn it down can succeed in switching it off. Her partner often needs to be re-educated to understand that sex doesn't have to equal penetration, and that it is possible to give satisfaction when he is not aroused himself. If he has a strong sensual element in his own nature he can discover that this is pleasurable for him too.

When Ms Sensual loses her appetite for sex she can usually find it again when she gives plenty of time to love-making. This works better for her than dressing-up games, erotic fantasies, or in-depth analysis of the basis of their sexual problems. Alternatively, an appeal to her senses generally can enliven her sexual response: a nude picnic in bed with wine can work, when they can have fun licking up any spillages. A holiday in which sun, sea and sand put her back in touch with the pleasures of her body can also revive her sexual appetite. Sport and exercise work in a different way. The rush of adrenalin is similar to sexual excitement, and she can find that with her system racing and her body stimulated moving into sexual arousal comes easily.

The Sensual woman who has been so damaged by past experiences as to deny her sensual nature can benefit from therapy that gives her 'permission' to trust her body and enjoy herself. If she has retained the capacity to find pleasure in the non-sexual aspects of sensual life she has the potential to find sexual fulfilment as well.

The Sensual Man

'Those who restrain Desire, do so because theirs is weak enough to be restrained.'

William Blake

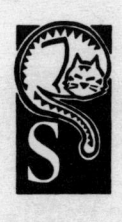

The Sensual Man

No one understands better than Mr Sensual the 'joys of the flesh': indeed in his purest form he would be hard put to think of joys that are *not* connected to the flesh. Anything to do with bodily pleasure is immensely satisfying to him: eating, drinking, sleeping and sex come high on his list of priorities. But his capacity for sensual pleasure is also more subtle than this. He can be very responsive to scents, and physical sensations that are pleasant but not sexual: the warm sun on his body; the soft 'give' of his favourite chair; the silky fur of an animal under his fingers. Unlike the Sensual woman, however, who can give herself uninhibitedly to the more gentle side of her sensuality, Mr Sensual will sometimes deem these pleasures unmanly, and lack of practise in developing them leaves them lying dormant. He feels silly deeply inhaling the scent of a rose. Anything connected to eating and sex, however, is compatible with his masculine image, so he's likely to develop the enjoyment of these aspects more enthusiastically.

Mr Sensual is not the only man to enjoy the satisfaction of his senses, but he is more seriously disturbed than other men when his physical needs are frustrated. The most astute Sensual businessman finds it difficult to concentrate in a meeting if his stomach is rumbling or his shoes hurt. While Romantic, Imaginative and Emotional men can forget about their bodies for long stretches of time when they are excited, interested or moved, Mr Sensual remains acutely aware of himself and what he is experiencing through his five senses.

At his best Mr Sensual is a *bon viveur*. King Edward VII, son of Queen Victoria, was a classic Sensual man. He came to the throne of Great Britain and Ireland in 1901, when he was 60, and had earned the nickname of 'Tum-tum' among his friends in recognition of his 48-inch waist. Good eating and good drinking was the cause. He loved his food, and was said to prefer hush at dinner so that he could concentrate on what he was eating and leave conversation to the intervals between courses. Observers said he could 'eat with impunity a wonderful quantity and mixture of dishes', which could include several dozen oysters at a sitting. He was concerned about his weight, but he could never deny himself. He had a large set of scales in the hall of his country residence at Sandringham, which he made all his guests stand on – delighting when he found anyone heavier than himself. He took annual trips to spa towns to 'take the cure' and diet.

Edward VII was equally dedicated to his sex life. His wife, Alexandra, was delicate, and after the last of their children was born sexual relations between them ceased. They'd been married eight years, and he wasn't yet 30. He had a number of dalliances, but he preferred long relationships which were almost like marriages. One of these, Daisy Brooke, said: 'He was indeed a perfect lover.' She was referring to his attentiveness: he *liked* women. Daisy was his mistress for a few years, during which time he visited her often, took her around with him, and wrote to her several times a week, addressing her as 'My own Daisy wife'. His last affair, with Mrs Alice Keppel, lasted 12 years until his death in 1910. He remained good friends with all his ex-mistresses, and reserved a pew for them at his coronation, which a wit named 'The King's loose box'.

Edward VII liked all his pleasures and comforts. He had the dubious honour of popularising cigarette smoking, and wouldn't give up cigars even when his health failed. When he acceded to the throne all the official residences were stripped of Queen Victoria's austerity and made more welcoming. 'The whole arrangements here are extraordinarily comfortable,' wrote a guest at Windsor Castle. 'They could not be more so.' He made sure that the servants' quarters were equally comfortable. Indeed, he was always concerned for other people to be as content as he was, and to have fun. He remembered the food and drink preferences of his guests, making sure that one always had a bottle of his favourite wine at his place setting, and that another, who had once asked for more fish at dinner, was routinely given a double helping. Winston Churchill said of him: 'He was naturally and genuinely kind-hearted.' The old-fashioned Lord Esher was more reproving: 'The King is kind and debonair and not undignified – but too human.' It was a humanity of which his subjects approved. He was known as 'Good old Teddy', and Lord Granville said: 'He is loved because he has all the faults of which the Englishman is accused.'

Edward VII is placed somewhere in the middle of the sliding scale of Sensual manhood. In their appreciation of the pleasures of life, Sensual men can be downright coarse at one end and show great refinement at the other. The rough-and-ready Mr Sensual will want large quantities of any tasty food; the cultured Mr Sensual will want a gourmet feast. The crude Mr Sensual will want quick, straightforward copulation when he's feeling sexy; the sophisticated Mr Sensual will want a more voluptuously prolonged session.

Sometimes the Sensual man's senses are equally developed, and each in its own way gives him maximum pleasure. For other Sensual men, however, one or other of the senses is dominant. For instance, there's the kind of Sensual man with a low sex drive who can go for long periods without sex, but who is a glutton, living from meal to meal. In contrast there is the Sensual man for whom sex is his most important drive and he pays less attention to what he eats, so long as he's not hungry. What all Sensual men have in common, however, is the urgency of their appetites. When their bodies tell them they crave something — be it food, sex, or anything else — there is no putting it off, no distraction great enough to divert their attention, and no logic or reason either. If they can't be satisfied they are uneasy, crestfallen, depressed or angry. Even the most generous-natured Sensual man is likely to be supremely selfish when in the grip of desire of one kind or another. Nothing is so important as what he wants or needs at this moment. On the other hand, the Sensual man who is well satisfied can be charm itself, as Edward VII was, and deem life perfect. Men of the other Sexual Styles need far more stimulation in their lives to be happy, and require far less material comfort before becoming dissatisfied.

In real life the Sensual man can be a hero and much adored, but he doesn't have the qualities that inspire the artists of literature or celluloid. He's too down-to-earth, too concerned with everyday reality and bodily comforts, too content with the woman in his life when their relationship is sexually satisfying. H E Bates's Pop Larkin, in the series of novels that started with *The Darling Buds of May*, is one of the few fictional portrayals of the Sensual man, and it's not surprising that he is a comic creation. Pop loves food, drink, nature, scents, sex — especially with the abundant Ma, his long-time (but unmarried) partner. In *When the Green Woods Laugh* the central comic setpiece is a dinner party, at which Pop in an extreme of misery has to contend with a chilly environment, poor food and minuscule quantities of alcohol. Pop adores Ma, and loves sex with her, but he is also unfaithful from time to time, while she, confident in his love, turns a tactful blind eye. Pop partly strays out of magnanimity. He thinks sex does you good, and that some women positively need a dose of his physical attentions to set them up. Indeed, this theory lands him in court in *When the Green Woods Laugh*. Even so, in common with many Sensuals, he prefers acting on his instincts to talking about sexual matters. When Ma tells him that his son-in-law is going to have tests to see why he hasn't been able to make Pop's daughter Mariette pregnant, he comes over coy: 'The subject of a test was so embarrassing that Pop felt both relieved and glad when Ma changed the conversation.' Like most Sensual men Pa is also good at making money. He made his fortune as a junk dealer and, like his Sensual brothers, what he most likes doing is spending it on his family, and building a home that is both secure and supremely comfortable. Having done so he is happy to stay put for life. Apart from one sortie to France, Pop prefers to live in his own little patch in the Garden of England, and never move from it. 'Perfick here,' Pop said. 'Wouldn't change it for nowhere else in the world.'

Mr Sensual has some similarities with the Imaginative man when it comes to his attitude to women. Like Mr Imaginative, he's not necessarily choosy about the type of women he prefers. When he's fond of a woman he usually would like to have sex with her. Sometimes he believes he only knows a woman when he *has* had sex with her. In his case what matters most is what she *feels* like when he gets her into bed. He might be attracted to a stunning, lean model-type, but if she's all hard edges when they are making love he will be disappointed. There might, in fact, be a discrepancy in the women he looks at and lusts after and the ones he ends up committed to. He's the man who usually likes some flesh 'to get hold of' even if the possessor of it doesn't look so good with her clothes on. Again, like the Imaginative man, sex is not naturally connected to his emotions. He doesn't have to feel anything at all for a woman he sleeps with except a desire to satisfy his lust. But where he differs from Mr Imaginative is that the *quality* of the sexual experience can be deeply moving for him. When the sex is profoundly satisfying, indeed, his emotions become engaged because *she* has made him feel this good.

Identifying Mr Sensual

Whoever said 'the way to a man's heart is through his stomach' was thinking of the Sensual man. At his most basic he will simply be out of sorts if he is hungry, and similarly be happy and amenable when he has had enough to eat. In many cases food means much more to him than this. The more discerning Sensual man has a fine palate and may even be an excellent chef himself. For some Sensual men their love of food amounts to an engrossing hobby: eating out or eating in takes up a large slice of their itineraries and is accorded great respect. When flavours and good cooking matter to him he can be even more put out by a poor meal than he is by having to make do with a simple peanut butter sandwich. A boring evening can be redeemed by good food, but it has to be very good company to make up for bad food. However talkative he is the rest of the time, when he is savouring the first mouthfuls of any meal he likes to concentrate all his attention on the sensations. Indeed, if he has cooked he will be annoyed by companions who appear oblivious to what he has served up, and consider it a waste of good food. Some Sensual men are relatively restrained in their eating habits, liking just enough of something exquisite. Other Sensual men are so carried away by the pleasure of the flavours that they eat too much. Most of them find it hard to pace themselves through a multiple course meal. When they are enjoying what they are eating they find it hard to stop and hold back room for what is to come.

Mr Sensual likes drinking, too. It's all part of having a good time. Whether he likes fine wines, or ice-cold beers, or the soft fire of good whisky, drinking is more than about satisfying thirst. Indeed he will sometimes drink too much simply because he is enjoying it so much. In the grip of any pleasure he finds it hard to say no. What's life for, he reasons, if you can't enjoy yourself?

With all this gourmandising you'd think he'd have a tendency to put on weight. You'd be right – though for many Sensual men this only happens if they become sedentary. His awareness of his body, and his pleasure in it, often means that he is quite physical – enjoying the feel of strength and speed, and muscles working as they should. If he has any talent he can be a professional sportsman, but even if he isn't he usually plays some sport in his spare time. Failing physical prowess is harder for him than for men of other Sexual Styles. No man enjoys ageing, or changes in his physical capacities, but it has an extra significance for the Sensual man. Because he is so centred in his body he finds it harder to feel compensated by, say, intellectual maturity or professional success. Even the most intelligent and thoughtful Sensual man tends to take great pride in what his body is capable of, and feels less happy in himself when this changes. While other men can continue to feel young while they are mentally vigorous or forging ahead in their careers, the Sensual man can deem himself prematurely middle-aged or old when his body refuses to obey him as it did before.

There is also the Sensual man who is far more lazy. This type might never have bestirred himself much, except sexually – but changes in his capacity in this respect can be depressing as well. Most men care about sexual prowess, but the Sensual man defines himself first by his sexual capability. All in all, he is not happy about putting on weight and slowing down. When he does, he finds it hard to stick to a diet, particularly one that is narrow and unappetising.

Fundamentally, when Mr Sensual is not at ease with his body he is not at ease with himself. Depression can follow physical decline or deprivation of any sort. Many men retreat into childhood when they are ill, but he is more babyish than most. Physical misery is the most acute misery he knows. Mr Sensual is often involved in a losing battle with himself over his pleasures – food, drink, tobacco – needing the immediate comfort while ruing the effects on his body. The more controlled Sensual cares more for his health than his pleasures, however, and will exercise greater will-power, though he may not be happy about it. Whichever, he's a stoic in the face of depression. The man who lives so intensely in his body, and in his interaction with the world is a realist at heart. While Mr Romantic can be caught up in his vision and hopes, Mr Imaginative in the world of ideas, and Mr Emotional in feeling-driven dedication, Mr Sensual understands best the here and now. When daily life is unsatisfying in any way he finds it hard to look beyond present troubles and find comfort. He's slow to anger, which can make him appear more easygoing than he is. But when he blows his top, you know it. Before that he might be depressed. But he's rarely paralysed by dark thoughts and misery. He's prepared to soldier on, putting in effort to make his existence more worthwhile, productive and pleasurable.

Perhaps that's why it's a rare Sensual man who doesn't work hard in his professional life, and see the value in it. Security is important to him, and making a secure niche in the world is part of this. Money assumes an immense importance for him because it allows him to buy the stable and comfortable life for which he yearns. He's often happiest in careers that have a tangible end product – something that can be consumed, held or measured. When this is not the case he is attracted to work that brings in the greatest financial returns. He might be concerned about ethics on an intellectual level, but he doesn't feel a pressing need to bring these considerations into his professional life. He has to live, he tells himself, and preferably to live well, so moral issues are a luxury when it comes to supporting himself and his family. The more altruistic Sensual can want work that contributes to the greater good, but he will usually still have an eye on the bottom line. He'd rather be a well-paid doctor than an aid worker. The Sensual man who is involved with the arts in some form is often most able to contact the range of his sensuality. In such a world he finds it easier to develop the more feminine side of sensuality without feeling less of a man.

When his job is not concerned with the practical and material world (and even sometimes when it is) he usually enjoys practical pastimes. He's the man who will spend Saturday putting up shelves, and will whistle while he works. His home is his base in life, and he will rarely begrudge time spent doing things to make it better and more comfortable. Even if he's not very good at DIY, he will usually be game to have a go – or will hover over workmen doing the job for him, offering advice, or 'overseeing' them. Similarly he will often enjoy looking after his garden. If it offends his sense of his masculinity he'll pretend not to be too interested in what is planted in the way of flowers, but he will like the heavy work, and if the scent of new-mown grass is intoxicating to him, no one need know. He'll often enjoy growing vegetables, or devising hedges of prickly shrubs to keep out intruders.

On the whole, he prefers activities centred on the home. This is the man who will suggest going to the movies and then say: 'It's so comfortable here, let's stay in.' Sometimes it's because he has ulterior motives: all that food, drink, and warmth has put more than fire into his belly – it has turned his thoughts towards sex. Sometimes, however, what he says should be taken at face value. He *is* comfortable. He's enjoying the supremely lazy feeling of a sensually replete man and having to get up, put his coat on and go out would spoil it. If you want to lure him out of the house it helps not to have food or drink *in* it.

He can, however, be an open-air type. Indeed, if he's not home bound he usually prefers to be outside than stuck inside somewhere that doesn't match his requirements for comfort. He prefers nature unadulterated: a good long walk, gulping clean air into his lungs, enjoying the sting of icy rain on his face – especially when he knows there's a bath, good food, and a warm and welcoming atmosphere at the end of it all.

Mr Sensual likes what he knows and is familiar with. This is true with friendships as well. He'll choose acquaintances who can be useful to him, but his best friends are his old friends. They know each other so well that they hardly need to talk.

Sexual Styles

However dynamic he is in his daily life, and however much he enjoys the cut and thrust of scintillating conversation at other times, the most gratifying social occasion for him is when he can look round with fondness at familiar faces. This liking for familiarity extends to his view of the world. He builds up a solid picture of how things are and should be according to his own experience. He sets more store by 'proof' than he does inspiration or speculation. The Sensual man draws comfort from his deeply held opinions, which can become set in stone. He finds people who think differently disquieting – another reason he prefers old, tried and trusted friends.

Comfort is always important to him – in where he lives and what he wears. Mr Sensual will rarely give a thought to fashion, what he looks like, or even sartorial propriety. He's the man quite capable of wearing grey loafers with a dinner jacket because his black shoes hurt. The most conventional Sensual man will thankfully embrace a stated dress code so that he doesn't have to think about what he wears. If he has the money he will go for the good-quality fabrics that feel nice: silk, soft cottons, wools and tweeds that are supple rather than coarse-textured and rigid. He can sometimes be a bit of a slob. He usually has an enduring fondness for old clothes that fit like a second skin, however shabby they might have become. At your peril do you throw out his old slippers, his gardening jacket, or that terrible jumper that smells of sweat and sawdust and which has 'gone' at the elbows. A Romantic male friend of mine closely examined a photograph of an eminent journalist whose shirt collar was frayed at the neck. 'What's he trying to *say* with that shirt?' he asked. If the journalist was a Sensual, he probably wasn't trying to say anything at all, except that it was his favourite shirt; he almost certainly hadn't noticed the fraying. The Romantic is always aware of image, while the Sensual is most concerned with comfort.

This lack of interest in style is often apparent in his choice of car. The Sensual man is much more concerned about what goes on under the bonnet than by the look of what he drives. He wants his car to do the job for which it was bought – get him from A to B without breaking down, and what anyone else thinks is irrelevant.

Like his female counterpart, the Sensual man is very tactile. He slaps his friends on the back, shakes their hands warmly, and perhaps for longer than they would wish, pats his women friends and kisses them in greeting. His liking for physical contact can make him stand too close – invading the 'personal space' of others. He can be a great fiddler: playing with the salt cellar, moving ashtrays, knives and butter-dishes around as visual aids to accompany an explanation he's making. If you show him something new you've bought he'll often touch it while he's admiring it. He touches himself too, quite unconsciously. He'll run his hands through his hair, hold the back of his neck while he's thinking, twiddle the buttons on his cuff. Sometimes he's downright off-putting – hoisting his genitals in a habitual gesture, biting his nails or even picking his nose. He's not motivated by nervousness so much as a need to be in touch with himself, check that he's in one piece and enjoy the vaguely pleasurable sensations he's creating. It would be cruelty to bind his hands. It's one of the reasons he drinks a little more than he should, takes a few more nibbles than he really wants, or finds it difficult to give up smoking – he's using his hands to touch in more or less acceptable ways.

The unattached Sensual man

The Sensual boy's nature is usually quite obvious from a young age. He is not the baby who splays his fingers in horror and cries when he is dirty. He's into everything – touching, tasting, smelling – even after most infants have moved on to a less physical stage. He loves cuddles, stroking his mother's face, the feel of the satin edge on his baby blanket. He responds passionately to the food he's given, spitting out unacceptable textures and flavours, and enthusiastically lapping up what he likes. He explores his own body with the same enthusiasm: finding comfort in touching his genitals and sucking his thumb. All these are normal aspects of behaviour in children, but his pleasure is more intense than most. He usually enjoys rough and tumble too — all the running, jumping physical games. If he's not reproved for unboyish behaviour, such as wanting to nestle on his mother's lap, or stopped from touching himself, he will usually grow up with a delight in his body and his physical capabilities. Indeed, the Sensual born into an uninhibited tactile culture will develop a rounded sensual nature happily. Growing up in a more reserved and controlled environment can make him uneasy with his natural desires.

As he grows into an adolescent his interest in sex becomes intense. Just as all developing girls show Romantic symptoms, so do all newly sexually aware boys seem to be Sensuals — concerned to get as much sex — or the nearest thing to it — as they can. It's what comes later that usually distinguishes the real Sensual from the others. It can take time, however, for his colours to show.

When his sex drive is high, he can change partners as frequently as the Imaginative — that's before he develops a sense of what he wants from a girl or a woman. In his case, the chopping and changing has more to do with finding a good physical match, and with discovering what he likes sexually. His investigations have an objective, whether he is aware of it or not. He wants to try everything he can sexually to see what suits him and what doesn't. While the Imaginative man is impelled to try new experiences for the novelty itself, in the Sensual man's case it is more a process of natural selection. He'll happily drop the less physically satisfying variations in favour of what feels really good to him. He may start off experimental but end up extremely conservative in his sexual habits.

He differs from the Imaginative in other ways as well, even though their behaviour can sometimes seem identical. The

The Sensual Man

Imaginative man can be quite cold-hearted in his dealings because he doesn't really connect with the reality of women. The Sensual man is more acutely aware of the individuality of the women he sleeps with, and to feel fond of them when the experience is good. Similarly, the Imaginative rarely looks back with regret. The Sensual man, however, is more likely to be sorry if his too enthusiastic investigations led him to ditch a woman who, in retrospect he realises, suited him sexually. When this happens he tends to slow down. Next time he finds such a woman he is much less inclined to let her go.

Not every Sensual man changes partners frequently, however. It is in his nature to fall in love when he is sexually satisfied. And it is the nature of male sexuality for satisfaction to come easily. A healthy man will always climax, even if love-making is over and done in a few minutes. Consequently the Sensual man is perfectly capable of falling for the first woman he makes love to. Lust, and especially well-satisfied lust, is what he wants from love. And not all Sensual men have a high sex drive. Some of them channel their energies into their sports, their hobbies, or their work. This kind of Sensual man will be even less inclined to play the field sexually. Once he's found his woman he's happy to settle down with her, with a sense of relief that he has that side of his life sorted out. Actually, too much chasing of women and changing of partners conflicts with his need for stability and certainty in his life. He often has a streak of laziness as well. If a woman offers herself to him he's unlikely to say no — indeed he'll say yes please with pleasure — but if he's getting the sex he needs already he's less keen to do the running.

Whether his sex drive is high or low, his flirting tactics tend to be rudimentary. Even a sophisticated, well-educated Sensual man has something of the cave-man in his seduction techniques. What he wants to do is get his hands on a woman, see how she kisses, get close enough to catch her scent and find out if it turns him on. At his most courtly, he'll help her on or off with her coat, make sure that he touches her hand as he passes her a drink, put his hand on her arm when he says something to her, lead her into a dance. Even so, if he reckons he's getting positive signals from her, he won't take long to make a pass. The shyer – or younger – Sensual man will manoeuvre himself as close as possible to her, and hope that she makes the first move.

Actually, the Sensual man usually likes women, if only because they are necessary fellow-players in one of his favourite games – sex. He likes the feel of women, and the smell of them makes him happy and languorous. Even the most dyed-in-the-wool man's man likes to spend some time with women for this reason. He has a generalised sense of gratitude to women because they are such a source of sexual pleasure. His physical appreciation of the softness of females can make even an oafish Sensual man behave with a certain courtesy in their presence. This is partly to do with his traditional outlook. Men are men and women are women. Such a body-centred man can't fail to notice the difference, or to respect it. In some cases, however, it can cause him to underestimate women. When he looks at a woman he imagines her soft and yielding in bed, and he misses the fact that she's a consummate businesswoman, or even that she's manipulating him professionally at that very moment.

Before he falls in love and settles down, the Sensual man will usually move on to a new woman when in his current relationship he isn't making love as frequently as he would like, or his partner doesn't derive the same pleasure from sex as he does. When the physical side of a relationship cools he feels that love has died. When a woman rejects him sexually he finds it hard to believe that she really cares for him, whatever she says. When he feels affectionate he wants to touch his partner, even if it's just to hold her hand, or have her lie against his chest while he's watching sport on television. It's the Sensual man who will say, 'I'm here, aren't I?' to the question, 'Do you love me?' and not see any irony in his response. Consequently, he interprets a woman's reaction in the light of his own. If she shrugs him off with irritation because she wants to concentrate on her book, or says 'not tonight' to his sexual advances, he hears, 'I don't love you.' On the other hand, a woman who delights in his body (his own great source of delight!) makes him feel loved for himself.

It's not surprising that Mr Sensual believes that the best way of making up after a quarrel is to fall into bed together. If he doesn't want to touch her after a row, indeed, it is a serious sign that the relationship is dying as far as he is concerned. It's hard for him to understand the woman who needs to make up first and make love later. Words are all very well in their place, he feels, but in matters of love they are redundant. Actions speak louder than words in his intimate relations, even when, in the outside world, they are his currency.

Sex and Mr Sensual

Only the most underdeveloped Sensual man sees sex as primarily a quick in and out activity focused on a brief spasm of pleasure – and even he has the capacity to change his ideas once he realises what else love-making can offer. The experienced Sensual man likes to take his time – to savour every caress, to explore every inch of his woman's body, and to give himself up to the pleasure of feeling her hands and mouth on him. Apart from this, he is usually quite straightforward in his sexual preferences. He likes his woman naked or, if she must wear something, it should be silky and easily removed. He doesn't want to have to wait too long to get his hands on her naked flesh. He loves everything about a woman's very differentness from himself – the mass of silky hair, smooth skin, the weight and softness of breasts, a rounded stomach, full buttocks and thighs, the wet slipperiness of an aroused woman. If a woman feels good to him he won't be too troubled by how she looks. The magic for him is the chemistry of skin on skin: he won't be checking on the pertness of her breasts or looking for traces of cellulite. He likes the smell of her, too. Sometimes he likes the sheer femininity of bottled perfume, but he often prefers her natural smell. A friend of mine had a Sensual lover she could only see occasionally. Whenever they met after a long gap what he wanted to do before anything else was to spend time deeply inhaling her unique scent.

What other men think of as foreplay – a sequence of ways to pleasure a woman and build her desire – he regards as a pleasure for himself. There's no sense of duty involved in stroking, licking, kissing, though the sexually expert Sensual man will try to touch in ways that arouse her most. And even though his most intense sensations are focused on his penis, he will love a woman who explores his body in return, enjoying the way his pleasure builds throughout his body, prolonging the moment of climax, making it more profound and deeply satisfying when it does come.

These seem simple pleasures, but he rarely tires of them. Much more tiresome to him is what he regards as unnecessary complication. Getting tied up in difficult positions, doing new things for the sake of it – anything that involves too much thinking and not enough mindless experiencing is a bit of a turn-off. Once in a while he'll have a go at something different, but what he really likes when he's feeling sexy is to do what he knows and enjoys best. His idea of exciting novelty is to pin his woman against the wall in urgent lustful copulation in a standing position. As far as variations go, his favourites are likely to be oral sex – him on her and vice versa. He usually likes the taste of a woman as much as the smell of her. If he *doesn't* like the taste of her it is usually because the 'chemistry' between them is wrong, or perhaps his refined palate rebels. Usually, though, a Sensual man who loves and delights in his woman tends to find her natural scents and flavours a turn-on. Neither does he usually find sex a messy business, as some men do. The over-fastidious Sensual man has usually had a severe upbringing that gave him an untypical horror of dirt and mess. When this hasn't been the case he actively enjoys the physical evidence of sex: the sweat, the mingling of bodily fluids.

When it comes to experimentation, however, he will often pass. He experiments most intensively at the beginning of his sexual career to find out what he likes. Then he knows. He privately thinks that all those sex books and videos on exotic erotic techniques and *outré* sex aids are for people who are rather jaded. Unadorned plain sex is good enough for him – better than good – he can't imagine anything else making it more wonderful.

All this is fine when he *is* experienced and has discovered the joys of extended body pleasuring. But some Sensual men have had less practice in love-making. If his only sexual adventures have been with an equally inexperienced woman he might never have gone beyond rolling on top of her once he has an erection and going straight into intercourse. Like other men, he finds this perfectly satisfying, even if his woman doesn't. But where he differs from men of other Sexual Styles is that once he has been introduced to more sensual love-making his pleasure in sex deepens further. The other Sexual Styles can prefer sex to be quick and efficient when they are no longer in love, or when the heat of first lust has died down, but the Sensual man will find his pleasure increasing, and his love deepening the more his body is awakened sensually.

One bar to him discovering the range and potential of his own sensuality is his traditional outlook. Mr Sensual tends to want to be 'the man'. He can think that there is something rather *un*manly about enjoying a woman's body unless he is inside her and thrusting vigorously. Similarly, he can feel a sense of alarm at his own pleasure when she is taking control. He can find it hard to lie back and enjoy her caresses – he thinks he should be *doing* something. Once he gives himself permission to relax and wallow in these sensations he is liberated to enjoy sex even more. It also stands him in good stead in later life.

When he realises that penetration is not the be-all and end-all of sex he can continue to enjoy his sex life when his erections are less frequent or firm, and even if he ceases to have them at all. All men feel challenged in their manhood when they can't get an erection, but for some men of other Sexual Styles once they lose potency they also lose all interest in sex. Because the Sensual man's sexuality is not exclusively centred in his penis he can continue to enjoy love-making till the end of his days. It remains important to him also because he has a deep need to be touched to feel loved. I know of one Sensual man in his late fifties who is married to a much younger and beautiful woman. They don't make love because he has erectile difficulties – but she also finds him physically off-putting, and they have no physical relationship at all. In common with other Sensual men it would take dynamite to shift him out of his marriage, even such an unsatisfactory one. Instead, he conducts an 'affair' with a plain and overweight woman of his own age. This is virtually sexless too, but it involves a lot of affectionate touching and cuddling, which he continues to need.

He is not alone. All Sensual men need physical closeness, and sex doesn't meet all their needs for it. This is not a man who enjoys sleeping alone, even when sex is far from his mind. He likes the warmth of human contact. He'll masturbate when he has no other option, but sex for him is about two bodies, and orgasm alone isn't satisfying enough for him. When he uses pornography to aid masturbation it's usually of the no-nonsense kind: close-ups of bodily parts and straightforward coupling. His alertness to his partner means that sexual enjoyment is increased for him when he experiences her pleasure too. Most men need to feel that they satisfy their women as a point of male pride. The Sensual man's need for her satisfaction is more complex. Sex is so profoundly important to him that he feels fundamentally rejected when she derives no pleasure from it. Perhaps this was behind the court case that Ronald Askew, a banker from California, brought against his wife for faking orgasms. She had admitted during counselling that she had never been physically attracted to him and had only pretended to enjoy sex to keep him happy. Although she said she still loved him, he was devastated and claimed he would never have married her if he had known. The jury agreed that his wife was defrauding him and awarded $242,000 in compensation (reversed by the Court of Appeal).

The Sensual man's delight in his partner's body and need for physical contact of all kinds can make him the world's best cuddler. He enjoys embracing, fondling, hugging, holding your hand and playing with your fingers while he talks to you. For other men this is part of courting behaviour, and once the relationship has settled down they touch their women far less. The Sensual man never stops. Again, however, a certain kind of Sensual man feels that this is an unmanly need. He thinks that all physical contact should lead to sex, especially if a pleasurable embrace causes the beginning of an erection. Indeed, this kind of man can feel threatened by a woman snuggling into him and touching him in an affectionate way if sex is far from his mind and he *doesn't* get an erection. He feels she is calling on him to perform, and he pushes her away. But the Sensual man with a lower sex drive, or going through a phase when he is off sex, needs cuddling and physical affection even more. A better understanding of his own nature is required so that he can allow himself the pleasure of gentle, aimless touching.

On the other hand, when his sex drive is high, prolonged physical contact of any kind turns his thoughts towards sex. When he holds his woman close his body takes on a will of its own. She might just have finished scrubbing the kitchen floor, her hair is a mess, she's wearing her oldest clothes, but suddenly she seems the most desirable woman in the world. This man doesn't need a woman to do a striptease in front of him, or to whisper erotic obscenities into his ear. She just needs to *be there*, with her accustomed scent and the familiar texture of her skin speaking direct to his senses. He needs no particular seductive atmosphere to put him in the mood for sex, which means that he might not understand when his woman feels differently. All he needs is to be relaxed – which usually means having eaten something first – and then he's ready to go. This is the man who can irritate his partner by being quite happy with last-thing-at-night sex, when they might not even have exchanged a loving word or look all evening. It doesn't matter to him that she has her hair in curlers, a layer of night cream on her face and is wearing an old nightgown.

This is partly because sex is a simple physical necessity to him. In some ways it's like a sport that releases tension and makes him feel good. At its best, however, sex means far more to him than this. Slower, more measured, more sensual love-making can be so deeply physically satisfying that nothing else in his life can compare with the way it makes him feel.

The Sensual man and marriage

Ideally the Sensual man marries a woman with whom he is physically compatible, with a matching sexual appetite. When he does, he can continue to desire her and enjoy their sex life together for the length of their relationship. It is the Sensual man who can most readily agree with the words of the French novelist Honoré de Balzac: 'Can one continue to desire one's wife? Yes, one can. It is just as absurd to pretend that it is impossible to go on loving the same woman as it is to say that a famous musician needs several violins to be able to play a piece of music and produce a splendid melody.'

But the Sensual man does not always find a wife who suits him so well physically. This is partly because other matters assume a greater importance to him when he is settling down. He wants a comfortable home, he wants all his creature comforts to be satisfied. His need for security and his traditional nature mean that he tends to reserve his commitment for a woman who is a good home-maker. He likes his slippers by the fire, his food on the table, his clothes clean and pressed. Actually, he's happiest with a wife who doesn't work and stays at home, particularly if they have young children. That's one of the reasons he works so hard, and is so dedicated to making money. He is much more generous after he is married than when he is courting. What he lavishes on his wife 'stays in the family' and is not lost to him. He'll provide the means for a good lifestyle, and he wants her to see to the details.

The Sensual man is quite content with a marriage like this, and is not easily bored. He is also very loyal. If his sex drive is high, and he's not getting the sex he needs at home, he might look for it elsewhere, but his commitment to his wife is supreme and unshakeable. This is especially so if they have children. He's content to live with a wife who is more a mother to him than a consort. Mothering makes him feel loved. Indeed, if he marries a woman with whom he is sexually compatible but she's not interested in looking after him he will ultimately be less happy than with a more domestic and less sexual woman.

His feelings of satisfaction might not be shared by his wife. So long as everything is calm and comfortable on the home-front, he can do without excitement in the way of shared interests or intellectual stimulation; he doesn't even need to feel strong love or passion — fondness or simple tolerance will do. He doesn't want to have to talk about things, especially their 'relationship'. Home is where you put your feet up and recover from the demands of the world outside. For some women this is hell, and he doesn't understand why.

His commitment wavers however if his wife is hostile. If she says 'get your own dinner', shrinks from his touch, won't let him get comfortable if it means dirtying or untidying her home, he feels rejected and unloved. Even so, and even if it is depressing for him, he will often stay longer in such a marriage than another man would. His realistic side tells him that another promising relationship could easily go the same way — and, he thinks, 'better the devil you know'. Neither does he want the upheaval, the shock to his system. He certainly doesn't want to leave the home he has lavished so much time, care and money on. She, in fact, may have to be the one to break up such an unsatisfactory marriage.

With a wife whose views of married life match his he can be supremely happy, especially if they are both equally keen to have a relationship that is physically affectionate. When they both feel the same way about sex their relationship can be the envy of much younger people. I know a couple in their fifties, who have been married for 15 years — a second marriage for both of them. They love their food, their house is warm and welcoming — and the sexual connection between them is palpable. A couple of times a week they retreat to their bedroom for some hours, taking with them nice things to nibble, and a bottle of their favourite drink. They don't go into details about what happens next — Sensuals rarely do — but it is clear that whatever it is it keeps them very happy.

When Mr Sensual will stray

The Sensual man who is well satisfied with his sexual relationship is unlikely to do much more than speculate on what it would be like to make love to another woman. He has no pressing need to know what sex is like with someone new when he is sexually content — he rarely imagines that it could be any better. Being unfaithful also takes time and planning, and involves a certain amount of energy that he thinks could be put to better use. On the other hand, Sensual men don't set great store by fidelity. Or rather, being unfaithful doesn't necessarily mean very much to them. If the opportunity of taking another woman to bed presents itself he won't be able to think of a very good argument against it. This is specially so, of course, if he is parted from his woman for any length of time. He needs sex, he reasons, so he had better take advantage of what's on offer.

It's another matter if he isn't getting the sex he needs in

his relationship, however. He will then put more effort into finding it elsewhere — though his preference would be for a long-term mistress rather than a series of shorter liaisons. He's not the world's greatest wooer, so it suits him better to have an understanding with a woman who doesn't oblige him to go through prolonged courting rituals, remember flowers, or to notice when she's had her hair done. On the whole he doesn't want to jeopardise his primary relationship, so he will even prefer a woman who has other commitments — she doesn't want a man around full-time, or is even married herself. He's not prepared to share her with a man she still finds interesting sexually, however, because his male pride needs to know that he is her most important sexual partner. In such a relationship he can be supremely undemanding, so long as the sex remains good. He has set things up so that he has everything he needs — home comforts on one hand and regular sex on the other. In such a situation his wife is in no danger of losing him for good — unless she kicks him out — and his mistress will know better than to give ultimatums, because he won't accept them.

The Sensual man and sexual problems

As he sees it, there's no sexual problem so long as he's getting as much good sex as he needs. His partner might not view it in quite the same way. Because he wants sex when he wants it, and needs little to put him in the mood, he can ride rough-shod over a woman who needs more preparation than an arm around her or a hand on her breast. If his sensuality is largely undeveloped, he might follow this 'seduction' with a quick coupling that leaves *him* satisfied, and *her* feeling even worse. The good news is that he can learn to take his time and enjoy it. Although he will never be brilliant at preparatory sweet-talk and scene setting, he can certainly develop his skills in gentle and more prolonged love-making.

A real sexual problem, to his mind, is if he suffers from

impotence – temporary or permanent. But as shown already, he is the man most likely to find that a new world of sensuality opens up for him when he is no longer concerned primarily with his penis. A number of sex therapists have told me of men with potency problems who, once they have learned other ways of making love, report that they have never enjoyed it so much before.

Getting him to a sex therapist for this or other reasons is the difficult part. He is deeply offended by the idea of having to talk about sex to a stranger – particularly having to talk about what he sees as his inadequacy. Strangely, though, once he overcomes his natural distaste, he often benefits more from the experience than other men. He is particularly responsive to sensate focus techniques, in which he and his partner learn to give each other whole-body pleasure. It is often said that sex is only part of a relationship, and when it goes wrong it is usually the symptom of other problems. This is generally true, but in the Sensual man's case his entire view of his relationship can be radically changed for the better when he is happier sexually. Other men might have to tackle the underlying problems first, whereas he is more motivated to tackle them *after* his level of sexual satisfaction rises. On the other hand, if Mr Sensual can't get an erection with his partner, but otherwise functions normally, his body can be trying to tell him something about the relationship that he is ignoring. Selective erectile difficulties like this can be the result of unrecognised anger or depression. The stalwart Sensual man can soldier along unaware of these 'abstract' issues until his penis rebels. Then he has to take notice.

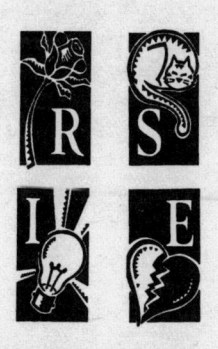

The Sensual Combinations

The Sensual Combinations

This section looks at Sensuals who have a strong subsidiary Sexual Style. It should be read in conjunction with the main Sensual chapter, and you should also look at the sections on sex and love for the secondary Style, or Styles. Each person will manifest their sexual combination in a unique way but, if you have identified your Sexual Style correctly, the broad themes will apply.

The SENSUAL-Romantic (S-R)

The pure Sensual is poles apart from the pure Romantic, so it is not surprising that the person who combines both elements is something of a split personality. The Romantic element in this Sensual's sexual personality can make for a certain unpredictability. The S-R has the pure Sensual's need for stability and earthy appreciation of physical pleasure, but also has the Romantic's demand for a certain amount of excitement and glamour in love and sex. Forced to choose between the two, the S-R will opt for comfort, security, regular sex — or at least an affectionately tactile relationship — but should the romance go, this Sensual will be far less contented than the pure type. The Sensual tendency to depression can be even more marked in this combination, because there is not the same ability to draw complete satisfaction from the Sensual's usual props: good food, good sex, a pleasant environment and cosy predictability. Without a regular dose of magic, fantasy, and being made to feel special, these Sensuals can over-compensate with Sensual indulgences: eating too much; drinking too much; becoming lazy and inert; or even becoming too focused on sex — hoping that the meeting of bodies will bring back that romantic exhilaration that represents the pinnacle of perfection to them.

On the positive side, S-Rs can be far more magnetic and outgoing than the undiluted Sensual. They usually take more care with their appearance, at least socially, are more likely to flirt or flatter, and like to have fun. But it is one of their contradictions that although they often try harder to attract, they need to feel that you are responding to the person underneath the image. The S-R woman with the padded up-lift bra will be wounded if you seem to mind the reality of her small breasts; and she won't want to wear her sexy underwear when your relationship is well underway. The S-R man likes you to admire his achievements and new car, but he doesn't want to feel that they are central to your feelings for him. Unlike pure Romantics, and even ROMANTIC-Sensuals (R-S) for whom image *is* part of their essential selves, for S-Rs it is a pleasing mask, which they like to be able to take off.

For this and other reasons, men and women of this Style can be somewhat deceptive. Their Romantic side can make them appear to be the life and soul of the party, but at home, with their partners, they often want to be able to switch off and plunge into pleasant domestic sloth. One of their characteristics is that in private they don't want to have to bother to pretend to be anything but their natural selves unless it suits them, but their Romantic streak demands higher standards from their partners. They want their lovers to continue to look good, treat them as special, and provide the romance they need. They need more refinement in their love-making and can be somewhat fastidious. They place more trust in their immediate responses to members of the opposite sex than purer Sensuals. While they still believe that love at first sight is mainly lust, it is necessary to their continuing attachment to have experienced it.

Successful courtesans of the past were often S-Rs. Diane de Poitiers became the mistress of Henri II of France, when he was 19 and she was 39 – almost an old woman in the 16th century. She had a Romantic dedication to retaining her looks, and she succeeded throughout her life – Henri remained her lover until he died, 21 years later. But Diane's Sensual enjoyment of sex was equally part of her secret, as Catherine de Medici, Henri's wife, found out when she spied on them. She saw Diane, 'caressing her lover with a wealth of charm and delicious folly, which her lover returned, until they slid from the bed on to the floor and, still in their chemises, pursued their gymnastics on the carpet.'

Henri himself was an S-R. He had a strong Romantic streak: he read countless romances and was attracted to the ideals of medieval chivalry. Diane was considered the foremost beauty of her day – intoxicating to a Romantic man. He had fallen in love with her at first sight when he was 11, and until he persuaded her to become his mistress she had never been unfaithful to her husband. But what marks Henri out as a Sensual first and foremost is his steadfast devotion to Diane thereafter. He neither took, nor wanted, any other mistress when, as king, he could have had his pick of women.

Some S-R women control their contradictory impulses by becoming the third party in a triangle. Most, true to their Sensual nature, however, prefer a more conventional set-up. But women of this combination can be more selective than their purely Sensual sisters – or at least they have more criteria that need to be satisfied. Good looks matter more to them. They are less likely to jump into bed with a man for lustful reasons alone. They need to feel that this is love – or could be love. They are consequently more hurt if it turns out to be a one-night-stand. They have the Sensual's ability to make a committed, long-term relationship, but their Romantic streak means that there is a hidden hazard. If romance is denied to them for too long, they may have an uncharacteristic break-out at some point. Dazzled by someone who reactivates their dormant Romantic side, they could well leave a steady, settled relationship with the same impulsiveness as a pure Romantic.

The S-R man is similar. He likes his pleasures; he wants sex when he wants it; comfort is supremely important to him. But he's not completely happy unless his partner continues to admire him openly, and he's less oblivious to the external attractions of his partner than a more completely Sensual man. Sex is better, he finds, if she looks good, and is in good shape. His Romantic streak means that he doesn't share the wholly Sensual view that being a woman is female enough. Femininity needs to be more obvious for his taste. Robin is an example of this. He hates women wearing make-up. He doesn't approve of them shaving armpits or legs. On the other hand, he only chooses naturally beautiful women who have no need of make-up, and are relatively hairless anyway. Despite this, they must take him as they find him — not minding if he's overweight, a bit smelly, or forgets to tell them how beautiful he thinks they are.

Like the woman of this combination, there is a weakness in the usual Sensual steadfastness for a man of this Style. While pure Sensual men are unlikely to be drawn away from their marriages by an affair, he is much more vulnerable to falling in love with someone new and leaving his wife if he is taken for granted, or his wife becomes less attractive to him.

Even so, both male and female S-Rs are Sensual first, and Romantic second. If the Sensual side of their natures is well looked-after they will tend to stick in a relationship even if the romance fades away completely. But they won't be as content as the downright Sensual, because part of them is being suppressed. Luckily they need far less romance in their lives than the pure Romantic, so only a little bit of extra effort will keep them happy.

The SENSUAL-Emotional (S-E)

There is a natural affinity between Sensuals and Emotionals, and as a combination it makes for a very intense person, as the instinctive qualities of both Styles are strengthened. The Sensual is most acutely aware of bodily needs and desires, and when combined with the secondary Emotional characteristic of being in tune with emotional currents (their own and another's) the S-E s are hybrids who know what they want and need – and also have an uncanny empathy with other people.

In the arena of relationships, the S-E is the most potentially passionate and loyal of all the Sexual Styles, with the obvious exception of the EMOTIONAL-Sensual (E-S). But unlike their mirror-image, with Sensual as their dominant Style they are more practical, down-to-earth, and less inclined to be swept away by strong emotions. The S-E feels deeply, and can be hurt more profoundly than a pure Sensual, but a stoical attitude carries this man or woman through.

Sex assumes a great importance for S-Es. Their Emotional streak fuels a strong drive to merge with others, and sex for them is the ultimate union. They can enjoy sex without strong feelings, but once they've experienced love-making with someone who powerfully affects their emotional responses, they don't want to settle for second-best. On the other hand, they are more likely to experience sex problems with an emotional cause than pure Sensuals. When they are unhappy their libidos can close down in sympathy. However, when good sex combines with a gut-wrenching connection to someone else, they hold on to that lover with a tenacity that a

Sensual or Emotional alone cannot match. Life-long fidelity is easy for them: in fact the reverse is harder — having to change partners often is disturbing. They need stability and emotional security. But that security can come in many guises — sometimes destructive power-play can be what they need.

Queen Victoria was an S-E, despite the fact that she gave her name to an era of straight-laced prudery. Her love for Prince Albert was distinctly earthy, leading to the deeper bond required by her Emotional side. Indeed, Albert's death after 21 years of marriage left her inconsolable. Without a fulfilling sex life and an emotional soulmate, her Emotional propensity to brood took over.

Even before Victoria married Albert, her S-E nature was obvious to others. As an 18-year-old Queen, she had a crush on her prime minister, Lord Melbourne, and Charles Greville, a contemporary, commented: 'Her feelings, which are *sexual* though she does not know it ... are of a strength sufficient to tear down all prudential considerations.'

During Victoria's short courtship with Albert, she filled her diary with descriptions of his beauty and their delightful canoodlings: 'He was so affectionate, so kind, so dear, we kissed each other again and again.' The day after their wedding night, she wrote coyly: 'When day dawned (for we did not sleep much) and I beheld that beautiful and angelic face by my side, it was more than I can express!' The next day she was even happier: 'His love and gentleness is beyond everything, and to kiss that dear soft cheek, to press my lips to his, is heavenly bliss!' On the last day of the honeymoon she wrote with pride: 'My dearest Albert put my stockings on for me ... I went in and saw him shave; a great delight for me.'

As Victoria's satisfaction increased her love deepened. She thought Albert was brilliant, and deferred to him in everything. As Greville noted: 'Her devotion and submission knew no bounds.' She hated being away from him for more than a day. She sometimes went to bed before him, and fretted when he wouldn't join her immediately. 'Tell Lord Alfred to let the Prince know that it is 11 o'clock. Tell him the Prince should merely be told the hour. The Prince wishes to be told, I know. He does not see the clock.' When their last child was born in 1857, after 17 years of marriage, Victoria was advised that it would be fatal for her to have another child. She is said to have enquired with much emotion whether that meant she could have 'no more fun with Albert'. Albert died during a bad bout of typhoid fever in 1861, after 21 years of marriage. She was wild with grief. For the remaining 40 years of Victoria's life she commanded that hot water and fresh clothes be laid out in Albert's room every evening; in the morning his chamberpot was taken away and scrubbed out with the rest. Shortly before her death, in 1901, she told her lady-in-waiting that she would be 'united with my beloved Albert very soon'.

Not surprisingly, S-Es are also creatures of moods, particularly melancholy. Sensuals have a tendency to depression, particularly when they are physically under the weather, or their desires are thwarted. Combine that with the Emotional propensity to be engulfed by emotional tidal waves, and you have the Style that can occasionally be paralysed by dark feelings, which they can't – or won't – explain. In some unfortunate cases, the Sensual's penchant for enjoying alcohol, allied with the Emotional's more complex need for it to drown sorrows, can cause problems in this situation. On the other hand, they can draw deep emotional comfort from the simple pleasures that appeal to the Sensual.

This combination of Styles has the Sensual's inclination to be home-loving, reinforced by the Emotional's similar – and greater – feeling that home is where the heart is. Paul McCartney is an example of a male S-E. As one of the richest, most talented and desired men in the world, he could indulge himself with an endless stream of women. As it is, apart from a pardonable sowing of wild oats when he was younger and a famous Beatle, he has remained happily faithful to his wife, Linda, since their marriage. They live the modest, homely style that suits Sensuals best, in an unostentatious five-bedroomed farmhouse. Their three children went to local state schools. McCartney is as likely to commute by train as he is to use his serviceable unflashy car, and his idea of a good evening is to stay in with his family, eat home-cooked vegetarian meals and drink mineral water. The Emotional component in his temperament is not only expressed in his commitment to Linda, but in his vegetarianism, passion against fox-hunting and injustice. He gives large amounts, anonymously, to charity — especially to causes that stir his social conscience.

On the whole, S–Es couldn't care less what their partners look like (Queen Victoria continued to admire Albert's 'beauty' when he became fat and bald). They might be attracted by good looks initially, but it ceases to matter quite quickly. The bond created by sexual and physical compatibility, joined by a powerful emotional connection, can survive the ravages of age and changing physique.

The emotional waters of this Sensual style run deep. Sensuals, on the whole, don't like scenes. This can often result in a fairly placid exterior that belies what is going on underneath. They don't like letting off steam, so a pressure-cooker effect is created. Every so often, and extremely rarely, they will blow up.

The S-E man or woman flowers when satisfying sex is fuelled by strong emotions. Nevertheless, Sensuality is paramount for them. They will doggedly continue in relationships that have cooled emotionally, so long as they are not too cold physically and because, in the end, they prefer what they know to the uncertain unknown. A close physical relationship will cheer them up, but to be truly complete they need to feel intensely bonded to their partners – as if, without them, they might not be able to survive.

The SENSUAL-Imaginative (S-I)

When a Sensual has a strong dose of Imaginative, the result is likely to be a person who approaches sexual matters with enthusiasm and curiosity, but with very little investment of his or her emotional self. Sensuals like the good things in life, and are driven by their sensual needs, be they for food or sex. But although they can become attached to anything or anyone that gives them pleasure, they don't necessarily have to feel emotionally connected to enjoy themselves. Imaginatives have a propensity to derive maximum thrills from what is interesting, novel, and different, and have little understanding of emotional undercurrents. Their hearts don't have to be touched – indeed, they operate best when they are thinking and analysing and not being troubled by feelings. Mix the two together and you reinforce the emotional distance: you have a ready-made potential heart-breaker, with apparently little conscience in relationships. It's not quite so – but they can move on without regret if their requirements for physical satisfaction and mental excitement are not met – without fully comprehending that it might have mattered very much more to the other person.

First and foremost Sensual, S-Is derive great pleasure from sex, and lean towards staying with someone with whom they have a fulfilling sex life, and with whom they feel comfortable and secure. But their Imaginative side does not allow the mindless wallowing in the experience that the true Sensual enjoys. There is restlessness too. Sex can't follow the same satisfying set pattern: experiment increases enjoyment. And the Imaginative in the S-I's nature has a roving eye. Men and women of this style can be exceptionally rewarding and skilled lovers as the Sensual's genuine enjoyment of long, slow, sensual love-making is allied to the Imaginative's technical expertise gained through the quest for variety. No wonder that they can leave a trail of broken hearts when they rarely give their own hearts in a relationship.

The Imaginative streak also adds a potent dose of sophistication to the Sensual's very basic seduction technique. This is a person who has a way with words. A woman being blasted by the full force of the attention of an S-I man thinks, 'He's really interested in *me* – not just my body.' He is, of course, but the interest won't necessarily last once her novelty has worn off. Both sides of his nature are also *very* interested in her body, and his dominant Sensual Style would feel deprived if all they did was talk. The S-I woman can also be very attractive to men. Rising from her like musk is the message that she really enjoys sex, and she clearly finds him *fascinating*. Indeed, she almost certainly does. The S-I woman needs a man to be mentally stimulating to increase her enjoyment of their sexual relationship.

In long-term relationships S-Is can be more constant than their similar counterparts, the IMAGINATIVE-Sensuals (I-S), or even their relatives, the SENSUAL-Romantics (S-R). They have the Sensual's need to put down deep roots and can be seduced into steady commitment by a relationship that is sexually fulfilling and generally cosy. Their secondary need for excitement and variety in partners could result in a certain amount of playing away but, because their hearts can remain completely untouched by the experience, their loyalties to their partners remain unaffected. Unlike the S-Rs, they think falling in love is simple lust and infatuation, and they wouldn't want to jeopardise their hard-won security for it. And, unlike I-Ss, for whom Imaginative concerns predominate, stability and comfort will always win out in the end. Many need interest and excitement *within* their relationship and will remain faithful to a partner who stimulates them mentally and sexually.

Edwina, the wife of the late Lord Louis Mountbatten (great uncle of Prince Charles) is an example of a female S-I. Rich, intelligent and privileged, Edwina was also excited by adventure. She was attracted by Mountbatten's good looks, and was even more dazzled by his well-travelled sophistication. When they met, in 1921, he was a 21-year-old naval officer, and she a 20-year-old debutante. She fell passionately in love with him, but although he returned her love, it was not with the sexual intensity she needed. The romantic novelist, Barbara Cartland, a good friend to them both said: 'Edwina was a complex personality because she had a man's brain in the body of a very beautiful woman.' She also had a masculine — typically S-I — attitude to sex and infidelity. Within three years of marrying she had embarked on a series of affairs, looking for the sex that her marriage couldn't give her. In common with other S-Is, Edwina had an emotional robustness, which her husband didn't share, and she couldn't understand his more sensitive nature. 'Rise above it,' she would say. 'Worse things happen at sea.' Edwina had a number of long affairs, which were important to her. Ultimately a Sensual, however, she never considered leaving Mountbatten, who gave her the security that she craved even more than the excitement she chased. Mountbatten was always there to comfort her when her affairs ended, and she was frightened of losing him. Edwina was inordinately jealous when Mountbatten paid attention to other women, despite the fact that she talked openly to him about her own affairs. When she died in 1960, they had been married for nearly 40 years.

For most S-I women, and for many men of this Sexual Style, Edwina's solution seems a poor compromise. What they would like above anything is to have stimulation, sexual novelty, and exciting interaction at home. Unlike pure Sensuals, to be really happy they need more than deep, quiet contentment. Ideally, they need to find their partners endlessly fascinating, a constant source of interest — to have conversations that are important and that make them think. Sex also continues to matter to them more than it does to the I-Ss, the reverse combination — but if it is to remain good in a lasting relationship it can't become too routine. Inevitably, when there are children, their options for making love around the house, and at times other than last thing at night, become limited. Erotic conversations, and new positions, however, remain an option. But although pure Sensuals rarely tire of their lovers' bodies when sex between them is satisfying, the S-I is programmed to retain a wistful wish for unexplored territory or some surprises at home.

Ultimately, with S-Is, however, Sensual considerations come first. They are prepared to tolerate relationships that have little Imaginative content. They can compensate by finding the Imaginative stimulation they need outside their relationships — and not just sexually: an interesting lifestyle and interesting friends will sometimes do instead. Unlike the Sensual with a Romantic streak, they don't absolutely have to find the missing element in another person.

What matters most is that their world is structured around their physical needs and is fairly stable and predictable. If their partners learn which buttons to press to make them feel comfortable and cherished they will relinquish excitement in the long run. For this reason they are not quite so demanding and restless as are their counterparts for whom the Imaginative Style is paramount. Even so, the person who wants to hold on to an S-I must learn that an element of surprise and challenge, both mentally and sexually, contributes to the success of the relationship.

Combinations of three or four

It is rare to have a genuinely equal balance of Sexual Styles. One will be dominant — in these cases Sensual — and the remaining two or three are also unlikely to be found in equal measure. In most cases one of them will combine most strongly with the main Sensual Style (in the ways described above) and the third and possibly fourth will add colour and subtlety, but little more. Most usually, aspects of the weaker Styles will be noticeable in other aspects of your personality — your attitude to clothes, career, loved ones other than partners, and so on. The following descriptions are therefore only broad guidelines to the possible ways the Styles can coexist.

The SENSUAL-Emotional-Imaginative (S-E-I)

When Emotional and Imaginative combine in the Sensual sexual personality, these instinctive people are given the means to express their complex and rich inner life. The Imaginative leavening of the intense S-E Style provides this person with a welcome alternative to being swept up by physical sensations and emotional drives. They can be more objective — and deflected from their immediate concerns by something new, interesting conversation, and the more detached world of ideas. The Imaginative input gives an outlet for some of their difficult or destructive feelings, too, so they are less likely to suffer in silence, or to explode in despair. Not surprisingly, this combination also has the potential to work with words and drama to reflect the human condition.

If the Emotional is stronger than the Imaginative, then the S-E-I is less likely to need sexual variety in terms of partners and positions, but instead will be more demanding about the intellectual qualities of a partner. Their emotions, in other words, will be evoked by someone who is interesting and mentally stimulating — but the sex will have to be good for it to endure. If the Imaginative is dominant, however, fresh bodies and new experiences assume more importance, yet the

Emotional need to bond will make this person less casual about relationships and therefore less inclined to discount the feelings of another.

But, in the end, these people are Sensuals. Ideally, they need to be stirred at a deep emotional and psychological level, and for this to be expressed in a carnal way. When they find this, the relationship can be richly satisfying and enduring. But ultimately this Sensual, like any other, can live without the deeper delights of a strong emotional and intellectual connection in the interests of long-term security, particularly if this includes a comfortable lifestyle and regular sex.

The SENSUAL-Emotional-Romantic (S-E-R)

The additions of Emotional and Romantic to this Sensual's Sexual Style, make for a more flamboyant openness in his or her emotional nature. The Romantic adds drama to the deeper waters of the Emotional. This can obscure this Sensual's basic nature. Less obviously phlegmatic, more tolerant of emotional extremes in others, their basic need for security, sexual satisfaction and comfort can take time to surface. Like any Sensual with a Romantic component they can be their own worst enemies. Their Romantic desire for thrills conflicts with their more fundamental need for stability.

In relationship terms it means that the most compelling attractions for these people result from a *coup de foudre*, which signals a deeper emotional connection. Looks matter more to them or, if not, there needs to be a more objective specialness or aura of glamour attached to the person who captures their attention and, consequently, their hearts.

When the Romantic is the stronger subsidiary element, there is a more enduring need to pay attention to feeding love with conventional displays of affection and admiration. Nevertheless, the Emotional tendency adds deeper commitment to this. If the Emotional side is stronger, there is less obvious need for regular reassurance, but the golden vision of continuing romance lingers as an ideal in the S-E-R's heart. For both, sex needs a certain refinement.

To feel that life and love are perfect, this Sensual needs to be thought wonderful — or to feel that his or her partner is extraordinary, and for this to activate more profound and long-lasting emotions. This combination can result in sex with a very special quality. But the practical side of this Sensual is prepared to put up with the loss of romance eventually, and even to feel less emotionally bonded over time. It's not ideal, but it's real life — a concept Sensuals understand.

The SENSUAL-Romantic-Imaginative (S-R-I)

This combination is the least stable of all the Sensuals. The Romantic and Imaginative elements in the cocktail exert a strong pull towards variety, excitement and drama, which can be disruptive to the deeper Sensual need for certainty and security. This is the Sensual Style most likely to cut off its nose to spite its face, forfeiting the Sensual's long-term commitment for shorter-term excitement, and then profoundly regretting it, or feeling unbearably insecure. It makes for a tendency to dissatisfaction whichever way the chips fall: boredom and a sense of disappointment in long-haul relationships when romance and interest have somewhat faded, or an uneasy tension when everything seems wonderful but is in a state of flux.

The S-R-I man and woman demand partners who are good-looking and interesting. It goes without saying that the sex must be satisfying too. If Romantic is stronger in the mixture then they give higher priority to the heightened feelings of infatuated love and the courting behaviour it entails. The lesser Imaginative element is then more likely to be expressed by needing a companion who is interesting to talk to. When the relative strengths are reversed, this S-R-I is likely to place more emphasis on variety of experience, including sexually, and the Romantic streak can be satisfied with less wooing so long as the partner seems special or good-looking.

In a perfect world, this Sensual hybrid wants interest, creativity and mutual admiration within a long-term, sexually satisfying relationship. Ticking off the pros and cons of Romantic and Imaginative concerns against Sensual needs, however, the S-R-I is most likely to take the surer, safer course of staying put in a relationship that has lost glamour and interest. When sex remains good it can be some compensation for the times of ennui, or being taken for granted.

The SENSUAL-Emotional-Romantic-Imaginative (S-E-R-I)

It is extremely rare to have all these elements expressed in your approach to love and sexuality. The Sensual who thinks he or she has them all is usually considering relationships in the abstract: 'What I really want to be happy is someone with whom I can settle down for life, with whom I can have an enduringly good sexual relationship, who will continue to interest me, move me deeply, and who will go on appearing as delightful and special as when we first fell in love.' These magical unions do happen and, of course, are intensely satisfying to representatives of all Sexual Styles. But in reality one – or possibly two – of the elements tend to be much more significant to you, and sometimes it takes the experience of a lasting relationship to make clear to you which these might be.

That said, someone who is predominantly Sensual has a better chance of making such a relationship than most. This is because Sensuals are more likely to withstand the natural lows in a relationship, sticking it out until matters improve. Elements that seem to be missing at one point can re-emerge at a later date, given time. Also if the elements appear to have equal importance, it is easier to bear the temporary disappearance of one, so long as some of the others still endure.

Sensuals who truly demand all these elements can find that it takes them a long time to find the perfect partner with whom to settle down. Being Sensuals, however, they might be prepared to compromise in the end – choosing a less rounded relationship in the interests of security and comfort, and because too much searching goes against the grain and their need for certainty.

The Imaginative Woman

'The brain is clearly the central erogenous zone for me, and he's got a big one.'

Marianne Wiggins, on her ex-husband, Salman Rushdie

The Imaginative Woman

Ms Imaginative was not invented during the 1960s, but she was liberated by what that decade represented more than any other female Sexual Style. She could come out of hiding at last. The 'anything goes with anyone' sexual climate, combined with efficient and discreet contraception, allowed Ms Imaginative to experiment sexually in a way which she had only dreamed of before.

'Dreamed' is the important word. For although Ms Imaginative can and does enjoy sex as much as any other woman, she is most turned on by the *idea* of sex, its infinite variations, and that sea of potential partners out there. She lives most comfortably in the world of ideas at the best of times. She has her feelings, but her head rules her heart. Indeed, if you want to capture her heart, the route is through her mind. She needs to be interested to feel alive.

In certain cases sex is not one of her interests, but merely an appetite that might be strong, or almost non-existent. When it's non-existent, sex will hardly concern her at all. If she *is* interested, however, she takes your breath away. This kind of Imaginative woman might believe she's Ms Sensual — after all, she doesn't know anyone else who has investigated sex and its possibilities so enthusiastically. But when Ms Sensual goes bed-hopping she is on a quest for the most satisfying sexual experience. Give her the man with whom she finds this and she's happy to stay put for a long time.

Ms Imaginative's quest is different: it is for the *ultimate* sexual experience. The trouble is that going to bed with a wonderful lover and having the most sensually fulfilling time ever is not enough. Before long, however good the sex, she becomes bored. That proves it can't have been the ultimate experience. It must still be *out there*. Without the excitement of the new, sex for Ms Imaginative loses its savour. An imaginative and innovative lover can hold her attention for a while but, eventually, her familiarity with his body, the sheer predictability of his *face* is enough to make her feel she is missing out.

In *Fear of Flying* Erica Jong introduced the quintessentially Imaginative heroine: Isadora Wing. This charming and sexually predatory woman was in search of the Zipless Fuck. 'Zipless because, when you came together, zippers fell away like rose petals, underwear blew off in one breath like dandelion fluff. For the true, ultimate zipless A-1 fuck, it was necessary that you never got to know the man very well.'

Isadora Wing was not just a literary invention. Erica Jong uses her to express many of her own thoughts and feelings about sex. For she too is an archetypal Imaginative. 'Sex, by definition, is something that you have with someone other than a spouse,' she writes in her autobiography, *Fear of Fifty*. A happily married Ms Sensual or Ms Emotional would beg to differ. 'Call it conjugal anything and the mystery withers,' she continues, convinced that mystery is the main exciting ingredient in sex. It is, for the Imaginative – but not necessarily for the other Sexual Styles.

Erica Jong describes another trait of the Imaginative woman: 'Odd people are attracted to me, and I find men with a touch of madness compelling.' In between her four marriages she had many lovers, a lot of excitement, but, finally, much disappointment. When the ultimate experience is always the next one, this is inevitable. Indeed, in her late forties Erica Jong went against type. She married a man she liked, but frankly admitted she wasn't attracted to him. They didn't even go to bed together for six months, and then it was disastrous. She resisted the Imaginative's impulse to move on, sex improved and their marriage settled down.

It is as a tamed or disappointed Imaginative that Erica Jong speaks this epitaph: 'The zipless fuck fantasy is better than the reality ... Generally women don't get a lot out of that kind of casual sex. A lot of women of my generation discovered that — to our horror.'

So, are all Imaginative women doomed to disappointment? And what did they do before the 1960s let them do their own thing? The answers to both are found in the complexity of Ms Imaginative. Remember that variety and novelty are important to her because they are exciting concepts. It doesn't matter if the physical reality is less satisfying than when she was thinking about it. When she is mentally stimulated she is sexually stimulated too. A man who can catch her interest, make her think, provoke her imagination, widen her horizons or even shake her certainties and beliefs — this is the man who is also most likely to turn her on. While some Imaginative women like the combination of sexual permutations *and* a mentally exciting man, for others the man and his mind is enough. The way he makes her think — and therefore feel — is more profoundly exciting than the idea of the zipless fuck, or an array of changing partners or sexually exotic variations.

So who is this mind-magician, with such erotic power over Ms Imaginative? He doesn't have to be Mr Mensa, or have a PhD, although some Imaginative women like this. Indeed, even those who prize measurable cleverness will lose interest in a pedant, or a man who starts sentences 'as I always say', even if what he always says is right. A touch of genius, however, is essential, and Ms Imaginative knows that this can equally be found in the drop-out whose career is a series of temporary jobs. He has an original way of thinking and expressing himself (Erica Jong's compelling 'touch of madness'), he is often idealistic, or even if he's somewhat cynical he can get worked up and passionate about an idea or what's happening in the world.

He has strong opinions: if you ask him what he thought of a movie he won't content himself with saying 'it was good', or 'it was crap'. He'll *tell* you. Ms Imaginative doesn't require him to share her opinions — in fact, so long as he doesn't offend her most deeply-held beliefs, she is more likely to be fascinated by a man who thinks differently. Because 'newness' is so thrilling to Ms Imaginative, anyone who makes her question or have to think in a new way is compelling and seductive. If, by chance, they do think the same way, Ms Imaginative will be irritated by a Yes man. But if he contributes by casting a new slant on her ideas, extending, illuminating and adding his own enthusiasm, she will feel she has found a soulmate, and this will deeply stir her sexually.

That is not to say that she is the only one to appreciate this kind of man. Most women, regardless of their Sexual Styles, want a man who is interesting, intelligent and lively company. But for other kinds of women these are only some of their shopping list of male qualities. Without other important characteristics they are not enough alone to invoke desire. Only the Imaginative woman who does not have strong elements of another Sexual Style can find these qualities in themselves erotic. She can literally be talked into bed: not by protestations of love, or by flattery, but by sheer mental pyrotechnics. The excitement of stimulating conversation is the most potent aphrodisiac.

There is also the Imaginative woman for whom the world of the mind generally is more fascinating than anything else. She might have no interest in sex whatsoever. Indeed she might be a bluestocking who devotes herself to ideas, research, travel, or an all-consuming cause that leaves her no time to think of men. Even when she does marry, sex is the least of her preoccupations. The writer Virginia Woolf, who was born in 1882, is an example of this type. She fell deeply in love with Leonard Woolf and married him, but their union was virtually sexless. The driving force of their marriage was encapsulated in the title of the biography written by George Spater and

Ian Parsons: *A Marriage of True Minds*. Virginia had a brief lesbian affair with Vita Sackville West, but the sex was the least important part – and homosexual affairs were the done thing in her circle. Writing was her passion, and she described it as almost sexual ecstasy. While writing *Three Guineas* she exclaimed: 'It has pressed and spurted out of me ... like a physical volcano. And my brain feels cool and quiet after the expulsion. I've had it sizzling now since ...' Certainly sex never moved her to such excitement.

Virginia Woolf suffered 'madness' throughout her life – a manic depression that eventually drove her to suicide. This is not exclusively an Imaginative's illness, but it is connected to a difficulty with handling powerful emotions – the flight into mental excitement, followed by being engulfed and paralysed by feelings at a later date. She wrote of her friend Carrington's suicide: 'A saying of Leonard's comes into my head ... "Things have gone wrong somehow." It was the night Carrington killed herself. We were walking along that silent blue street with the scaffolding. I saw all the violence and unreason crossing in the air: ourselves small; a tumult outside: something terrifying: unreason. Shall I make a book out of this? It would be a way of bringing order and speed again into my world.' 'Unreason' and 'order' are the important words. There is nothing ordered or reasonable about strong emotions, and they can't be analysed away. Like many Imaginatives Virginia Woolf was only able to cope with feelings when she could make sense of them – attach words to them – and when she couldn't she experienced it as 'madness'.

Identifying Ms Imaginative

We know more about Ms Imaginative's sexual lifestyle than all the other female styles put together. This is because she not only likes to think and talk about it, but if she has any talent at all she will also write about it. Many journalists who make a career writing about their own sex lives for magazines are Imaginatives. Airport sex novels, whether aimed at men or women, often feature Imaginative heroines. These protagonists rarely have to be in love; they never have the kind of sexual experience that is boring to describe but intensely fulfilling to experience. Romance is an optional extra. Their sexual encounters are usually weird, wild, kinky, with every combination of partners (multiple, same sex), and sex aids – animal, vegetable and mineral.

The fictional Ms Imaginative is, of course, a caricature. Her real-life counterpart often has a job to hold down, the housework to do, family and friends to consider. For all sorts of reasons she might be reluctant to experiment sexually, or find the wilder reaches too bizarre – although she will always be exceedingly curious. This is one clue to her nature. While talking about sex is no big deal these days, and most women, whatever their Sexual Style, enjoy these conversations, Ms Imaginative is the keenest to open the subject, and the one who wants to go on talking about it longest. She is not a traditional gossip, in the sense that she is not specially interested in character assassination or analysis of emotions and motive. But she loves juicy tit-bits – new information about what other people have been up to. She is fascinated by anything you tell her about your own sex life, and, on the whole, is prepared to tell you about hers. While the other Sexual Styles might want to know about *your* sex life, they are, usually, for different reasons, more reluctant to talk about their own. Ms Romantic feels it destroys the specialness. She'll hint it's wonderful, and leave a row of dots. Ms Sensual would rather do it than talk about it. Ms Emotional, if she's happy with her partner, may well feel it's a betrayal to go into details. Ms Imaginative may be no less in love, may feel intensely romantic about her man – but all that is separate and irrelevant. It is no more difficult for her to tell you what they have been getting up to sexually than it is for her to describe her recipe for chocolate cake.

The Imaginative Woman

Whether she is talking about sex or not, the character of Ms Imaginative's friendships and social life are usually indicative of her basic nature. What she likes is to have an interesting time. She likes her brain to buzz, and the conversation to be fast and furious. The people she chooses to see most often are those that she can spark off. This doesn't mean that she can't be very fond of old friends with whom she feels comfortably at home, but if their company is merely cosy she won't feel a pressing need to see them more than occasionally. Indeed, if you are interesting she will automatically like you. It is a quality she values above almost anything else.

While Ms Imaginative can enjoy an evening in which she just has a good laugh, or a quietly companionable time if she is feeling tired, neither of these really satisfy her. If she can't be fascinated she'd rather be startled, outraged or forced into an argument with someone who challenges her ideas. A fresh thought, or an old one expressed in an original or articulate way, excites her more than anything. Because she can't really understand people who feel differently about this, she sometimes feels it is her duty to liven up what she considers a dull gathering by being controversial, or entertaining. Her idea of misery is for one week to be socially identical to the last, which means she's out at movies, exhibitions, adult education classes, and prepared to try anything once – roller-blading, bowling, perhaps that seedy little back-street club someone told her about. Because of this she often pushes herself beyond her limits. She has no sense that she has done too much until she comes down with a cold, or she can't raise herself from her bed in the morning, or her brain becomes woolly with tiredness.

The more home-bound Ms Imaginative won't be quietly vegetating in front of the television. Her brain will be active, even if her body isn't. She'll be reading, studying or writing. When she reads she can be intoxicated even more by the writer's use of language than she is by the details of the plot. She doesn't feel herself when her brain is idle, and it will make her restless or guilty. At the very least she'll be having an hour-long conversation on the telephone with a friend. For other Imaginative women, however, life at home and at work, however stimulating, makes her impatient after a while. She needs to stretch her brain with exotic experiences. Sometimes she works just so as to make enough money to travel. She lives for her holidays — not as other women do, for the restful contrast with work — but because she thirsts for new experiences. If she can arrange it, her work itself will involve travel, or she will take to the road without any idea of how she is going to finance herself, driven by the more compelling need for adventure.

As with all the female Sexual Styles, the way Ms Imaginative dresses does not give the most reliable information about what she is really like. It would be a mistake for a man to decide on the basis of a woman's outfit that she's going to be available for a particular type of sexual experience — a mistake that lands some men in court. All women can be strongly influenced by prevailing trends, and are as likely to dress to suit their body types as they are their secret sexual identities. Ms Imaginative isn't an exception. However, when she is fashion-conscious she will be at the leading edge of fashion. She won't wait for new styles to hit the high street, but will be wearing her own version while it's still on the Paris catwalks. She can occasionally be a fashion victim: as 'new' is synonymous with 'wonderful' in her vocabulary she can occasionally be blinded to whether what she is wearing suits her or not.

Not every Imaginative woman, however, cares about what's in or out unless she is still young enough to want to impress her contemporaries, or is in a business where it's important. The idea of following *anything*, including fashion trends, offends her sense of uniqueness. Whatever she wears, however, tends to be individual. An Imaginative woman I knew used to wear ordinary, inexpensive clothes, but always topped her outfits with a different, beautiful shawl. She was constantly draping and rewinding it, so that your eye was drawn to its exotic colours and patterns rather than what she wore underneath.

The Imaginative Woman

Meeting Ms Imaginative over a meal or a drink can provide more positive indications of her deeper nature. Unless her Imaginative core is much tempered by another Sexual Style, or she is on a diet for health or weight reasons, her interest in what she puts in her mouth is likely to be negligible. She will like to try different cuisines, or the most unusual items on the menu, or a brand-new cocktail, not because she really cares what they taste like, but more in the interest of experimentation. Indeed, if the conversation is engrossing she's likely to forget what's in front of her until it's too cold to be edible, or the ice has melted in her drink. Contrast her with Ms Sensual, who might be equally fascinated by what is being said, but can't really concentrate until her hunger is assuaged. Ms Imaginative can be a good and inventive cook, as her experimenting nature finds expression in the kitchen too – but the look, the presentation and the unusual ingredients interest her more, ultimately, than the flavour.

Ms Imaginative can also be spotted by her body language when interacting with other people. She finds boredom hard to tolerate, and it shows. Whereas some people express this by looking glum or resigned, she is more likely to be impatient. If she can't move away she will be on the simmer, a mass of involuntary movements. She'll tap her foot, play with her hair, look away, cough nervously – perhaps even nod too much with what looks like enthusiasm but is really irritation. When her interest is caught, however, she is likely to be motionless, poised to catch every word, her body inclined towards the speaker. Some Imaginative women are listeners by nature, but they always have to be intrigued. Many prefer talking. All of them find silence somewhat disturbing. The more peaceable Imaginative woman enjoys most having conversations with people who think the same as she does – either sharing ideas, or simply exchanging memories. Others are more comfortable with the clash of voices, whatever they might be saying – even if they are arguing – than the stillness of a pause, however companionable or loving.

The unattached Imaginative woman

You would expect the archetypal Imaginative woman to play the field more enthusiastically and intensively than any other Sexual Style. It's not quite as simple as that. All the Sexual Styles have the potential to be promiscuous, depending on the strength of their sex drives, and whether they are successful in their search for having their needs met. The Imaginative woman who finds the idea of sex over-rated can be as happily chaste as a nun. It's not the number of partners she has had that indicates her Sexual Style, so much as her attitude to them – sex alone does not have the power to move her emotionally. The Imaginative woman's libido is no higher than another woman's, and sometimes it can be low. Her curiosity about sex might rarely translate into a desire for action. While she is going through adolescence she might also be unaware of her true nature: most adolescent girls are exceptionally romantic, and these strong feelings can obscure her understanding of her basic Sexual Style. Conditioning, family values, religious training, as well as other outside influences, can cause her to check her natural impulses, and it might only be much later in life that she is able to identify what makes her tick.

Nevertheless, if she is a true Imaginative, with little or no dilution from the other Sexual Styles, by her mid-twenties she is likely to have had a number of partners, without guilt or anxiety – and discovered a desire to continue to extend her sexual horizons with more men and more interesting sexual permutations. Even if she is fundamentally heterosexual, she is the most likely of the Sexual Styles to have dabbled in same-sex encounters, as she doesn't like to feel that there is something she hasn't tried. Because the route to her sexuality is through her mind, she might also find herself in bed with another woman who has dazzled her mentally, even if she continues to prefer men. As Angie Bowie said about her marriage to David Bowie: 'The conventional concept of marriage would not have suited my style; I was a bisexual butterfly ... I loved the creative intimacy of our marriage, but I have to say the sex was pretty lousy.'

A good example of an Imaginative woman on the loose is 'Jeanette', who once used a woman's magazine as a confessional. By the age of 31 she had slept with over 150 men, sometimes five in a week, and even two in a day. 'When I was young I was fascinated by sex,' she says. 'My family never really talked about it – when love scenes came on the TV we'd all go red and look away. It was this big taboo subject. When I was about nine years old I found a soft-porn mag in the woods near my house. I couldn't believe what I read about masturbation, penetration and oral sex. I wasn't disgusted, more intrigued – and I felt a weird warm feeling inside. From that moment on I suppose I had an interest in the whole business of what went on between men and women.'

Jeanette is not the sort of Imaginative who is necessarily attracted by what a man has to offer mentally. Variety is all-important. What distinguishes Jeanette's experiences as those of an Imaginative is that they are almost empty of any emotional content. 'I feel I operate like the traditional man – my sex life doesn't necessarily have to be bound up with my emotions. I'm pretty physical anyway and feel quite happy about being intimate with men physically – but not necessarily emotionally.' The strongest thing she feels, apart from desire, is a contempt for many of the men. 'Sometimes when I've had a one-night-stand I want the man to leave. If they get stroppy I say, "Look you've had what you want – I don't want to share a coffee and a chat with you tomorrow, so sod off."' When sex means little more to an Imaginative woman than a meaningless romp, she can't conceive of it having more significance to the man, or believe that he will be unduly hurt by dismissive or cruel behaviour.

Jeanette has sought to explain her attitude. 'My father was a notorious sleep-around and used women, while my mother didn't like sex. Sometimes I do feel I am avenging my mother for his behaviour. In the way that my father shat on women sexually, I do the same to men.' This is clearly a contributing factor in Jeanette's contempt for men and her anger, but it is only because she is at heart an Imaginative that she chooses this way of acting on it. An Emotional woman who has a similar childhood experience, for example, will play out her reactions differently when she becomes an adult. If she is very damaged by it, her response might be unhealthy – she could find herself drawn to a powerful, woman-hating man and stick to him through thick and thin, despite her misery. A Romantic woman with a similar father could grow up frightened of men and untrusting. If she did decide to wreak revenge on other men she is less likely to use them sexually than to lead them on and then reject them – denying them the sex her father had taken so easily from other women. Only the Imaginative woman can use sex as a weapon without any emotional consequences rebounding on her.

Jeanette can see another motivation when she looks back. 'I also think that in my younger years I was seeking approval. I didn't feel very attractive as a student and I didn't fit in at university. Sleeping around then was a way of making me feel sexy and alluring – it gave me some kind of status in my own mind. Half the time I'd have sex and not even enjoy it, feeling a bit miserable afterwards.' A Romantic or Emotional woman would not find her self-esteem enhanced by sleeping around. Both of these would be more likely to feel worse about themselves if all their encounters were so casual and uncaring. A Sensual woman would feel despairing that the sex itself was so unenjoyable.

In common with many Imaginative women, Jeanette believes that she is driven by sensuality. 'I have practised being good in bed and I demand equally good sex from my lovers. I have moved on from doing it for security to doing it because I honestly enjoy it. There are loads of reasons why I've had so many lovers. But the main one is that I really enjoy sex.' But when she elaborates on what she enjoys, her Imaginative nature is revealed. 'Nothing beats that incredible feeling when you want someone really badly, when you're pressed up against the wall kissing passionately *with all the expectation of what's about to happen. I don't think I've ever found a thrill that excites me so much.*' They are my italics: the expectation is the thrill, and, as she has said, after it's over her greatest desire is sometimes to kick the man out of bed.

An Imaginative woman with more happy memories of her parents' relationship is unlikely to have had quite so many lovers, or treat them so badly. He casualness about sex will be more blithe, and will usually leave both of them feeling good afterwards. While she won't be too troubled if an encounter turns out to be a one-night-stand, she is less likely to seek them obsessively. I know of a woman who works part-time as a sexual surrogate: having sex with men who have sexual problems and who are seeing a psychiatrist who 'prescribes' her. She is a warm-hearted, loving and uninhibited woman whose deeper emotions are not touched by sex. It seems no more intimate to her than shaking hands. She has been living for years with a man who accepts her work, and also accepts that she takes lovers for pleasure from time to time. Neither of them is concerned about this, but the lovers often are. She is confused and upset when they accuse her of playing games with them. To her it *is* a game – a healthy, uncomplicated one for two players, but she never sets out to hurt. The Imaginative woman of this kind will often number ex-lovers among her friends, and may occasionally go to bed with them for old times' sake when she is in between relationships. It's just good fun, and she feels in no danger of rekindling a dead love.

The Imaginative woman who is more concerned with a man's mental equipment than she is with sexual experimentation can be more disturbed by brief encounters. While the mental connection retains the power to excite her, her desire will remain high. If she's still turned on by his mind she will be upset if he wants to move on. She will be more bothered by his rejection of their intellectual rapport than by any sexual betrayal. After all, she is better equipped than women of other Sexual Styles to understand the erotic attraction of a fresh body, and not believe it means anything personal.

In some cases Ms Imaginative is prepared to deny a call from her emotions and her sexual instincts if the man in question doesn't fit in her mental landscape, or challenges what is deeply important in her views on life. Beatrice Webb (née Potter) was an example of this. Born in 1858 into a rich and privileged family, she was a great beauty and an intellectual. She turned her back on her family's values to fight for the 'people of the abyss' as a socialist. She fell passionately in love with Joseph Chamberlain, the handsome leader of the radical wing of the Liberal party, and President of the Board of Trade. He wanted to marry her, and she yearned to be with him, finding him magnetically attractive. But that would have meant giving up her work and becoming the little wife in the background. Chamberlain also made it clear that she would have to subordinate her opinions to his. For more than six years she fought her passion for him. Eventually she married Sidney Webb, a man she found physically repulsive, because they shared the same socialist vision and could work as equal partners as writers and founders of the London School of Economics. Only an Imaginative woman could exercise such a control over her instincts and sacrifice physical and emotional happiness for principle.

Sex and Ms Imaginative

If people were uncomplicated it would be possible to sum up Ms Imaginative's sex life by saying 'she will try everything once with anyone or anything'. But sexuality defies such over-simplification. What makes sex good for an individual is affected by personality, emotions, thoughts and preferences, as well as by upbringing, background and life experiences.

The Imaginative Woman

Even an undiluted Ms Imaginative will have different sexual tastes and preferences from a woman who is an equally typical representative of this Sexual Style. There are going to be some things she finds revolting to contemplate, or boundaries she will never breach. Indeed, the unrestrained sexual adventuress let loose by the Sixties might even now be receding into the past since the advent of AIDS.

But she will adapt, as she always has had to before. After all, her mind is even more important in her experience of sexual pleasure than her bodily sensations. Telephone sex, for instance, which has a limited appeal for the other Sexual Styles, can be exquisitely erotic for her.

While she might be much more conservative in her sexual tastes than the Imaginative in fiction, nevertheless she is likely to enjoy sexual experimentation more than average. She'll rarely be content with a small number of basic sexual positions. She's usually game to try an exotic or complicated one, and even if it turns out to be uncomfortable or unsatisfying, the difference will be enough to make it intensely exciting for her. Whether or not she physically enjoys sex acts such as giving or receiving oral sex, or anal sex, she will usually want to have a go to see what it's like. Unless it is part of her psychological make-up she won't be drawn to sadomasochistic practices as a personal preference, though she will see them as part of the rich tapestry of sex — and therefore worth sampling. Tie her to the bed too often, or use the same old jackboots and whip, and she will become bored or angry. If you are lucky, she'll laugh: she is the woman most likely to enjoy sex as light-hearted sport at times. Indeed, unless she is in love, bringing in romance, emotions or repetitious sexual needs can dampen her ardour — introducing what seem like unnecessary complications. Dressing up, on the other hand, might strike her as an essential complication. She won't be especially drawn to the texture (like Ms Sensual) or the atmosphere she's creating (like Ms Romantic). What she will like is the opportunity to try on a different personality and express her sexuality through it. Sex toys can appeal to her sense of fun as well as her need to experiment.

When she's not testing a new position or sex act, she will at least want to be in a different location. The bed has its limitations, and she will need to vary it with the kitchen table, half-way up the stairs, the bath, the rug by the fire, and so on. The sexual mood needs varying to suit her too. If it's always soft lighting and gentle romantic caressing she'll find it a yawn. She likes to be surprised. Sometimes she can find a fast, furious 'quickie', over in minutes, exhilaratingly arousing. As the thrill of the unknown and unexpected intensifies her passion, she may also like the danger of semi-public sex: in the back of the car, behind the filing cabinet at an office party, outdoors. The thought that they could be disturbed, spotted, even prosecuted, adds a sensational edge.

These sexual games and preferences aren't unique to the Imaginative woman. Other Sexual Styles can also be turned on by them. The difference is that while other women might return to what they find exciting time and again, Ms Imaginative will find constant repetition kills the pleasure.

Fantasy usually plays a big role in the Imaginative woman's enjoyment. Indeed if she is nervous, inhibited, or her Sexual Style conflicts with her moral values, she might fantasise more than she performs. In some cases, when physical satisfaction is a low priority, the arousal created by fantasy is pleasure enough. For other Imaginative women it is a masturbatory aid, or an enhancer of an otherwise dull sexual encounter. Unless she is a very shy version of this Sexual Style, she can also relish sharing fantasies – talking about her own, and hearing about her man's. For some Sexual Styles talking about fantasies robs them of their erotic content: not so for Ms Imaginative, who can find that the thrill increases. She can find pornography more stimulating than women of other Sexual Styles – it gives her ideas and feeds her fantasies. Even if she isn't turned on by what her man likes reading or watching she is often prepared to put up with it, and may even enjoy finding out what is so exciting about it for him. This ease in talking about sex is often helpful. She is more willing to say what she wants and would like to try (and listen to what he has to say) than many other women. She can often enjoy talking dirty, and may be very voluble when she is making love.

All this, of course, is a generalisation. It is not a blueprint for sex with Ms Imaginative. Some Imaginative women need much less sex than others. Some have little interest in sex, experimental or not. Some will only find a new man exciting, not a new position. For various reasons some will find certain sexual variations absolutely taboo. For others the ultimate turn-on will always be the man's mind, and the love they make will be secondary. Indeed, when she finds sex itself a bore she can be happier in a relationship that does not require it. When it means nothing to her she will find it almost impossible to understand why her partner keeps wanting to do it. Because her own emotions and sensuality are subordinate to her logical, thinking mind, she finds it hard to understand people who are differently motivated. Sometimes the more intellectual and controlled Imaginative woman will despise a man who, as she sees it, lets his body master his mind.

The Imaginative woman and marriage

Just because Ms Imaginative is able to separate sex from love doesn't mean that she can't fall wildly, deeply and romantically in love. For it to be more than a passing passion he'll have to be the kind of man already described: someone who interests her overpoweringly, out of bed more than in it. Sometimes her choice can seem odd to her friends. He might not look anything special or be obviously successful. Her nature doesn't demand this – although perhaps when she is making a 'sensible' choice of life partner she will be somewhat concerned about his economic prospects. Even when she genuinely falls in love with a man who is obviously successful he is unlikely to be a cautious businessman who has merely speculated well, or someone who has inherited wealth – there must be brilliance or creativity too. Power or solvency alone aren't enough.

Sometimes they can seem to be startlingly incompatible: he's much older or younger than she is, intellectually leagues above her, or from a different culture or background. While women of other Sexual Styles can also be attracted to men like this it is not necessarily for the same reason. It is their very differentness that draws Ms Imaginative to these men: the feeling that there is so much to know and learn about them, or from them. Knowing someone inside out is not a desirable concept to her – she'd always prefer to believe that there are further depths to plumb. When she is an intellectual Imaginative looking for a soulmate, she will only be attracted to men with classy minds, and be unable to see good qualities in any man who is less than her intellectual equal.

Nevertheless, in common with other women, Ms Imaginative can marry for all sorts of reasons, not just love or desire. The older she is before making the decision, the more likely she is to bring extra considerations to her choice. If her biological clock is ticking she might become less choosy. If, like Erica Jong, she has become disillusioned with her Imaginative lifestyle, she is less likely to trust her desires and instincts exclusively. Or, like Beatrice Webb, the only important consideration is how they harmonise intellectually.

Whether she marries the first man she falls for, or the man she sees as her last chance, settling down is harder for Ms Imaginative than for other women. For some Imaginative women the idea of a long-term commitment can cause terror, and be a turn-off sexually. The Oscar-winning actress Emma Thompson said about her marriage to Kenneth Branagh: 'Marriage is an extremely dangerous step ... I mean, how stupid can you get? You put all your eggs in one basket and say you are going to stay with this person for the rest of your life.' At the same time she reminisced about her Imaginative past: 'I had everyone before

I was married. I was very fortunate in having belonged to the pre-AIDS generation that could sleep with everything with a pulse. I enjoyed a varied sex life from the age of 15.' The Branaghs split up after six years of marriage.

Most people pause on the threshold of marriage and wonder if they are doing the right thing. But it is a rare Imaginative who doesn't have more than a moment of bleakness at the thought of having to spend the rest of her life with just one man. Fortunately, once she gets past the fear, she can have many happy years before it begins to pall. If she has a family to bring up, a lifestyle that challenges and involves her, a husband she respects and finds good company, marriage will not seem too confining.

On the other hand, the Imaginative woman does not value highly the elements that can make marriage so rewarding for other women. Routine, habit, certainties, security, the comfort of being loved, homely pleasures – all these have only limited charm for her. They are not *interesting*. Sometimes, indeed, she feels more committed and vital in a marriage where there is dissent or financial insecurity. While she's battling with creditors she knows she's alive. If she argues with her husband at least she feels they are engaging on the mental level.

One of the things that makes marriage hard for her to tolerate is her Sexual Style. As we have seen, it is novelty and mystery that make sex intensely exciting for her. With the best will in the world – and the best lover – there is a limit to how long she can find the man she lives with mysteriously exciting. If the sex they do have is enjoyable, and they do not lapse too readily into routine, then, everything else being fine, she will not mind too much. Over time, however, her desire for sex will lessen. She might find it enjoyable while they are making love, even have regular orgasms, but no sense of anticipatory pleasure. If she gets to the point where she never feels desire for him, always starts love-making from 'cold', then it becomes increasingly hard for her to come anywhere near orgasm.

While continuing to find her husband interesting can keep

her desirous for longer, even this won't last forever. If her natural sex drive is low she might be genuinely happy to live without sex and take pleasure in her unwavering interest in what other people are doing (although she might develop a prudish streak, she'll always want to *know*). Her attitude to sex can become a practical matter of 'been there, done that'. When she's had her fill of experimentation she can consign sex to the past with barely a thought. If her sex drive is higher, or sex became too habitual too soon, then she will be restless. Whether she acts on her restlessness or not – by having an affair, or leaving her husband – depends on whether she still finds him mentally admirable or exciting. As in all Sexual Styles there is a bottom line: she can tolerate a marriage without a strong emotional connection; romance is pleasant but not essential; even a non-existent sex life is bearable. But if she finds him boring and they have little to say to each other in friendship or in anger then she will reach breaking point. The surest way a man can hurt her deeply is to shut her out of his thoughts, or refuse to talk to her. If she stays in a marriage like this out of fear of the alternatives she will become nervous or depressed.

The pure Imaginative who is somewhat disconnected from her own emotions can find the undercurrents in marriage difficult to handle. One Imaginative woman I know admits to talking to herself because, 'I only know what I feel when I hear myself say it.' This kind of woman can eventually come to understand some of her own emotions by talking about them, but will usually find it harder to understand her partner's. If it is not something she has identified and classified for herself, she can't accept the reality of it. She can simply block out or ignore her man's distress when it is foreign to her, thereby leaving untouched issues that need to be addressed about their relationship. Even when she has a good grasp of emotions intellectually (she might even be a psychologist!), she can still have trouble with the reality of them. She has a horror of feeling deeply – retreating into 'explanations' instead.

When Ms Imaginative has a long and happy marriage this is usually because she and her husband share concerns and a vision beyond bringing up the family and making a home. Sometimes working together is what does it: when they have business and strategy to discuss there will always be something to say, and seeing him interacting with colleagues or clients keeps him from seeming predictable. It can work equally well if they share an interest in an absorbing hobby, or enjoy learning things together. Working for causes: political, environmental, charitable, can also provide a focus, mutual respect, and endless issues to discuss, worry over and argue about. The Imaginative woman who has always been more interested in her man's brain than in sex can feel committed forever to a man with a challenging complex mind, particularly if he is similarly unconcerned about sexual matters.

Another force for stability, although the marriage itself can be less satisfying, is when they live fairly independent lives, and the family home is merely a base. This does not necessarily mean an open marriage in which they take other sexual partners, although it can. Before Emma Thompson split up with Kenneth Branagh she was asked her reaction to Hugh Grant being caught with a prostitute. She said: 'If Ken were to go strolling down the boulevard looking for a cheap thrill, I'd think, "That seems a perfectly reasonable thing to do if you had the urge".' The point of marriages like this is that they give each other rope, knowing that the more flexibility there is the more likely they are not to leave each other.

When Ms Imaginative will stray

If she knew it wouldn't rock the boat, the typical Ms Imaginative could be tempted to be unfaithful even when she feels she's found the perfect man. One who is fully aware of her sexual predilections might even warn her husband or partner of the possibility. Jeanette, who was quoted earlier, had been involved in an exclusive relationship with a man for two years. 'I've finally managed to be monogamous,' she said. 'I haven't gone off sex or changed my ways because of any outside pressure – it's more that I have a lovely relationship with a special man and I don't want to ruin it. But I have explained to him how I feel about sex and he knows that perhaps in the future I may be unfaithful to him. I don't think he's happy about it but he's trying to accept that it's part of my make-up.'

Infidelity for Ms Imaginative need not be a big deal. She can satisfy her curiosity, get a thrill from the experience (secrecy *plus* mystery is a big turn-on) and return to the marital bed emotionally unaffected, guiltless and refreshed. *Not* being unfaithful is a conscious choice she makes as an offering of love, and because she doesn't want to hurt her partner. Even Mr Imaginative, who understands the impulse, can be wounded in his male pride by a woman who feels the need to find sex elsewhere. Whereas for Ms Emotional, Romantic or Sensual, being unfaithful is usually some sort of statement about their feelings for their partners, for Ms Imaginative it is quite separate. She can even have a sexual dalliance with her best friend's man and not feel she has betrayed or hurt either by so doing, as long as it remains a secret.

Nevertheless, if Ms Imaginative has lost respect for her partner or finds him tedious, or if their sex life has never been inventive enough to hold her interest, she might be tempted into a pattern of chronic unfaithfulness designed to punish him for being a disappointment. She becomes careless of whether he knows about it or not. When his brain has lost its charm for her she might, like other women embarking on an affair, be looking to set up his replacement.

This can also happen to the Imaginative who has no interest in sex whatsoever. She won't merrily sleep around, but if the intellectual connection with her man has gone she will be susceptible to a more interesting man. If the circumstances are right she might even leave her current partner without having had sex with her lover first.

Ms Imaginative and sexual problems

It must be obvious by now that boredom is the main challenge to Ms Imaginative's sexual satisfaction. If she is bored or irritated she can't be put into a good mood by sweet-talking (like Ms Romantic), stroking (like Ms Sensual), or protestations of love (like Ms Emotional). If her man has ceased to inspire her she is extremely unlikely to want to make love to him at all.

But, like other women, Ms Imaginative can sometimes have sexual problems when her relationship is otherwise fine. Sexual difficulties caused by deep psychological problems are not the province of this book, and, of course, Ms Imaginative can be damaged like anyone else by past traumas. An unusually inhibited Ms Imaginative, however, can sometimes be helped by unpicking early conditioning and 'messages' about what is good or bad about sex to discover why it is that she finds it hard to act in accord with her nature, or feels guilty when she does so. Occasionally, knowing that she has accepted opinions as facts can liberate her to enjoy her own Sexual Style.

Sometimes it is only when Ms Imaginative is in a settled relationship that she begins to understand her Sexual Style. If her previous experience has been with short-term partners, she might never have had time to become bored or to realise that she has a great need for variety. She might be disturbed and perplexed by her failing sexual interest in the man she loves. If she never experimented much sexually, she might even be unaware of the untapped possibilities in love-making. Despite the name, not every Imaginative woman has an inventive imagination.

If this is the case, her partner often needs to be the one to open her mind and lead her to explore different experiences. If she is otherwise well-adjusted she will usually take the hint quite quickly and soon start making her own suggestions.

Imaginative women are often good candidates for sex therapy. With encouragement they can thoroughly enjoy talking about themselves and their sex lives. Whereas some women of other

Sexual Styles can find this painful or difficult, she will often feel released and motivated. The pure Imaginative is able to operate without reference to her emotions, and talking about them is often preferable to experiencing them. She will tend to find it deeply interesting, as well as illuminating and exciting, to dig deep into every area — emotional, sexual and physical. But if, during the course of therapy, she discovers that it is her partner himself that she finds dull, not their sexual routine, little will help.

On the other hand, if this is not the case, and they are simply stuck in a rut, the sex therapist can help them out of it. While the touching exercises of sensate focusing won't in themselves be enough to revive Ms Imaginative's desire, if she has never tried them before she may well be turned on by the different approach. Much more useful in her case will be a therapist who is full of ideas and suggestions, or who can point them in the direction of books that offer others.

When sex itself has ceased to be interesting for her almost nothing will revive her interest. When she feels that she has done everything she ever wanted to do it's hard for her to see the point in doing it all over again. This is especially true when the sensual side of sex has been its least interesting aspect. If her partner is similarly disinclined to make love there is no problem, so long as they find the rest of their relationship rewarding. When he needs their sex life to continue she will think he's being a bore.

It is hardest of all for the happily-married Imaginative woman with an enduring sexual appetite who has tried everything she ever wanted to with her partner, and now feels doomed only to repeat herself. If she values her marriage, and knows that being unfaithful can jeopardise what she prizes, she may have to accept that sex can never be so exciting for her again. The fortunate Imaginative woman discovers this sufficiently late in her life and in her marriage for it not to cause her more than a passing wistfulness.

The Imaginative Man

'The sensation of having "arrived" has never been a comfortable thing for me. Flirting with a woman has always been more exciting than *being* with a woman.'

Richard Dreyfus, actor

The Imaginative Man

The phrase 'bored to death' might have been invented by an Imaginative man. He needs to be active mentally to be happy. What's going on in his head is what matters most. A life that is predictable holds little charm for him. If there is nothing new to discover, explore, or think about he becomes restless – sameness is intolerable. For a certain kind of man this relentless inquisitiveness is expressed in his love life. Women are uncharted territory, with an infinite variety of types to experience and classify. He is not a man to think 'all cats are grey in the dark' – in other words, that all women are the same once you get them into bed. He is fascinated by their different shapes and sizes, varying likes and dislikes, their odd quirks and predilections. His sexual pursuit of them is almost scientific, and once he has satisfied his curiosity with one woman he is eager to get on to the next. The anticipation involved in flirting is tantalising. Where will it lead? What will she be like? Sometimes having his curiosity satisfied is much less rewarding than the expectancy that precedes it – or, in effect, the *idea* of a woman matters more than what he does with her.

Actually all Imaginative men have the tendency to want to have as many women as they can, though with some it is confined to a stage in their lives when they are young and randy and full of energy. Indeed, most men have an interest in experimenting with different women, but for the Emotional, Sensual or Romantic male their curiosity is usually diverted by a woman who holds their attention for longer. Some Imaginative men long to change partners frequently, but don't have what it takes to attract them. They make do with talking about sex, reading about it, or – in extreme cases – becoming voyeurs, watching other people doing it. And there are, of course, Imaginative men who find women of limited interest. Their curiosity takes a direction other than sex. All Imaginative men, however, need to have their interest engaged, to be fascinated, or to be involved in something that keeps their minds ticking over.

'Walter' was the pseudonym of a Victorian Englishman who wrote an erotic autobiography, *My Secret Life*, and had it privately printed in 1882 in a limited edition, when he was probably in his sixties. Sex interested him above everything else. Written from copious notes he had kept since his early twenties, his work details all his sexual experiences from boyhood upwards, with over 2000 women of all nationalities, 'except a Laplander'. Most of these were prostitutes, but a good number were servants or 'respectable' women of his acquaintance or whom he met on his travels. Many such books rely heavily on fantasy, but Walter's has the ring of authenticity. He liked women of all kinds – from young virgins to the much more mature – and of all shapes and sizes, good-looking and ugly. Unlike Casanova, he genuinely enjoyed the company of women. When a woman captured his imagination he saw her often, sometimes for years. Happiness, for Walter, however was new sexual experiences. A couple of times he felt himself to be genuinely in love, but: 'Such was my weakness and fondness for the [female] sex, that I never could keep faithfully to any one woman absolutely, however much I loved her. I have wished and intended to do so, have tried hard to avoid infidelity, but surrendered at last to the temptation. The idea of seeing another woman naked ... seemed to foreshadow to me voluptuous pleasures never tasted before with any other woman.' In his introduction to the Grove Press edition of *My*

Secret Life, G Leghorn wrote: 'His inability to maintain any deep emotional relationship with the women he makes love to ... [means] he is searching for something in his sexual life with many women which he is fated never to find, because what he is searching for – what he is dissatisfied with – is in himself.' This is debatable. Walter seemed not so much dissatisfied as enjoying the search itself. In common with other Imaginative men he *needed* new experiences: he was impelled to investigate the unknown. Indeed his Imaginative nature is most clearly shown not by the fact that he couldn't be faithful to the women he loved, but that he couldn't conceive of emotions being naturally attached to the sex act. He was a man who seemed genuinely to like women, and treated them, on the whole, kindly – but on the occasions when he had forced a virgin or an unwilling servant girl, and she had been frightened or upset, he couldn't believe that it really mattered to her that much. Sex was natural and fun. It didn't touch his deeper feelings so he couldn't comprehend that it did for anyone else.

Walter was fascinated by different bodies, and couldn't get his fill of them. He had a strong dose of Sensuality in his nature, and actively enjoyed the physical side of sex more than the purer Imaginative. His sexual personality was dominated by Imaginative concerns, however. 'I had from my youth an excellent memory, but about sexual matters, a wonderful one. I recollect even now ... the face, colour, stature, thighs, backside, and vagina of well nigh every woman I ever had.' He also enjoyed watching other couples make love and, later in his sexual career, had threesomes with other men and women. As Leghorn says: 'His principal form of sexual experimentation or search for novelty is not in sex technique – as it must be with monogamists – but, as with all Don Juans, in *varietism*.'

In this day and age there are very few men with the time and means to devote themselves to sexual exploration as Walter did. When sex is important to Mr Imaginative it is more likely to be a hobby than a full-time pursuit. And then it is very much a sideline. At his most basic, Mr Imaginative invests little of his emotional self in his sexual dealings. Making love to a new woman can be erotic and intriguing, but it doesn't necessarily have any more profound significance for him. This can continue to be so after he marries, or seems to have settled down in a stable relationship. He won't see it as important if he takes the opportunity to bed another woman and it won't affect what he feels for the woman he loves.

Some Imaginative men are much less promiscuous, and are less interested in sex altogether. This can be because sex seems a repetitious activity, and the possible permutations of women or positions are not extensive enough to fascinate him. Sex is less exciting for this kind of man than an absorbing book or a passionate exchange of ideas. In this case he won't find it too hard to limit his sexual attentions to the main woman in his life, and then only when his libido demands it. When it doesn't, he's content to swear off sex for long periods. If women themselves hold little interest for him this is even more likely. So it was for the eponymous hero in Kingsley Amis's novel *Jake's Thing*. Coming up for 60 he discovers he has lost his sex drive, which is disturbing for him – and for his wife. In the past he had been to bed with more than 100 women, and had had a number of affairs. Examination shows that there is nothing physically wrong with him, so he and his wife embark on sex therapy. When sensate focusing is suggested, he dutifully does what he's told – caressing his wife, and submitting to her attentions in return. This sensual experience leaves him quite unmoved. Like most Imaginatives, if his interest is not stimulated neither are his sexual feelings. When Jake is touching his wife his mind wanders onto irrelevant matters. 'In itself each motion he made was unequivocally if only by a little on the pleasant side of the pleasant/unpleasant borderline,' he realises. And when it is his turn to lie back and be stroked by her it is little better: 'Twenty minutes of an experience I wasn't looking forward to and which has turned out to justify such ... mild forebodings.' At the end of the novel the doctor tells Jake that perhaps there *is* a physical cause – a chemical imbalance – and hormone supplements might be the answer to restoring his libido. He mentally runs through all the women he has ever known, with their irritating female natures and habits. The last words in the book are Jake's to the doctor: '"No thanks," he said.'

For another kind of Imaginative man the intellectual connection he has with the woman he loves is what activates his erotic nature. He finds himself sexually unmoved by women when there is no mental rapport. When they can talk or argue passionately, when she delights and surprises him with the way she thinks, his emotional and sexual nature becomes engaged. The way to reach this Imaginative man is through his brain.

This, in fact, is the key to all Imaginative men. They live most vividly inside their heads. Feeling is subordinate to thought, and needs to be connected to it to be understandable. Indeed they are uncomfortable with emotions that they can't analyse. When he 'thinks' he should be happy, he can be disturbed by not being able to understand why he isn't. In extreme cases Mr Imaginative can be switched off from his feeling nature altogether, only knowing if something is wrong when he becomes ill, or can't work. Jake's impotence depressed and perplexed him until he was able to justify it to himself by realising that he no longer liked nor was interested in women. When the problem was solved he no longer felt bad. What it amounts to is that Mr Imaginative doesn't trust feelings so much as logic or inspiration. On the other hand, it is fairly easy for others to change his mood by making him laugh, diverting his attention or planting an intriguing idea. His brain racing is the most uplifting feeling he knows.

Identifying Mr Imaginative

You can often hear Mr Imaginative before you see him. He likes to talk — and to listen too, so long as what is being said captures his attention or his imagination. A good argument invigorates him. Indeed he is quite capable of arguing passionately against his own beliefs if the mood so takes him. Even when he is talking about something that concerns him most nearly, such as his current obsession or a cause that has caught his attention, he can be quite crestfallen if you merely nod and agree with him. Duelling with words lights him up. In certain circumstances he can be verbally violent, as he attempts to bend you to his way of thinking. He is genuinely surprised when others are hurt or alarmed by this. Some people can become distressed during a war of words, but it is his lifeblood. He usually likes the last word, however, and he can be better than most at having it. His idea of a hellish night is when the only conversation is a perfunctory exchange about the weather or the latest sport results. If there's nothing interesting to say he believes something is seriously wrong.

Some Imaginative men are more reserved in company, but one to one are equally loquacious. For a certain kind of Imaginative man the need to find a soulmate is paramount. 'Soulmate' to him means mental compatibility. He will look for people who reflect and amplify his views on life. He doesn't want to argue, but he does want energetic mental interplay which confirms and validates himself.

Even if Mr Imaginative isn't a great talker his mind will be busy. It's no pleasure for him to let his mind drift into vacancy — some people find this relaxing but he feels restive. He may be a voracious reader. If not he'll want to be doing something that gets his mental wheels turning. When he's not specially interested in intellectual matters he'll be on the look-out for new experiences, or will enjoying plotting and planning what he's going to do next.

The Imaginative Man

If he is intelligent and well-educated, Mr Imaginative often works with words — as a writer, teacher or researcher. The academic finds ideas more powerfully involving than people and other life experiences. The teacher can be excellent at conveying what he knows, or he can just enjoy sounding off — some Imaginative men have butterfly minds that rove indiscriminately over what currently interests them. This type of man often becomes drunk on his own words, admiring his own verbal ability rather than being concerned with what he is getting across to his audience. The more focused Imaginative man has immense powers of concentration — whether he is a mathematician, a chess-player or a lawyer, when in the grip of his current mental obsession he will not be deflected by a beautiful woman stripping off in front of him, hunger, or news that his mother has died. What he is thinking about is always more real to him than a call from his body or his emotions. The clever Imaginative will also be drawn to insoluble problems. He might want to change the world in some way or popularise arcane principles. Unlike the Emotional man, who can seem to be driven by the same motives, in his case it is the complexity of the problem that intrigues him most. Mr Emotional is powered by intense emotional conviction — Mr Imaginative, instead, has an almost lordly need to impress his own ideas on others. The more peaceable Imaginative man will want colleagues with whom he can work in harmony towards a goal. He feels most happy in himself with people who think like him and agree with his aims.

Not all Imaginative men have great brains, however. If this is so, he will look for work that provides variety of experience — as a commercial traveller, for instance, or anything that gets him out and about in a way that is not routine. His interest in others can lead him into work that involves meeting new people. It suits him because once he has learned what makes someone tick he loses interest and wants to move on. When he knows a person's idiosyncrasies he will be bored if he has to see him too often. If he can't find a career that indulges his curiosity, he will need to invest far more energy in his off-duty life. A man with a run-of-the-mill job, or no work, is much more likely to turn his attention to women or to an extra-curricular life that offers novelty and variety. He will want to be doing something different most evenings. If he enjoys standing at a bar with a drink in his hand it will be somewhere that he knows has a changing clientele which will provide him with new people to spark off mentally. Like Mr Romantic, gambling appeals to him. But while Mr Romantic dreams grandly about what he'll do when he becomes a millionaire, Mr Imaginative is exhilarated by pitting himself against others. He'll prefer poker to the turn of the roulette wheel: he trusts himself more than Lady Luck. Losing is almost as compelling as winning: not knowing what the next half hour will bring shakes him out of a boring rut. Similarly he likes to travel. Seeing new places and experiencing different cultures is brain food for him. He won't want to go to the same old holiday cottage abroad, he's more interested in somewhere he hasn't been before — in his fantasies *no one* has ever been there before.

Imaginative men always want to be trying new things. They are the first to see the latest play, read the current book, or try out a newly-opened bar before the workmen have finished packing away the scaffolding. Mr Romantic is sometimes like this because he's concerned to be fashionable — for Mr Imaginative it's the newness itself that appeals. He'll derive less pleasure from seeing a movie everyone else has raved about, even if it's brilliant, than from being one of the first to see the new art-house offering that turns out to be terrible. Variety is important. He'd rather have a badly cooked meal in a place he's never visited before than return time and again to the reliable restaurant on the corner. He'll want to try different activities as well. Action follows thought, often at the expense of his capacities. No one is more likely to push his body beyond its limits, with the exception of Mr Romantic.

The Imaginative Man

Both of these men can be oblivious to signals of tiredness, incipient illness, or muscle strain when they are driven to do what they want. If there's a new sporting craze among 12-year-olds, Mr Imaginative won't rest until he's tried it. He might not go on to master it if it takes too much dedication, but at least he knows what it's like. In this way he can seem as childlike at times as Mr Romantic occasionally does. In the Romantic man's case, however, he has an optimistic view that life will be better round the next corner. Mr Imaginative, in contrast, retains a youthful enthusiasm for anything untried and unusual.

The older or more sedentary Imaginative man won't go in for roller-blading, but he will have an eye for a new gadget. Brochures of strange little objects that help you do something you never even knew you wanted to do are his weakness. He's likely to change his corkscrew regularly as new improved versions arrive on the market. The more intellectual Imaginative will be similarly fascinated by new ideas, even if they are confined to his narrow area of specialisation. This mental flexibility can make him an innovator. When it is linked, as it can be, to original, inspired thought, he may be years ahead of his time, sometimes dismissed as a crank – only to have his ideas resurrected after his death.

He is not intrinsically interested in what he wears, drives or eats. The Imaginative man who finds these matters dull will be quite unconcerned about them, and equally dismissive of what other people think. If they do intrigue him, however, he will be at the cutting edge of fashion. If clothes have an appeal, he will want to shock or intrigue others with what he wears. He might even be a dress designer, who ignores bodily shapes in favour of introducing novel ideas and concepts. Similarly if transport captures his attention he is unlikely to become attached to a vehicle that suits him well, but will be looking to change it often, or become an expert in adapting his current model to make it different from anything else. Like Ms Imaginative, what interests him about food is unexplored sensations — he's the man who will try the sheep's testicles because he wants to know what they taste like. If he's moved to become a chef he'll want to put flavours together that have never been tried before — like the futurist poet Marinetti, who astounded Italy in the Thirties with his weird food combinations designed to assault the palate, such as salami cooked in black coffee flavoured with eau-de-Cologne. Otherwise the Imaginative man's interest in food can be remote. Indeed, if it doesn't capture his imagination he'll often need to do other things while he's eating. If he's not having an involving conversation he'll want to be reading, watching television, or making notes for a forthcoming project. When his attention is riveted by something else he can literally forget to eat.

Some Imaginative men live in an ivory tower, quite happy with their own company and thoughts. Most, however, enjoy the demands of a social life. They like to have people to talk to. Indeed, they often collect people — not, like Mr Romantic, people who are famous or admirable — but anyone interesting. This can include the bum who lives in the shop doorway if he is not a repetitive bore. Parties appeal because there are more people to talk to, and some of them might have something different to say. In the extreme he likes to be with people simply because it gives him a chance to talk. He likes the sound of his own voice. He often has a need to put his thoughts into words to confirm them as real. This is most helpful for him when it comes to analysing his feelings. He needs to label and identify them before he can accept them. This is what his old and trusted friends are good for — especially women, who like these sorts of conversations. On the whole, though, he has less need for the security of long-standing friendships than do other men. He won't automatically seek your company because he's fond of you. He'd prefer, on the whole, to be stimulated by new acquaintances. When mental powers are important to him he will be something of an intellectual snob. Then he'll find it hard to value or like someone whom he sees as an intellectual inferior.

The unattached Imaginative man

When the Imaginative boy's sexual feelings first awaken, his curiosity about sexual matters will be kindled. Sometimes this happens long before. Most little children like to explore each other's bodies, but he might be more dedicated than most. Seeing one little girl's bottom doesn't stop him wanting to see another. He'll listen with eager fascination to grown-ups talk – particularly when they don't want him to. He'll pick up snippets about this adult activity called sex and wonder what it is and what it's like. When he reaches the age that makes it possible for him to find out he'll embark on his investigations with enthusiasm. If his basic nature is low on sensuality he might actually enjoy playing with his computer *more*, but the testosterone pumping round his body will heighten the interest value in the girls of his circle. When he 'gets lucky' he might wonder what all the fuss was about and temporarily lose interest in the other sex until the next hormone surge.

Like many adolescents he will usually play the field. But he's likely to continue to do so more than average in later life, as long as his interest in women and sex hold. Of course he can fall in love – but until he does his emotions will be untouched by the affairs he has. He can be fun to be with, interesting and unusual as a partner. You can find yourself caught up in a whirl of different activities and spend evenings having memorable conversations. But if you are expecting more from him you might be hurt. Just because you're hanging around together, just because you're having sex, doesn't make the relationship *important* as far as he is concerned. A woman who feels differently will perplex him. If she cries, or becomes angry at his treatment of her he will be bewildered or think she is playing mind games. It's hard enough for him to understand his own emotional state – well nigh impossible for him to put himself in the position of someone experiencing feelings that are foreign to him. Similarly, even when he does fall in love he finds it difficult to comprehend his partner's sensitivity to his continuing interest in other women. Because he can separate his sexual nature from his emotions he expects his lover to understand how supremely unimportant such interest is. This could well be the reason behind the actor Hugh Grant's seemingly inexplicable dalliance with a prostitute in June 1995. The international press gasped in amazement that the man who lived with Elizabeth Hurley, one of the most beautiful women in the world, should be caught by the police in his car having oral sex performed on him by the prostitute Divine Brown. In fact, many of Grant's quoted comments before this event show him to be an Imaginative. He told one reporter that he and Elizabeth Hurley used to like to book into hotels as brother and sister, and then scandalise the staff by sharing a double bed. This is a typical Imaginative strategy for pepping up a sex life that has become routine. He has also said of sex scenes in films: 'If I do them early on in a film, I find it very sexy. The thing is, I've always found *strangers* sexy, so if an actress is still a stranger, then it's real sexiness.' As an Imaginative, he would find it hard to understand why his woman would mind his dalliance with a prostitute.

An Imaginative man might run through many relationships before he finally settles down, and chase one-night-stands more enthusiastically than other men. While men of the other Sexual Styles may take the opportunity to go to bed casually with a woman they never intend to see again, many of them actively prefer a relationship to have more to it. The Imaginative man finds the thrill of the new conquest and the brevity most satisfying to his nature. It doesn't terribly matter what happens when they are in bed together, the novelty of the experience is enough.

Mr Imaginative has his own way of flirting. He won't flatter a woman so much as dazzle her. Because he values his thought processes above anything, he will display them to attract. If he's clever he'll start a stimulating line of conversation. If not, he'll tell witty anecdotes or try to make a woman laugh. Walter, the Victorian erotic adventurer, often talked dirty to women he wanted to seduce. As thinking about sex aroused him, he assumed it would do the same for all women. Even the most uneducated Imaginative will have a way with words and a good turn of phrase. When he's witty, charming and interesting he can have great success with women even when he is not particularly physically attractive. When he's determined to make a conquest he will use his way with words to tell them exactly what they want to hear. He can't see that it matters if it's not the truth – after all, it's not *important*.

There will always be Imaginative men who, like Walter, find everything to do with women and sex interesting throughout their lives. The financier Bernie Cornfeld, who died in 1994, was like this, and had the means to build his lifestyle around this predilection. He had what amounted to a harem of women, dividing himself between as many as 12 at any one time. Among his conquests were famous beauties, such as the actress Victoria Principal, the model Alana Hamilton (who later married Rod Stewart) and Princess Ira von Furstenburg, as well as the 'Hollywood Madam' Heidi Fleiss. He boasted of once having sex with eight of them in a single day. Typical of the Imaginative, he never became deeply involved with women emotionally. The only one he loved was his daughter, Jessica, who has said that she only had to tell him that she didn't like one of his girlfriends for her to disappear from his life within weeks.

Cornfeld was an outright Imaginative in other ways, fascinated by people generally, not caring who they were so long as they were interesting: 'He never judged a person by his station: [at his parties] actors would sit with mechanics, judges with hustlers, and gardeners with harlots,' said Jessica. She also remarked on his Imaginative love of company and talking: 'If

I had a party, he would turn up with bottles of liqueur and candles. He would sit and enthral my friends with anecdotes.' His financial career was the legitimate face of gambling, with the same cycles of wins and losses – he was a millionaire at times, but died nearly penniless.

More usually, the Imaginative man will discover that his interest in sex is directly related to the strength of his sex drive. In other words, when he feels the need to make love he will find women fascinating, and sometimes any woman will do. When he doesn't, he'll hardly give them a thought.

The Imaginative whose sex drive is not strong and whose mind is most taken up with other interests is far less likely to waste time chasing new conquests. In some cases he will have very few relationships before he settles down, and could even be a virgin when he marries. On the whole, though, he won't like feeling that there is an experience he has missed out on, so these days this is less common.

Some Imaginative men think women have less interesting minds than men. Or they find the way women's minds work irritating or confusing. Because the quality of mental interaction is so important to these men they will have less respect for women generally. These Imaginatives will be most casual in their encounters, preferring not to have to spend too much time in women's company. They can leave women feeling distressed – not valued for themselves, and hardly valued for the sexual experience they share. The man of this kind with a lower sex drive may have little to do with women at all until he decides it's time to marry, if he ever does.

In contrast, the Imaginative man who is looking for a mental soulmate will be far less casual in his dealings with women. He will often prefer to get to know a woman well before he takes her to bed. As their mental intimacy increases, so does his desire. When he finds a woman like this he wants to keep hold of her, and other women have far less power to attract him. When this Mr Imaginative is in love with you he'll look beyond your outer form to the beauty within – you feel loved for yourself. Indeed when he falls in love with your mind you will be beautiful in his eyes.

However, in common with other men, some Imaginative men split off their sexuality from what is profoundly important to them. In some cases he will believe that their mental connection is tainted by his baser sexual needs. In these circumstances he may have purely sexual encounters on the side, while cherishing the unique compatibility with the woman he loves.

Sex and Mr Imaginative

When Mr Imaginative is interested in sex and his sex drive is high, he'll want to sleep with as many women as possible. As one Imaginative quoted in *Elle* magazine said: 'It's all about collecting the set, wanting to experiment. It's men with no imagination who only go for one body type.' This young man insists that most men think the same way 'if they are honest' – he sees life through the lens of his own Sexual Style so he can't conceive of another man feeling differently. Other men can be much more specific about the physical type they most desire – particularly Romantic men. Mr Sensual might have no particular preference as far as women's bodies go, but when he finds someone with whom he is physically compatible he will be less inclined to 'collect the set'.

When the Imaginative man's interest is caught by a particular woman, however, or he is in love, he might temporarily lose interest in other woman. But when the erotic fascination starts to wear off he'll become bored unless they vary their sexual routine and begin to experiment with new ways of making love. This is the man who will avidly embrace sex books filled with different positions and techniques from around the world and will try as many as he can. Mr Imaginative's most erogenous zone is his brain. Looking at complicated positions, and thinking about trying them is as sexually arousing for him as naked body-to-body touching is for Mr Sensual. Even when the imagined position turns out to be more uncomfortable than pleasant he will enjoy the experience. The physical enjoyment of sex is usually secondary to the erotic build-up. Indeed, although gratifying his lust and having an orgasm is satisfying, it is rarely enough in itself to make the experience worth repeating. It is a feature of human sexuality to be aroused by thinking about sex, but for Mr Imaginative it is almost the most exciting aspect. Good sex, for him, is not so much about sensations as it is about erotic expectancy. The most explosive orgasms do not come through effectively targeted touching but through the thrill of his erotic imaginings. When he is more conservative, or less knowledgeable about the possible sexual variations, he will need to spice things up for himself by fantasies − perhaps to do with other women.

Fantasy always plays a big part in his sex life. He'll rarely go from cold to excited arousal without some mental preparation. If the woman he has been with for years undoes his zipper without warning, he is unlikely to be turned on − whereas Mr Sensual would be, and certain types of Emotional men would be too. If a new woman does so, or a stranger, it would be different. The erotic shock would then be exciting. Mr Romantic or Mr Emotional in similar circumstances might be aroused but put off. Indeed, if Mr Imaginative is not a specially adventurous lover he can only find the novelty he craves with new women or in illicit or dangerous circumstances. It is easier for him to satisfy his need for variety with someone else than it is for him to continue to find new things to do in a long-lasting relationship. Sex that becomes routine, even if it is pleasurable on a physical level, eventually saps his sex drive. He can't begin to feel desirous when he knows exactly what is going to happen. When the actuality of sex does little for him he may get most intense enjoyment from erotic conversations, and even find talking sex over the telephone with a woman he never sees most exciting. Because the mechanics of sex can seem boring to a minority of Imaginatives, giving himself quick, masturbatory relief is more desirable for this type than having to spend time attending to the needs of a woman. At its most extreme his interest in sex can be purely intellectual: he might collect pornography or even become a researcher into sexual matters, rarely needing to put his considerable knowledge into practice.

More usually, Mr Imaginative will see sex as good, clean (or dirty) fun. It doesn't necessarily touch his heart and, if his sensual nature is not especially pronounced, neither are the sensations overwhelming in themselves. What's left is a sportive 'let's see what we can do that's interesting'. He'll be amused by multi-coloured or speciality condoms, dressing-up games, sex aids, or designer drugs to intensify orgasm. Meaningless sweet-talking will do little for him; building an elaborate fantasy together is much more in his line. He can also enjoy talking during sex – exciting himself by using obscene language, or commenting on what he is doing. He might well like his woman to tell him in detail about other lovers she has had and what they got up to. He is the least likely of the Sexual Styles to suffer from retrospective jealousy. The exception to this, of course, is the Imaginative man who feels that he is above things sexual. Then he might find it coarse and disquieting to know that the woman he is involved with attaches more importance to it.

Whereas many Imaginative women find one-night-stands ultimately unsatisfying, they remain very exciting for Imaginative men. Both male and female Imaginatives find the idea of them erotic, and neither feels emotionally troubled by having a purely physical encounter. But there is a physiological difference. A man can almost always climax however brief or unexciting the sex, whereas a woman's needs are more complex. The Imaginative woman often tires of quick casual sex once she has satisfied her curiosity about it, but the Imaginative man will usually continue to find it compelling. At their most basic his encounters are more like masturbating on a body. Young men who worked in bars on the Greek island of Kos were interviewed by *Marie Claire* magazine. Their job is to entice women into bars. Most of them also use the opportunity to have sex with as many as they can. One said: 'I don't bother to make love to them properly. It's more "Thank you very much. Bye".' Another said: 'You don't know how long you'll live, so you might as well shag anything that's going: big, small, round — just turn them round, do it doggy-style and think of someone else.'

His need for novelty means that Mr Imaginative will find love-making that is confined to the bedroom ultimately dreary, especially in a longer lasting relationship. He'll want to try other parts of the house — or outside, or at the office, in the cinema, the car, at a party — and other surfaces apart from the mattress. It's not that he is exploring what it feels like so much as enjoying the wonder of a new experience or the idea of being caught out. He's usually game to try anything once and, if he isn't particularly inventive, he will appreciate a woman who has ideas of her own. If he is drawn to investigate the outer reaches of sex, such as little-known perversions or orgiastic sessions with multiple partners, it is his interest that is titillated rather than a compelling emotional or physical need. In the end he might find these things disgusting or unpleasurable, but he will be delighted to have had the experience. Often he will enjoy thinking about them before and afterwards more than doing them at the time, and will add them to the repertoire of mental images he uses to arouse his desire. For one reason or another, some Imaginative men will never try the more bizarre sexual practices, but will still be turned on by the idea of them. He often enjoys pornography for this very reason — it offers him the images without him having to go to the trouble of sampling the reality.

All this describes Imaginative men who are interested in sex, and for many it is descriptive of a stage in their lives when sexual needs are urgent. When their sex drives wane they become more interested in other aspects of life. Some Imaginative men reach a point where they consider their investigations complete, and are no longer so fascinated by sexual concerns. They've done it all, enjoy their recollections more than anything, and perhaps remain unmoved by the prospect of sampling further sexual pleasures.

The Imaginative man who is most captivated by a woman's mind will be somewhat different. He may well enjoy sex with her, but what counts for more is the mental interaction between them. Indeed, he is turned on most by the kinds of conversations they have, and the feeling of mental intimacy. She doesn't necessarily have to be his intellectual equal, however. He can be drawn to a woman to whom he acts as a teacher — passing on his knowledge and ideas to an eager, receptive partner. Or perhaps she is the stimulating thinker, who opens up his mental horizons by what she has to say to him. In his case, sex follows most naturally from a period of intense talking and sharing of ideas. His heart opens, and so does the channel to his sexuality. He enjoys sex most profoundly with a woman who engages his brain and his interest. Sex, for this kind of Imaginative, becomes most meaningful when it is connected to an inspiring mental sympathy. If he is low on sensuality, however, what they do sexually will matter less than the way she has made him feel in their mental relationship. Indeed if sex itself matters little to him, then even if their sex life is not very frequent or satisfying he will not feel the same need to seek variety or new partners as a more sexually interested Imaginative will.

The Imaginative man who is most concerned with the world of ideas is likely to have the least curiosity about sex. Even when he has a high sex drive he won't be bothered to divert too much of his thinking time towards sexual matters. In his case sex will be something to be got over as quickly and efficiently as possible when the need arises, and he will be relatively content to confine his sexual demands to one woman. If he doesn't have a partner he will take his opportunity where and when he can, and will be irritated by a woman who thinks it should mean something. Sexual needs can seem an annoyance to him: they simply need attending to so as to free his attention for more important matters. When an Imaginative of this type has a lowish sex drive sexual considerations will hardly trouble him at all.

The Imaginative man and marriage

Whereas the Imaginative woman often finds marriage difficult because she usually needs a lot from her husband in terms of mental stimulation and perhaps sexual variety, the Imaginative man is often more content. When the main focus of his intellectual life is his work or other considerations he can even bear boredom at home – and while sex is important to him he is perfectly happy to find it elsewhere, so long as his wife continues to look after him in other ways. The writer H G Wells is an example of this. He married his second wife, Jane, in 1894, and after their second son was born in 1903 their sex life ceased. It was agreed that he could look elsewhere for sex, which he did – and he told Jane about it. Sex was important to him, as biographer Gordon N Ray commented, as a way of 'assuaging the physical itch that would otherwise distract him from his writing'. Wells saw Jane, he said, as 'the wise, calm, and practical good woman of the Proverbs' and, as Ray added, 'a symbol of purity to be revered and cherished, if usually at a distance'. His most important and enduring affair was with Rebecca West, also a writer, with an intellect to match his. It started in 1913 when she was 20 and he was 46, and lasted ten years chiefly because, as an Imaginative, he fell in love with her mind: 'I loved your clear open hard hitting generous mind first of all and I still love it most of all because it is most of you.' Despite this, he wouldn't leave his wife, who attended to all secretarial and practical matters. When his relationship with Rebecca ended, Wells was concerned about keeping his sexual needs satisfied, and concluded he should look for a 'body slave'. A later mistress showed understanding of his Imaginative nature when she wrote to Rebecca: 'It's only a pose of his that he needs people, he only needs them to elaborate his ideas and spread them and, so long as he can work, he'd master every kind of shock, however sorrowful.'

Mr Imaginative who is less interested in sex will bury himself in his work or anything else that fascinates him if his marriage is monotonous, rather than having affairs.

The Imaginative man who is looking for a soulmate will demand more from his wife. He will be most happy in a relationship that continues to be mentally stimulating, in which he and his wife have lively conversations and mutual interests. The wife who wants to hold him should pay more attention to what she offers his mind than what she does his body in terms of food, sex and general homely comforts.

For any kind of Imaginative man, emotional intimacy is likely to be the problem area in marriage. He's not very good at getting in touch with his feelings, particularly when he can't explain or justify them. If he experiences jealousy, for instance, but there is no apparent cause, he will not know why he is disturbed or angry but feel impelled to make his wife suffer for it. Anger in general can be perplexing. He fastens on the obvious cause – she didn't listen when he was explaining something to her – unaware that the anger is connected to deeper, more painful reasons, such as early rejection from his mother perhaps. Unless he has an interest in psychology, indeed, most attempts to explore the source of strong emotions will seem like mumbo-jumbo to him. He can talk so lucidly about his thoughts that he is often unaware that he hasn't begun to understand his feelings. It is therefore difficult for him to sympathise with a woman who has more ready access to her emotions. He can often be exasperated by the 'illogicality' of it all. A patient wife, with a better grasp of these matters, can help by enabling him to find words to attach to what he feels, and guide him into talking about events in the past. In some cases hearing himself explain his own experiences will lead him to make the imaginative leap to his present circumstances and emotions, and thereby increase his understanding of his emotional world.

When Mr Imaginative will stray

It has already been seen that Mr Imaginative doesn't attach much importance to fidelity. While his interest in sex is high he won't think it does any harm to have the odd fling, and if he isn't getting the sex he needs at home he will not be troubled by guilt. Because of this his partner might be quite oblivious to what he has been up to. However, if he believes that as it means nothing to him it shouldn't matter to his wife, he might make no attempts to cover his tracks. He can get himself into hot water by casually seducing the next-door neighbour, assuming it's casual for her as well — and then be bewildered when pain or unpleasantness results. He's the man most likely to think wife-swapping is a good idea. While other men might want to go to bed with the woman next door, they don't like the idea of their wife doing the same with the man next door.

When sex is very important to Mr Imaginative he might have more long-term affairs, as H G Wells did, without it changing his feelings for his wife one bit. Sex with someone else will rarely lure him away from his marriage. The woman who is able to accept this can be fairly sure that she will not lose him. It sometimes helps the tolerance of a woman with a man like this to realise that the other woman is not 'better' but merely 'different'. This can be hard if she is going through a period of self-doubt, or is worried about failing attractiveness and ageing.

The exception is the Imaginative man who seeks a soulmate. Should his relationship with his partner become disappointing in this respect he will be profoundly dissatisfied. In this case he is more likely to leave her for another woman who promises intellectual satisfaction than is the Imaginative who is less concerned about the quality of his relationships.

The Imaginative who is uninterested in sex, or becomes so over the years, is far less likely to bother looking for it outside his marriage. He will wonder at other men who waste so much valuable time doing so and will be unable to see the point.

Mr Imaginative and sexual problems

The root of any sexual problem the Imaginative man has is usually boredom – either with sex itself, or with the dullness that results from routine. When he likes sex, long-term commitment can be a turn-off: 'Is this what I'm going to be doing for the rest of my life?' he wonders. Trying new ways of making love is the most effective antidote, and he usually welcomes a partner who finds opportunities to keep his interest focused on her. It could be as simple as calling him at the office and saying she is thinking about sex – starting his mental wheels turning sexually in her direction. Or it might mean that she is the one to come up with new ideas. It works for some couples in this situation to play elaborate games: they pretend they don't know each other in a bar – and she picks him up, or vice versa. Or they role play in the privacy of their own home, developing scenarios that involve a lot of titillating talking and to-ing and fro-ing before they end up in bed. Even this can pall eventually – and they might cast their net wider, bringing in other couples or individuals. This has dangers of its own and can ultimately destabilise the relationship if his wife finds sex more emotionally involving than he does. While his interest in sex and his sex drive remains high this can be a particularly difficult problem to solve, and even an inherently good relationship can suffer. Therapy that helps them add acceptable variety is often most useful. Sometimes concentrating on developing a rich fantasy life together can help bridge the gap and keep interest alive.

A different sort of problem arises when his need for variety and new experiences doesn't match hers. Constant experimentation is somewhat unintimate, and a woman who needs a more reliable sexual routine to be happy can be put off by it. She can be upset by the fact that his interest is in sex, and not in her or her body specifically. When his sensual nature is undeveloped, he can be irritated if he is expected to satisfy her particular sexual requirements. Again, more fantasy can help dovetail his needs with hers: he gets the necessary mental excitement and in return gives her what she wants. Even so, both might feel short-changed by this compromise.

The man who has never been much interested in sex, or has lost interest once he has experimented to his satisfaction, poses another problem. He is rarely inclined to make efforts to revive his sex life, and can live quite comfortably without sex. If his partner is less happy with the situation they can clash about this, but he will find it hard to understand why she is disturbed. In these circumstances he is less likely than the Imaginative woman to agree to any form of counselling or therapy. While Ms Imaginative will try to solve a problem that bothers her partner, her male counterpart can feel that it is not deserving of his attention.

What often works well for the Imaginative man and his partner is to have sex less often than perhaps one or both of them would like, but to make every effort to make it as different and stimulating as possible when they do. The anticipation and planning involved in this can be just what Mr Imaginative needs to hold his interest and increase his desire.

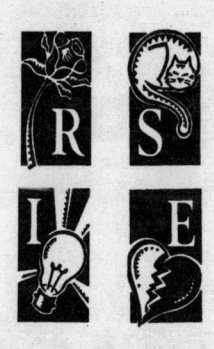

The Imaginative Combinations

The Imaginative Combinations

This section looks at Imaginatives who have a strong subsidiary Sexual Style. It should be read in conjunction with the main Imaginative chapter, and you should also look at the sections on sex and love for the secondary Style, or Styles. Each person will manifest their sexual combination in a unique way but, if you have identified your Sexual Style correctly, the broad themes will apply.

The IMAGINATIVE-Sensual (I-S)

When Imaginatives have a strong dose of Sensual in their natures they have the potential to be the foremost sexual explorers. The Imaginative's restless search for different experiences (whose very novelty gives them meaning), allies to a genuine pleasure in the world of the senses. Sexual journeying offers perpetual excitement, deepened by the Sensual capacity to enjoy the adventures for their physical satisfaction as much as their curiosity value. Both Imaginatives and Sensuals have the capacity to separate their sexual feelings from their deeper emotions so that even difficult or unpleasant situations can be chalked up to experience without causing lasting damage or hurt. These are the people prepared to sample the more arcane sexual practices that other Sexual Styles leave to the realm of fantasy.

The 1960s and '70s were littered with I-Ss, or people pretending to be. More interesting – and certainly completely authentic – are the examples of this Sexual Style that fell outside this period, when typical I-S behaviour was frowned on. One such person was Jane Digby, an aristocrat born in England in 1807. Her emotional and sexual career was extremely chequered. As one summary put it: 'She had married at 17, her first husband, a man 20 years older than herself; eloped with an Austrian prince; married a German baron; had an affair with the King of Bavaria; fallen for a Corfiot count, then an Albanian brigand general; and slept with a good few other men of different nationalities and social standing before marrying at almost 50, the Bedouin chieftain 20 years her junior. Various children were strewn along the way, abandoned as she trod the wilder shores of love.' That she enjoyed sex in a sensual way is clear; she wrote in her diary on her 62nd birthday, 'Sixty-two years of age and an impetuous romantic girl of 17 cannot exceed me in ardent and passionate feelings.' But the roving Imaginative in her always dominated, needing to sample new experiences and new men – especially of different nationalities.

Jane Digby was also interested in the sex lives of others. She told Richard Burton, the explorer, the sexual secrets of Arab harems, having learnt to read and write Arabic. The Imaginative quest for the new often results in people who develop their intellect through education. Burton thought she was, 'out and out the cleverest woman ... She spoke nine languages perfectly, and could read and write in them. She painted, sculpted, was musical and her letters were splendid.'

Certainly few I-S women would be so cavalier about their children. The Sensual in their natures, for one thing, tends to ground them more firmly and gives a preference for some stability in family life and its pleasures. Yet the I-S combination definitely endows an emotional robustness. Happier in the worlds of ideas and physical sensation than they are with emotions, this Sexual Style also has scant talent for understanding people around them who feel more deeply and suffer for longer.

Whether I-Ss act on all their impulses, or merely wish they could, many would consider the archetypal I-S, Jean-Paul Sartre, to have had the best of both worlds. This French left-wing activist and one of the greatest philosophers of his age, managed to have a life-long attachment (Sensual), while having all the new experiences, sexual and otherwise that he could want with intelligent partners (Imaginative).

Sartre met Simone de Beauvoir in 1929 at the Sorbonne, when he was 24 and she was 21. They remained lovers and friends for the next 50 years. Early on they had decided that they wanted to become a role-model for modern couples: they wouldn't marry, and neither would they even attempt to remain faithful to each other. What was much more important was to tell each other everything, to be 'transparent' — which, for the Imaginative, represents the height of intimacy. This included telling each other about their sexual adventures — and both of them had many other affairs, long and short.

Sartre was both fascinated and alarmed by his sexual appetite. 'I've never known how to conduct either my sexual or emotional life,' he wrote to de Beauvoir. 'I feel deeply and sincerely that I'm a bastard. And a small-scale bastard, a kind of university sadist and a sick-making civil service Don Juan.' Their union lasted so much longer than that of many Imaginatives because they continued to interest each other intellectually. Sartre's Sensual side was also gratified by de Beauvoir, although he continued to have the Imaginative need for other women. 'My dear love, you've given me ten years of happiness,' he once wrote to her. 'You are the most perfect, the most intelligent, the best and the most passionate.'

The most obvious exceptions amongst the free-loving I-Ss, are those for whom their Imaginative nature is expressed more strongly in a pressing need to find an intellectual soulmate. In this case the desire for novelty and interest is focused on the more enduring pleasure of finding it in one electric and fascinating personality. Then the Sensual side of them gives the will and ability to make this a lasting union. Sex with such a person is a pleasure to them, and their gratification is increased and stimulated by their satisfying mental interaction. Sometimes they come to this realisation about themselves later in life: they do their sexual adventuring first so that their curiosity is satisfied, and then are able to confine their passions to one particular person.

More usually, however, this Imaginative is closely focused on sex and its pleasures, and will find it easy to shop around for exciting partners without concern for those left behind. Sex must be physically rewarding, but if a partner becomes a bore, or sex becomes predictable – even if pleasurable – this I-S will find it hard to tolerate.

As Imaginatives first, however, it is ultimately most important to them that their lives – and their partners – should be generally interesting. They can be content for long stretches with a partner who shares their interests, with whom they can have continuing stimulating conversations and a lively and varied life. It is a feature of the Imaginative nature that they can ultimately lose interest in sex once they've done all they wish to do. This is less likely when there is a strong Sensual streak, but they are still prepared to put up with less fulfilling or frequent sex if their interest is engaged. If sex continues to excite their curiosity they might be unfaithful if sex at home is disappointing, but it won't affect their loyalty to a partner to whom they can talk about everything. The lines in W H Auden's poem perhaps sum up their need for loving closeness and variety: 'Lay your sleeping head, my love,/Human on my faithless arm.' Often it is concern not to hurt their loved ones, rather than lack of desire or opportunity, that stops them seeking new partners.

The best chance of long-term happiness for I-Ss is with partners who think as they do, with whom they can build a stable, comfortable home and enjoy a mutually satisfying sex life.

The IMAGINATIVE-Romantic (I-R)

This Sexual Style glories in the heightened emotions of new love. Combined with the usual Imaginative's need for stimulation and variety, this can make for a person with little natural staying power in relationships. One thing is sure, however, a relationship with this person, however short, is guaranteed to be thrilling. This is the live-wire – the person with immense capacity for enjoyment and an endless hunger for new ways to have fun. For the I-R, life is a giant *smorgasbord*, which seems annoyingly short – there's certainly no time to waste doing the same old things, or staying with someone who has become predictable.

For the I-R, the normal Imaginative tendency to be greatly interested in sex and its variations is given a Romantic twist that means he or she derives greatest satisfaction when in an unreal state of besotted admiration. This gives the I-R formidable powers of seduction. The Imaginative way with words has a compelling urgency when the Romantic in the I-R believes this is love. What they say is genuinely meant, as well – despite the fact that they might not mean it any more in a few weeks' time. The problem is that this combination has a rather refined sensibility, a fastidiousness that can make the reality of a relationship, including sex, seem not just dull but also somewhat distasteful. For the I-R there is no greater thrill than the thrill of the chase. The intoxicating love (Romantic) often turns out to be all in their heads (Imaginative), and there is little in their natures to make them want to stay around when this has been proved to be so. This combination can also make them the greatest 'teases' — male or female. Erotic flirtations that go nowhere can be immensely titillating and satisfying to them.

On the other hand, because physical sex itself is less important to them, and because they are able to rationalise or totally reject the more disturbing deeper emotions, some I-Rs can exhibit enduring loyalty in ways that flabbergast onlookers. When they find a partner who continues to embody what they need in terms of fascination and glamour they can tolerate flagrant infidelity and bad behaviour.

One such person is Jane Clark, the wife of the British Tory ex-minister Alan Clark. Miles of column inches were devoted to their apparently strange relationship when his diaries were published. In amongst the political gossip were details of all his affairs, and at the time of publication three ex-mistresses popped up to complain about their inclusion. The interest value was heightened by the fact that these three were a mother and her two daughters. Columnists speculating on why Jane Clark had put up with this for decades of married life tended to conclude that she was either too down-trodden and scared or simply didn't want to give up the home and lifestyle to which she had become accustomed. No one seemed to believe her when she said, loudly and consistently, that it was much more than that. Of course she didn't like him having affairs. She despised the women. But, she insisted, he was the most fascinating person she had ever met. Life with him was constantly interesting and stimulating. She had contemplated leaving him once, and had even done so for a day — but the prospect of life without him was dull and featureless so she had come back. He suited her I-R nature down to the ground. Despite — or perhaps because of — his infidelities, he was still a glamorous, romantic figure to her. Her Imaginative nature had found its soulmate, the perennially intriguing idol, and she was not going to let that go for such unimportant reasons.

More usually, however, the I-R finds it impossible to derive all the interest necessary from one other person. Then the Romantic in him or her craves to find it in someone else. I-Rs can be beguiled into believing that it has indeed been found. The I-R is the marrying kind. Often. When a person seems distinctively Imaginative, yet has been married more than average, there is generally a strong Romantic streak as well.

Timothy Leary, professor of psychology at Harvard from 1959 to 1962, whose famous slogan was 'Tune In, Turn On, Drop Out' is an extreme example of a male I-R. In one interview he gave, aged 74, he said with the pride of an Imaginative, 'My career has been dedicated to chaos ... My own life is extremely unpredictable and disordered.' His view, he said, coincided with Marshal McLuhan's: 'He only knew what he thought when he heard himself say it. To do that, you need people to play mental tennis with.' In common with many other Imaginatives, Leary's life had been dedicated to trying the range of experiences — pushing himself and his brain to the limit. Tellingly, however, he had been married 'five-and-three-quarter' times — once for 15 years to Barbara, 'an extremely elegant woman ... From her I learnt everything I need to know about social graces.'

At 74 Leary seemed a pure Imaginative, with little Romantic concerns left. He was host to streams of visitors of all kinds. He freely admitted to taking cocaine and other drugs, as he always had: 'I try all the new designer drugs that come along.' The chaos of his life was evidently satisfying to him: 'Every rule I make I break.' Most nights he was out clubbing: 'I like to be where new things are happening so I can put my receptors out.' This Imaginative receptiveness to new ideas was also giving him a fascination with the Internet: 'I'm infatuated by digital technology because it's brain food.' Nevertheless the Romantic in Leary was internalised. He was more than interested in the working of his own mind, he had romanticised it. At one point he said with some excitement that he was becoming senile: 'For me it's a thrilling adventure. I'm fascinated by the changes in my own brain.' More than that, he wanted other people to share his passion: 'I'd like to get some institute to do a thorough evaluation of my mind.'

In the final analysis this Imaginative, like others, can't bear to be bored. Sex can be a passion for a while, but is rarely a life-long concern. Emotional undercurrents, they feel, are best ignored — indeed, they are classified under the heading of 'too dull and amorphous to be worth attention' or, even, 'frightening'. The heady excitement that accompanies Romantic feelings are quite different, and can hold their interest in a relationship for as long as they last. But, as Imaginatives, I-Rs are prepared to continue in a relationship once the romance goes, as long as it involves open and interesting communication.

The IMAGINATIVE-Emotional (I-E)

Less fickle than many Imaginatives, this combination needs their emotions to be touched for their interest to be piqued, and they find it harder to be casual about sex. In many cases, indeed, I-Es find sex an irrelevance. When their sex drive is high it lends an added interest to sex, but gives it little power in their lives. When their sex drive diminishes they don't feel the loss of a sexual life. They can feel very passionately about a relationship that has little or no sex in it — sometimes, indeed, sexual feelings that have no outlet contribute to an intensifying of the emotional quality in the relationship. Often the Imaginative predominates when they are younger, and they have a full and varied sex life. But sooner or later they make a relationship with more fundamental emotional connections and they become more able to live on their sexual memories if this partnership is less fulfilling in that respect.

Nevertheless, people who have both Imaginative and Emotional in their natures find the contradictions difficult to live with at times. The Imaginative thrives on newness of experience and uncertainty and rejects what it sees as boredom and routine. The Emotional feels a need for deep commitment and bonding with another, and the concept of boredom is meaningless. Understandably, these different needs can conflict. In the quest to reconcile them, however, I-Es can make relationships that seem highly unusual to other people, *especially* when they appear deeply satisfied with them.

Dora Carrington was an example of how sex can be an irrelevance in the passionate life of an I-E. One of the Bloomsbury group of artists, Carrington preferred to be known by her surname. She was born in 1893, and met Lytton Strachey, the writer, 22 years later. Initially she found him physically repellent, but she soon fell in love with him. This love grew in passion and intensity despite the fact that he was homosexual and did not want a sexual relationship with her — despite, indeed, the fact that although he loved her in his way she was far less important to him than he was to her. 'When you read me your work [I feel] more delighted than at any moment in my life,' she wrote in one of her early letters to him. 'Forgive me if I express what I want to say so vilely. Only I had to write immediately to tell you that I was in love with you.' Most of all she loved and admired his mind, as an Imaginative would: 'Sometimes with Lytton I have amazing conversations. I mean not to do with this world — but about attitudes, and states of mind, and the purpose of living. This is what I care for most in him. In the evenings suddenly one soars without corporeal bodies on these planes of thought. And I forget how dull and stupid I am — and travel on also.'

Carrington had affairs, but even when she enjoyed the sex it meant little to her, and did not touch her emotions — it did not make her 'soar' as exciting conversation did. She even married someone else — Ralph Partridge — as much as anything because Strachey was in love with him, although she, too was fond of him. Her attitude to sex is summed up in something else she wrote: 'Do you know even at the most intimate moments, I never get the feeling of being submerged in it. I find myself outside, watching also myself and my workings as well as [Ralph's] from the detached point of view.'

When Carrington agreed to marry Partridge, at the age of 28, she wrote to Strachey: 'You are the only person who I have ever had an all absorbing passion for. I shall never have another. I couldn't now – I had one of the most self-abasing loves that a person can have. You could throw me into transports of happiness and dash me into deluges of tears and despair, all by a few words.' She shot herself two months after Strachey died of cancer, dying herself in Partridge's arms. She was 39, and she had loved Strachey devotedly for 17 years.

When an Imaginative has a strong Emotional element the wish for a soulmate is heightened – someone who combines the interesting mind necessary for an Imaginative, with the capacity to touch deep emotional chords. Then a great love is born, even if the relationship has difficulties or is uncomfortable and unhappy at times. This kind of Imaginative is not so blithe about being unfaithful, but can rationalise that so long as affairs are with people who don't touch them emotionally then they don't count. They'd prefer, ideally, to have a good sex life with their partners, but their dominant Imaginative nature means that they are programmed to find this somewhat boring over the years, even when they feel deeply.

D H Lawrence is an example of a male I-E. He was famous for writing about sex, particularly in the then shocking *Lady Chatterley's Lover*, but his interest rarely translated into action. His marriage to Frieda was characterised by the stormy passages that often can be found in relationships where one or both have a strong Emotional streak. It had, as Humphrey Carpenter commented in a review of a biography of Frieda, 'passionate mutual loyalty which grew out of, rather than being destroyed by, the conflicts'. Lawrence's Emotional needs were also connected to reproducing his relationship with his mother, and Frieda's attitude to him was aggressively maternal.

Lawrence stole Frieda from her husband, and she ran off with him, leaving behind her three children. He was terribly jealous of her love for these children, and the fact that she missed them badly. One time he tore up her photographs of them and stamped on them. He didn't mind her being unfaithful to him — that gratified his Imaginative passion for hearing about the sex lives of others — but he wasn't prepared to share his 'mother' with any other children. Their own sex life was practically non-existent, but he pumped her for details of her affairs and used these in various guises for his heroines.

Looks, or anything that they consider superficial, are of minimal importance to I-Es. They can, of course, be attracted to good-looking people, but they are quickly turned off if there is little else of substance to them. These Imaginatives set greatest store by having an interesting and varied life, and they want this interest and variety to be reflected in their interactions with their partners. The combination of Imaginative and Emotional also endows great powers of analysing and expressing the complex world of feelings. The worst slight partners can deal I-Es is to shut them out of their thoughts. An I-E who is neglected in this way feels deeply unhappy. Then, even if there is still a strong emotional bond, and their partners move them deeply, life becomes insupportable. This is when the Imaginative in the I-E asserts itself, and he or she will move on.

Combinations of three or four

It is rare to have a genuinely equal balance of Sexual Styles. One will be dominant — in these cases Imaginative — and the remaining two or three are also unlikely to be found in equal measure. In most cases one of them will combine most strongly with the main Imaginative Style (in the ways described above) and the third and possibly fourth will add colour and subtlety, but little more. Most usually, aspects of the weaker Styles will be noticeable in other aspects of your personality — your attitude to clothes, career, loved ones other than partners, and so on. The following descriptions are therefore only broad guidelines to the possible ways the Styles can coexist.

The IMAGINATIVE-Sensual-Romantic (I-S-R)

Good and varied sex in an intoxicating relationship that is intellectually stimulating is what this type requires. The Sensual in this Imaginative's nature accentuates the pleasure and interest in sex, and the Romantic increases the longing for the relationship to have the heady thrills of new love. Although a Sensual streak usually adds stability to any combination, in this case it is much more likely to be expressed as an earthy appreciation of sex, and do little to reduce the Imaginative and Romantic's strong combined urge towards delicious novelty in sexual and emotional adventures.

Sensual and Romantic tend to fight in combination. One wants a mindless wallow in tried-and-tested pleasures, with an unbroken vista of more of the same in prospect. The other needs drama and glamour and, especially, a sense of heightened tension between two people who believe each other to be wonderful. When this conflict is played out in an I-S-R temperament, the Imaginative resolves the clash in its usual way — by taking flight and trying to find the new experience that promises to offer it all.

It's hardly surprising that this can be an attractive combination, if emotionally devastating to others who have allowed themselves to become attached. Someone who has been involved with an I-S-R may retain a wistful sense of loss for many years after the fling is over. Because it usually does end – sooner rather than later.

On the whole these Imaginatives will find that relationships hold their attention when they find their partners deeply interesting, and when this is backed up by good sex and an infatuated sense of being special. When the intoxication passes or the sex grows stale the relationship can still survive if a lively mental rapport remains, but without this it stands little chance.

The IMAGINATIVE-Sensual-Emotional (I-S-E)

A relationship that delivers satisfying sex and a strong feeling bond can hold this Imaginative's attention for a long time. The I-S-E is the Imaginative with the greatest potential for staying put in a relationship, and not feeling hard done by for doing so.

Sensual and Emotional together deepen the feeling nature of the I-S-E, both physically and emotionally. This dilutes the Imaginative's usual need to escape from anything too heavy or predictable. The satisfying sex the Sensual enjoys can often deepen the connection demanded by the Emotional.

Because Imaginative and Emotional needs are so different, I-S-Es can sometimes find their own drives disturbing. With Sensual in the mixture, the urge for physical closeness and security adds weight to the Emotional need to feel connected at a profound level to someone else. That is why finding the right partner is so essential. This combination, indeed, sometimes results in a person dedicated to pushing back the boundaries of conventional sex as far as they can go, and finding a deep and enduring emotional gratification in this. With a partner who wants the same, therefore, a unique bond of complicity and mutual need is formed.

When the right partner can't be found, the Imaginative and Sensual combine to drive I-S-Es on a sexual quest typical of IMAGINATIVE-Sensuals, but the Emotional streak can make them unhappy even while feeling impelled to go on. In effect, they punish themselves with guilty thoughts, or make their conquests suffer for not being what they need.

In common with all Imaginatives, they are most content with partners who remain interesting and challenging, and, in the case of the I-S-E find it easier to commit when sex is good and fundamental emotional needs are met. But good sex, and even an emotional bond will not be enough in themselves to hold the I-S-E if the relationship loses other elements of variety and interest.

The IMAGINATIVE-Romantic-Emotional (I-R-E)

This Imaginative needs to feel deeply about someone within a relationship that has an aura of specialness and excitement. Romantic and Emotional together usually make for a somewhat unpredictable combustibility, as the Emotional's usual deep, slow burn is brought to the surface by the Romantic's more showy flare. As part of the Imaginative's make-up, this can result in people who enter and exit relationships with much more drama and turmoil than is usual for the cooler pure Imaginative.

The Emotional in the I-R-E temperament deepens the attachments that these people make, and the Romantic requires an element of enduring admiration. Being Imaginatives, this admiration is likely to be for the mental qualities or interesting personality of their partners. Their Romantic streak, however, is also likely to call for partners with a greater degree of good-looks or success — possibly both. The Romantic need to have pride in their partners will, in the case of the I-R-E, translate into deeper commitment. Alternatively, profounder emotions will be touched when the Romantic need to be adored is met.

Sex is less important to I-R-Es — or, rather, they will tend to have the Imaginative fascination for sexual matters, but the quality of their sex lives will not be a deciding element when they give their hearts.

Imaginative and Romantic together dilute the Emotional need to bond intimately. The first two combine more easily, and therefore their similarities are strengthened. The result can be a person who flits as often as the IMAGINATIVE-Romantic, but who does so at some personal cost, or who is more careful with the feelings of others when doing so.

At best, the I-R-E can be shiningly loyal to a partner who is an interesting and romantic figure. Being interested is the most important element, however. Some elements can be relinquished — yet the relationship will not be doomed if mental sparks continue to fly.

The IMAGINATIVE-Sensual-Romantic-Emotional (I-S-R-E)

With this uncommon mix, the Imaginative purports to demand a relationship with glamour, good sexual communication and a strong emotional connection. What happens in reality, however, is that the Imaginative's great ability (and even greater yen) to move on to new experiences leads him or her to have a series of relationships in which different needs are met at different times. The more the I-S-R-Es demand, in other words, the more likely they are to operate like pure Imaginatives, moving on in the hope of finding the elusive perfect combination. This is the person who is to be found looking fondly back and describing past relationships in terms of the needs they met: 'I had great sex with that one; I really felt deeply then; that was the most stunning-looking person I ever dated,' and so on.

Actually, like most people who feel that they are an equal combination of all the Sexual Styles, experience in relationships can give them deeper insights into their real needs. More usually the purported I-S-R-Es will find that one or two elements represent more insistent demands, and they can settle for relationships that might seem, on the face of it, a compromise.

But whether they are truly such a combination or not, as Imaginatives first there is one compromise they can never make. They can stand a certain diminution in almost every aspect, but cannot put up with a relationship that becomes predictable and where communication has become perfunctory.

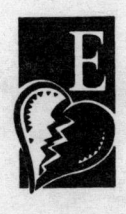

The Emotional Woman

'Anger and jealousy can no more bear to lose sight of their objects than love.'

George Eliot (Mary Ann Evans)

The Emotional Woman

It should be easier to be an Emotional woman than an Emotional man. Women are expected to be emotional: they have a right to cry, to give themselves devotedly to love, to show their suffering openly. The Emotional man might have to maintain a white-faced outward rigidity while seething inwardly with powerful turbulence. Ms Emotional, on the other hand, is free to let the world know what she feels. But it's not that simple. Weeping can be acceptable in a woman, but consuming violent rage might be less so. An uninhibited outpouring of love is expected of her; cold revenge, calculatingly planned, is not. The Emotional woman sometimes places a lid on the volcano of her emotions when she perceives them as unfeminine or too frighteningly powerful.

Ms Emotional can be the softest and most gentle creature in the world, caring even more for someone else's sufferings than she does for own, instinctively connecting direct to other people by locking into and sharing their joys and their sorrows. Or she can be most acutely aware of her own emotional state and less responsive to others, seeming to have no capacity to protect herself healthily from life's experiences. Whereas most people toughen as they mature — not becoming hard, but resilient — this type of Emotional woman retains a child's openness and vulnerability. Every harsh word or bitter ordeal makes a direct hit on her heart and leaves its mark. Alternatively she is so terrified by her natural lack of defences that she tries —

sometimes with great success – to erect an impenetrable shield against other people. There is also the Emotional woman who is much less battered by her emotions. On the contrary, she glories in being swept up in a powerful flood of feeling. When she hates she's implacable, when she loves she's passionate. She doesn't enjoy being hurt, but she is galvanised by it – energised and swept along by the changing currents of her emotions.

Whether she is a sweet and caring nurse or a terrifying Valkyrie, Ms Emotional can be summed up by the words 'her heart rules her head'. All men and women have to grapple with strong emotions on occasions, and can be transported by powerful love. Women of other Sexual Styles have weeks or months when they are ruled by their emotions: when they are in the middle of a crisis of love or pain. But for the rest of the time (most of their lives) their feelings are less noticeable, more governable, less generally relevant. What marks out the Emotional woman as different is that she is always at the mercy of what she is currently feeling. The clamour of her emotions drowns logic, reason and sense. Indeed, emotion *is* logic as far as she is concerned. Where another woman in the grip of jealousy might be aware that it is causing her to behave badly, the jealous Emotional woman is quite convinced that her behaviour is justified and rational. Whether she shows what she's feeling or not, all her actions and decisions are affected by it.

Inevitably, being a woman, she is usually destined to reveal her greatest capacity for intense emotion in her love life. Like her male counterpart she can also be dedicated to a cause or a profession that moves her profoundly, but when she meets the man of her life she can give up everything to focus herself wholeheartedly on him.

Her love for her man can be a source of the greatest joy, but it can equally be a constant supply of grief, turmoil and pain. This is because her emotional requirements are far from simple. What stirs her most deeply, and therefore draws her most irresistibly to her love object, is defined by her formative experiences as a child. You'd think a woman who had been sexually abused, or had to live with a violent alcoholic parent, would do everything in her power to steer clear of men who reminded her of these experiences. Indeed many do: any hint of these characteristics in a man fills them with repulsion, and they fall in love with men who are very different. But not the Emotional woman. The events of early life seem to create a sensitivity and a fascination for the very experiences that harmed her so badly. The man who awakens her passionate nature is the one who touches this mysterious, damaged place in her heart.

There is usually a pervading emotion attached to Ms Emotional's childhood experiences: it could be sadness, fear, rejection, sacrifice, self-doubt, shame, anger, revenge — or the more positive emotions such as compassion and, at best, unconditional love. Whichever it is, there must be something in the man she loves that brings this element out in their relationship. In the uncanny way that Emotional women have of picking up subliminal signals, she recognises the man's nature even if he appears, on the surface, to be completely different. Sometimes, even, she is impelled to behave towards him in such a way as to draw from him the very qualities to which she is secretly attracted, even if she believes she hates them.

An Emotional woman who meets her match in this way feels so intensely about the man that she commits herself totally. Many of these relationships can be rewarding, particularly when her motivating emotion is not self-destructive or violent. But even if it is, she can put up with a lot. Other women find it hard to understand her — they certainly don't classify her feelings as love. They can be appalled when their kind, gentle friend remains locked in a relationship with a brutal man for years. Other Emotional women don't stay the course with these compelling men. After a while they will leave — and sometimes harbour an implacable hatred for the man who caused their suffering. But somehow or other the next man they fall for is fatally similar. It is hard for Ms Emotional to learn from experience, as other women do. Feeling is the most profound experience she knows, and when caught up in the vortex of strong emotion she is quite out of touch with common sense. She must be cool to be logical, and only when the fire goes out of her feelings can she act with reason. Indeed, when her feelings cool towards a man it *is* logical for her to think of leaving him.

Yet she longs to be loved and treated well. This yearning can mean that eventually she does the right thing, and chooses a man who has good, solid qualities. Nevertheless, sometimes she is compromising with her nature. She'll love him in her way, and strive to make it work, but her feeling for him is never so profoundly, gut-wrenchingly affecting as it was for Mr Wrong.

Oprah Winfrey, the brilliantly successful talk show hostess, bears many of the hallmarks of the Emotional woman. She has talked freely about the sexual abuse that marred her childhood and marked her relationships well into adulthood. 'I had such a sorry history of abusive relationships with men. I needed everyone to like me, because I didn't like myself much. So I'd wind up getting involved with these cruel, self-absorbed guys who'd tell me how selfish I was, and I'd say, "Oh, thank you, you're so right." I had no sense that I deserved anything else.' She has talked equally frankly about how awkward she found it when she eventually changed this pattern by forming a relationship with the steady, loving Stedman Graham, who has been described as 'the most reliable person on the face of the planet'. For a long time she found him too nice, too good, too reliable.

Oprah was able to fall for a 'nice' man at last because she uses her Emotional nature in her work — and by so doing has come to understand herself better than the average Emotional woman is able to do. Changes are most likely to follow genuine understanding. Her most successful talk shows are the emotional confessionals, where people cry, spill their guts, and rage – and Oprah is often one of them. The fact that she does this so effectively and has won such huge audiences is because, as an Emotional herself, she is well able to elicit emotions from others: 'I really, really understand people's pain.' The Emotional who has this compassionate understanding is usually also motivated to help others: 'I look on the show as my ministry. I want it to free people from their fears and constraints. I want it to teach them.'

Oprah has another distinguishing Emotional characteristic: her relationship with food. She says: 'I have used food in the past to suppress my feelings, rather than confront them. Even now, it's hard not to.' Before she became secure in her success it was even more obvious: 'It was a perfect way of cushioning myself against the world's disapproval. I thought I was handling the stress just fine. At night I'd sit up alone in my room and order French onion soup by the gallon. "Oh, and could you fry up a cheese sandwich to go with that?" That's how I was "handling" things.'

But the feelings never just go away for Ms Emotional. They have to be rechannelled in less harmful ways. It's not surprising that Oprah replaced a passionate attachment to food with an equally dedicated passion for exercise. She works out twice a day, running up to eight miles at dawn, and it is said that nothing keeps her from this programme – not meetings, interviews, nor illness. She claims to have transformed her unhappiness, but the Emotional never fully shakes off the legacy of the past: 'I'm happier than I've ever been, and healthier. My first thought when I say that is, "OK, when do I get hit by a truck?"'

Oprah is an example of an Emotional woman who wears her heart on her sleeve. Many are far more circumspect, feeling intensely inwardly, but showing little on the surface. A brave smile might be the only sign of a deep reservoir of pain. It takes a more penetrating observer to pick up the clues that reveal her essential nature.

Identifying Ms Emotional

Ms Emotional doesn't immediately stand out in a crowd. Unless she has a strong element of Romantic or Imaginative in her nature she is too taken up with what she is feeling herself – and the feelings she is picking up from the people around her – to be aware of the impression she's making. Other Sexual Styles can be largely oblivious to the emotional state of another person unless their noses are rubbed in it, but for Ms Emotional it is often palpably obvious. She can almost see the cross-currents of emotional interaction between people like beams of light connecting them. She can certainly sense them. When she walks into a room she often instinctively knows if there has been an angry exchange, even if everyone is behaving in a friendly manner now. Sometimes, however, she is more noticeable. That's when she is the open Emotional woman and someone has angered or upset her. Caught on the raw she might react quite violently, although she is more likely to file the insult away to brood about later.

In a smaller gathering, or when you get her on her own, she'll certainly grab your attention. It's not so much what she says or does, it's the quality of attention she fixes on you. She really listens. She might not, actually, be taking in every word of what you say, but she's listening for the sub-text – what you are feeling and what motivates you. Emotions, for her, are what real life is about and if she is to connect to you as a human being she needs to understand what makes you tick. Only a very shy Emotional woman, paralysed by feelings of fear and insecurity, or a very self-obsessed, sorry-for-herself type will not be fascinated by the emotional lives of other people. You might be explaining to her the laws of thermodynamics and she'll suddenly say: 'You're very sad about something, aren't you?' You don't know how she guessed. Even if she doesn't say it, she might well be thinking it, and while she nods gravely at your words, she'll be speculating privately about your secret sorrows.

The Emotional woman who is more self-absorbed, however, will often read non-existent meanings into what you say. *She's* angry, so she thinks you are, or *she's* feeling paranoid, so she believes you're out to get her.

She's much more openly interested in these matters than is the Emotional man. Indeed talking about people's feelings and motivations can be her preferred social pastime. A jokey, chatty evening, or one in which people swap ideas and talk about principles or abstract concepts can seem curiously empty to her, however intellectual or well-educated she is. You haven't touched the core of life as she sees it unless you consider the human dimension. Mind you, it's a different matter when it comes to talking about her own feelings. They're far too raw and powerful – indeed too intimate – for her to want to talk about them. Neither does she find it easy to put them into words, even if she is highly articulate about other matters. As her best friend you can be shocked and surprised when she mentions something that happened ten years ago that upset her profoundly or made her furiously angry. You never realised before. It's not so much that she was being secretive, but it took all this time for her to be able to look at the feelings dispassionately enough to be able to talk about them.

If she does tell you, even only ten years later, you should regard it as an honour. She might have many acquaintances, but she has few real friends, because she needs to feel very trusting. Once she has taken you into her heart it would take a bomb to dislodge you – and she doesn't have to see you often to keep her feelings topped up. She can be downright suspicious of other people – or vacillate between opening her heart to new friends and then casting them off angrily or freezing them out the moment they put a foot wrong. She tends to be a creature of moods anyway – she's helplessly enslaved by them. Whether she acts them out or simmers and suffers in silence, if you are close to her you have to be prepared to take the rough with the smooth. With some Emotional women 'the rough' can be painful. Her own inner torment can sometimes lead her to be cruel — hitting out so that someone else feels as bad as she does. She may, indeed, use against you what you have told her about yourself in happier times, although if she loves you she will be very remorseful afterwards.

This type of behaviour is one of the reasons she finds trusting hard: knowing what she is capable of leads her to suspect that others operate in similar ways. The more secretive Emotional woman can also harbour resentments about things you have said or done to her — sometimes quite innocently — but she doesn't confront you directly because it makes her feel even more vulnerable. On the other hand, her talent for empathy can make you feel more deeply understood by her than by anyone else you know.

Ms Emotional is not readily identifiable by the clothes she wears. In common with all women she is likely to be influenced by fashion and the feminine view that clothes are important, as well as an understandable desire to look her best. Left to her own devices, however, she would not consider dress an important matter. She might unconsciously match clothes to her mood — wearing black when she's sad and primrose when she's feeling joyous. She doesn't care too much about comfort — physical discomfort generally seems a minor matter compared to emotional angst. At the extreme, she's the type who in the past would have worn a hair shirt or pebbles in her shoes if she felt she needed to atone for something. Nowadays, if she wants to look good, she'll not mind pouring herself into something tight, or suffering shoes that are half a size too small. If she's not in the mood to worry what she looks like she might well wear a synthetic blouse that makes her feel a bit too hot and doesn't have a particularly nice texture because it's easy to wash and she doesn't have to iron it. When nothing about clothes interests her she'll have an interchangeable wardrobe based on one colour with a lot of identical items so that she never has to think about what to wear.

There are some exceptions to this, however. One is the Emotional woman who has discovered that clothes have an ability to affect her mood for the better. Then she'll treat herself through her wardrobe when she feels she deserves it. Another is the Emotional woman who expresses her artistic nature through her personal appearance, in which case she will always be exquisitely dressed. It is also impossible for her to be dispassionate about any area of her life, and she either considers clothes beneath her attention, or is passionate about getting them right.

Food tends to figure large in the Emotional woman's life. One of the reasons is that her nurturing nature is expressed through feeding the people she loves – and to this end she can be a good and creative cook. It's when it comes to eating that her attitude is more complex. She often has a love-hate relationship with it. You might see a spasm of anguish cross her face when she's offered something delicious. She might eat too much for comfort, or, like Oprah, as a way of blotting out her emotions. After all, food was the first 'love' Ms Emotional experienced as a baby and it might ever after have this connotation for her. Equally, she can reject it because it makes her fat, or because in some way she feels compelled to punish herself by withdrawing this 'love'. Many anorexics, bulimics, or bingers and starvers are Emotional women. They can subdue and control their bodies, even if they can't do the same for their emotions. Two of the most famous women of our time have suffered from eating disorders: Diana, the Princess of Wales, and Elizabeth Taylor – both Emotional women who show endless compassion for humanity at large through their charitable work, but far less for themselves, or for people who have hurt them. Even Emotionals with a more balanced relationship with food find it hard to be neutral about it: they may be vegetarians, vegans, or health food fanatics.

Ms Emotional can fight a similar running battle with alcohol, or other mood-altering substances. Sometimes her emotions are so unbearably intrusive she literally doesn't know what to do with herself. Drink or drugs can appear to offer blessed relief for a while, but she knows they are false friends. It's hard for her to moderate her consumption, as some substance-abusers are eventually able to do. When she finds the will-power to deal with addiction she will usually give up entirely. She has most success if she finds another way to handle her emotions – through therapy, art, or putting her energies to the greater good. Exercise is one healthy way of channelling the energies of suppressed emotions, which is why it often appeals to her (as the Princess of Wales's newly muscled and toned body shows). It also helps her avoid another pitfall connected to her nature. Emotions with no obvious outlet can turn against her – giving her ulcers, migraines, or contributing to a health breakdown which leaves her susceptible to more serious illnesses.

The Emotional woman is often drawn to work that involves her with other people and allows her to help them. This is excellent for the more emotionally robust type, and can also take the more sensitive introspective out of herself. She might also be a musician or artist of some kind, or work with human psychology, where her intuition adds depth to her scholarship. Sometimes she is torn between the need to work for and with other people, and the distress she feels at office politics or the normal cut and thrust of professional life. She can be terribly hurt by colleagues who are difficult or rude, or she may be paralysed by unfounded suspicions that other people are out to do her down. She is less well equipped to deal with all this than the Emotional man, and her righteous anger can turn inwards into a debilitating depression. On the other hand, she can be a consummate office politician when she tries, with a better than average feel for manipulating those around her because of her subtle grasp of exactly the right way to approach each individual.

As life out in the world can seem cruel, it's not surprising that her home is very important to Ms Emotional. She wants to feel safe and reassured. It is often cluttered with loved objects and photos that hold special warm memories for her. She might surround herself with animals – they are more reliable and unconditionally loving than human beings. She can be a superb hostess, but she also needs to retreat and she might not invite guests over very often. She needs time on her own, or with a trusted partner, so that she can recover from the bombardment of other people's emotions, and the hurly-burly of the kinds of interactions she inspires.

Her need for safety and passionate attachments can also turn her towards religion, especially when it makes her feel there is a universal love out there that she can contact, or a benign, all-loving being looking after her – or even a harsh and judgemental god, if that accords with her view that life is hard. Stigmatics – who spontaneously bleed from the places where Christ was wounded during crucifixion – are almost certainly Emotionals. For instance, St Mary-Magdalen dei Pazzi, born in 1566, was said to have 'suffered acute trials and tribulations' when she became a nun at the age of 17. She would regularly whip herself to subdue her spirit and desires. She first showed signs of the stigmata when she was 19. The fact that stigmatics happen to be passionately committed Emotional women does not, of course, belittle the spiritual aspect of the manifestation.

Even when she's not religious (and then she is often passionately contemptuous of those who are) she needs something to take her out of herself. Sometimes this is films or literature – nothing insipid, but work that deals with great themes, where people suffer. She loves music for the way it is able to express all that she feels and more. She also responds to nature of the wild and tempestuous kind – high winds, strong waves, forbidding mountains, open spaces. A neat formal park with pretty flowers doesn't move her especially – what she wants are the elements and vistas that match or exceed in strength what is going on in her inner landscape. These have the power to calm her more than anything, and put her own turbulence into perspective.

The unattached Emotional woman

Little Ms Emotional often enters adolescence feeling bruised. Even when, on the surface, she had a perfectly normal and stable upbringing, with good enough loving parents, her acute sensitivity has caused her to suffer. The usual ups and downs of childhood affect her more strongly than most. She can harbour bitter memories of punishments she received that other children would have long forgotten. Indeed, the memories continue to fill her with the exact emotions they created at the time, causing her to cry or feel furious or shamed throughout her life. Her uncanny attunement to the feelings of others means that she is likely to have 'taken on' her mother's sorrow, sexual disgust, repressed anger, and so on, and to have been buffeted by subtle undercurrents in her family that might have been missed by a less emotionally impressionable child.

Not surprisingly, she steps cautiously into the arena of relationships and sex. She has a longing for love and an almost equal fear of being hurt. It doesn't suit her to play around in sexual experimentation with an assortment of boys. Actually, it never does suit her to have a variety of partners, even later on in life. She can't approach anything she does blithely or superficially and sex is too powerful an activity for her to take casually. The Emotional teenager (or grown woman) who sleeps around has sometimes been damaged by sexual abuse, leaving her self-esteem too low to say no. Or she is desperately seeking love through sex, or is in rebellion against an over-strict or sexually repressed background. She can also have a high sex drive, and her desires make her easily seduceable. Whatever motivates her, however, casual sex will inevitably lead to heartbreak, leaving her feeling bad, disgusted or rejected.

The Emotional Woman

Like all teenage girls, she is usually intensely romantic — hoping for great things from love, and idealising the boys or men that capture her attention. It takes some sophistication and experience to differentiate between infatuation, lust — and love with more enduring qualities. She can continue to be mixed up about this for a long time, sometimes throughout her life. After all, she is always powerless to fight strong feelings, and is impelled to follow where they lead — and few are stronger than infatuated new love or sexual attraction. This can mean she has more relationships than really suits her nature. She's really looking for an emotional connection that endures: once new love passes she can realise that there's very little there. She can seem similar to Ms Romantic, but underneath she is different. Ms Romantic is at her happiest when in love and on cloud nine — the stronger ties of mature love fail to excite her in the same way. Ms Emotional might be ecstatic when infatuated, but she is most profoundly content when tied by bonds of a more complex emotional nature.

The precise nature of the love she is looking for varies from one Emotional woman to another. The timid Ms Emotional who felt brow-beaten by powerful parents can feel she has found a soulmate in an autocratic man who provides for her but also creates an undercurrent of fear that she can find erotic. The compassionate Ms Emotional who willingly looked after loved ones in her childhood, or felt enveloped in loving tenderness, will need to recreate this atmosphere in her most significant relationship, and so on. Indeed people of other Sexual Styles have similar tendencies to reproduce patterns from the past, but in her case this replication of her strongest emotional imprinting causes the greatest outpouring of emotion and can bind her loyally and obsessively to the man who evokes it.

There is usually an essential element of power play in her most important relationships. In its most benign manifestation this can be expressed as a great need to care for her loved ones, who depend on her. Another kind of Emotional woman wants

Sexual Styles

to feel dominated in some way or, as she might put it, to be looked after. However, she can be extremely strong herself – particularly the more openly passionate woman – and although she is attracted to a powerful man she is also impelled to fight him. Power play becomes power struggle, and in some cases the very unhappiness this creates is also the source of an enduring sexual interest and erotic charge. Even the more passive Emotional woman can insidiously bid for power against the very man whose strength and dominance attracts her. This can take the form of moods, martyrdom or subtle undermining. The problem with this is that if she succeeds in her largely unconscious attempts to dethrone him, she might also find that she can no longer love him in the same way.

Change is usually hard for her, because it makes her feel insecure. If it also changes the nature of her emotional interaction with her partner it can threaten her love for him – or, at least, what binds her to him. In another of my books I told the story of Fiona, which had in turn been told to me by a counsellor. Fiona sought help because she was so unhappy with her husband, Harry, who bullied her relentlessly. Eventually Harry joined the counselling process, and it was clear that everything the counsellor had heard from Fiona was true. Fiona was a bad manager and a poor housewife, but Harry made matters worse by his criticism and unpleasantness. Over the course of counselling he experienced a change of heart, and felt deep remorse. They worked on ways that he could help rather than condemn, and ways that Fiona could learn to manage better. But over the weeks as Harry strove to keep to his part of the bargain Fiona reneged on everything she had agreed. Indeed her behaviour deteriorated so that she drove Harry into bewildered rages. She would weep in the counselling room about his cruelty and her terror, oblivious to her contributory provocation. In the end she took a job that made it impossible for counselling to continue. In common with other unaware Emotional women, Fiona was driven by an emotional need whose origins were obscure to her. She said she hated the unhappiness and the bullying, but she helped perpetuate it. It was what she knew 'love' to be. A kind and helpful Harry seemed profoundly wrong to her. Indeed her commitment to the marriage seemed to depend on his tyrannical behaviour, and her obsessive though miserable attachment to him was jeopardised by a change in him for the better.

Fortunately, most Emotional women have more healthy emotional requirements, and their relationships can be models of strong and enduring love. But if she goes through a series of attachments that all fail in similar ways, there tends to be a pattern that goes back to her formative years. If she had an absent father or rejecting mother she can be uncomfortable with men who offer love and security. Instead, she falls passionately for the inveterate Casanovas who leave her high and dry. Or if she was made to feel most valuable and loved when she was denying herself for the sake of others, she will tend to be drawn to needy men, whom she can cherish and nurse. If her cherishing works too well, however, and they no longer need her loving attention, she might be driven to undo her good work by undermining them – thereby chasing them away.

When her emotional needs are less self-destructive she can be the most womanly of partners, combining unflinching loyalty with warm nurturing ways. The man who captures her heart will be in no doubt that he is the foremost priority in her life with the exception of her children – even the intellectual high-flyer will place her relationships first. Nothing, in the end, gives her so much satisfaction as intimacy with another human being.

Sex and Ms Emotional

Sex can never be uncomplicated recreation for the Emotional woman. When circumstances are right for her it can be profoundly meaningful. When physical pleasure is allied to emotional fusion she understands the phrase 'the earth moved' in a way few other women do. On the other hand, sex in other contexts can be disturbing or downright distressing. When she doesn't feel strongly for the man, or her partner is casual, she finds it hard to feel good about the experience, even if the sex itself is pleasurable. She can't relate to the concept of sex for fun, or 'no strings' sex.

The point is that every aspect of sex has significance for her, starting with taking off her clothes. Most women agonise to a degree about whether their bodies are good enough, particularly at the start of a sexual relationship, but for her it means more than this. She feels intensely vulnerable, which immediately opens the floodgates of her emotions. From that moment on she connects to a man with her feelings, which makes it unthinkable to pretend that nothing of importance has happened. Sex itself, particularly when she enjoys it and is highly sexed, also releases the emotions that she usually likes to keep private. Because she is so adept at tuning into someone else's emotional state she feels she is laying herself bare in all senses of the word. She believes a man will 'know' her more than carnally when they make love. She can't conceive of him being unable to see into her soul and understand the depth of her feelings. This can sometimes cause her to freeze, sexually as well as emotionally – and then feelings of failure as well as self-consciousness add to her misery. No wonder she feels humiliated – even fundamentally rejected – if it turns out to be casual for him.

When she lives in an environment that treats sex lightly she can worry that there is something wrong with her. No one else seems distressed by casual sexual encounters. She might think she just needs more experience, and should loosen up. She might worry that she is frigid because she can't let go with virtual strangers. But this is her Sexual Style, and she needs to value and respect it. When she accepts her nature she knows that before she can enjoy love-making and reach her potential for great sexual satisfaction she needs time to get to know a man well, to feel emotionally drawn to him and trust him — and to feel sure that her feelings are reciprocated.

When she finds such a man Ms Emotional has the capacity to enjoy sex hugely. Her sexual pleasure is usually directly related to the strength of her emotions, and the more strongly she feels for him the more responsive she is physically. The kind of love-making she enjoys is then partly dependent on the defining quality of her most important emotion. If this is strong but tender love then she likes love-making to match — gentle, sensuous and slow. Anything else feels wrong, and therefore her desire and her responsiveness are affected.

In contrast, if power is what turns her on she will like a man to dominate her, be masterful, ravish her gently or even somewhat roughly. If fear or humiliation are the emotions that make her feel most completely herself she might like him to show a little cruelty, hurt her just enough for it to be erotic. In extreme cases she will only become turned on by sadomasochistic sex or real pain. Sometimes she prefers to create the *atmosphere* of these more worrying emotions rather than to experience them through sex. In this case she responds well to sharing fantasies — or dressing-up games in which they act out roles or mini-dramas to excite each other, and then make love in the normal way.

Sometimes the Emotional woman's preferences are directly traceable to her first sexual experience, for good or bad. One sex therapist told me about a woman who, as a young teenager, had become involved with a much older man who had initially raped her, and then used her shame to blackmail her into continuing to have sex with him over a period of months until finally her family moved out of the area. In a way, it was continuation of treatment she was accustomed to. She was a neglected child, disliked by her parents, and had no sense of personal worth. The abusive man was ugly, smelly and violent and she had been frightened of him and repulsed by him. Nevertheless, she couldn't help becoming sexually aroused when he forced himself on her. She consulted the sex therapist because over the years she found it impossible to enjoy sex unless it was as violent and humiliating as this first experience. After a series of abusive relationships in which she had been unhappy but sexually satisfied she was now involved with a loving and gentle man for whom she found it impossible to feel desire. In certain cases early experiences such as this — or even much milder but nevertheless devastating ones — have the effect of blocking her sexual feelings. If arousal is connected to her most unpleasant emotions she prefers never to become aroused at all. Similarly, she can take to heart her parents' views on sex — whether they were explicitly stated, or she simply picked up their attitude in her intuitive way. If they disapproved of sex generally, or she deduced, perhaps, that it made her mother unhappy, it can affect her own feelings. She might find sex frightening, sordid, or be disgusted by her own sexual drives.

These, of course, are examples of the worst kind. Most Emotional women have far better experiences in childhood, and far less traumatic initiations into sex. Many of their sexual pleasures are truly pleasurable, and the connection to the past is benign. She can be turned on by certain textures and scents that remind her of happy times, if only subliminally. She can like using creams and talcum powder for sensual massage, echoing, as they do in a pleasing way, that sensual time in her childhood when being physically tended by a loving carer made her feel so good. At her most gentle she can enjoy sex in which she is babied, or find her own desire much increased when she treats her man in such a way — perhaps bathing him, washing his hair, giving him a long, slow massage, and then letting him take charge of the proceedings.

Ms Emotional also needs to be in the right mood to enjoy sex. She likes to feel needed by her man, important to him, that her strength of feeling is matched by his. Like Ms Sensual she often needs a lot of physical attention — affectionate hugging, kissing, holding his hand, or feeling his arm round her. In her case it is because she is moved when she knows that he wants to be close to her, is impelled to touch her, cares enough to care how she feels. When her sex drive is not particularly high this will be even more important to her. If he only holds her for sexual purposes she might find it difficult to become aroused, even if he is a good lover and knows her body well. The more combative Ms Emotional can find a row or a fight gets her sexual juices going, as well as her heart pumping. For many Emotional women, though, this can be off-putting. When he has been angry with her, or has upset her, almost nothing will switch on her sexual feelings until everything has been made right again. If he thinks that sex is the cure-all for disagreements she will feel violated and outraged. When sex is the ultimate expression of love for her it can seem a defilement to use it for less exalted purposes or as a way to say sorry.

Ms Emotional can, however, need sex for reassurance that she is loved. She doesn't trust words at the best of times — she knows that they can be used to twist meanings and hide emotions. When their bodies are naked and close together she feels that she can see into his heart. This is even more important than the physical ecstasy of love-making when she is feeling insecure.

Sometimes, too, sex is where she exercises her power in the relationship. When his desire for her has been a strong element in their lives she might feel his commitment and love is measurable by how much he wants to make love to her. Sometimes this means she's unhappy about making the first move sexually. She doesn't want to have to *make* him desirous, she wants it to be spontaneous. When she does make the first move it will usually be in the early, most lustful, days of the relationship, when it is sometimes hard to tell who *is* making the first move. If she is prepared to initiate sex it is usually when prompted by an upwelling of love, and almost never without this feeling.

Music has great power in her life. She can find it profoundly soothing. It can also be the most subtle of sex aids – there might well be a particular tune that acts on her like an aphrodisiac. Like Ms Romantic, she also likes soft lighting, a calm atmosphere, and a sense that they are two people who are important to each other. She finds it difficult to give herself uninhibitedly to love-making if there's a chance they might be disturbed. How can she listen to her body and her instincts when she is listening out for the children? Indeed she might be hypersensitive to discordant noise of any kind. The wailing of a police siren breaks the erotic spell. Sex is a serious business for her and she tends to give herself wholeheartedly to it or not at all.

The Emotional woman and marriage

Ms Emotional craves to be Mrs Emotional. How could she want anything else when she loves? The man who moves her most profoundly becomes part of herself, and she can't conceive of letting him go. Whenever she loves and loses it's like amputating a limb. That's why she's so loyal; that's why she's so obsessive and tenacious. Indeed it suits her to marry fairly young, because the pain of too many failed relationships accumulates and makes it hard for her to be happy.

She has the potential to make an excellent wife. Nothing is too much trouble for the man she loves, and it makes perfect sense to her to devote herself to looking after him. It's one of the ways she proves how much she cares. At her best this nurturing is generous-hearted, and her husband realises how lucky he is. Less healthily, she can be more craven, making it clear what she is sacrificing to make him happy at the expense of her own happiness. Of course, this has the opposite effect, making him feel uncomfortable, guilty, and possibly trapped.

Her heart rules her head in terms of choosing a husband, as it does in every aspect of her life. Sometimes, though, it looks to others as if she has been more calculating. This is because he can be conspicuously successful, rich, or even famous. To give her credit, she's rarely as attracted by the trappings of success as by what they symbolise: the successful man is the powerful man, and she is truly bewitched and in love with him for this reason — never mind that he is far too old for her, or seemingly unattractive — to her he is perfect. If she is driven by a different pressing emotional need, however, the man she finds irresistible could just as easily be the incipient alcoholic who is always out of work. She'll do everything in her power to make this relationship good, and the frailest, most ethereal Emotional woman can call on great reserves of strength when motivated by love and the need to keep her family together.

Children are usually very important to her. Babies, particularly, move her profoundly, because with them communication is pure — it's all about emotion, touch, and words have little relevance. Indeed, the love stirred in her by her children can eclipse what she feels for her man. This sometimes suits him fine, particularly if he is a traditional man with a full and interesting life outside the home. He might be less enthusiastic if it means that as the power of her attachment to him becomes less intense so their sex life also drifts into nothingness. She also maintains a strong attachment to her original family. Sometimes she thinks they can do no wrong and wants to see them constantly. Her feelings can be more mixed: her parents treated her badly but she still feels bonded to them out of a sense of duty and guilt. Even when she hates them they are still vividly present in her life. I know of a 40-year-old woman who loathes almost every member of her extended family — but she is still fighting them, locked into obsessive feuding first with one and then another.

The main problem area in her marriage is connected to precisely what can make it so good — her strong emotions and her vacillating moods. When she is deeply hurt she can retreat into herself. It's that problem she has with attaching words to what she feels. A sensitive man will know that something is wrong, though he might not be able to get out of her what it is. A more busy and word-oriented man can be less attuned to the undercurrents. If she's not complaining, he thinks, there's nothing to worry about. Nevertheless, her feelings will out in one way or another. She might be ill more often, show signs of irrationally obsessive behaviour, put on a lot of weight, or lose it drastically. These may not be conscious cries for help — but cries they certainly are. If her husband loves her he needs to help her find more healthy ways of expressing what she's feeling — especially when he might be the unwitting cause — or to find new outlets for the emotional energy she is turning against herself.

Ms Emotional is capable of putting up with extremes of bad behaviour from her man in the interests of keeping her family and the security of her home intact. But if you lose her love she will make you pay in one way or another, and is prepared to bide her time. Make her jealous with another woman and she will appear to cope, but once the affair is over and she feels secure with you again she can exact revenge in numerous quiet ways. If you leave her for another woman, indeed, her revenge can be more dramatic and blatant. This is the woman who sells your prized antique car for a song through the small ads, takes the scissors to your collection of rare bank notes or cuts the crotch out of all your trousers. The Princess of Wales's televised interview in which she talked of her marriage and Prince Charles's inadequacies as a husband, years after they had officially separated, is an example of this. Particularly telling was the way she implied he would not, or should not, be king. The Emotional woman finds it hard to forgive and forget, and if she can hurt those who have hurt her she will do so — even if she must wait a long time for the opportunity. Her empathetic understanding of what makes others tick also means she knows better than anyone else what will hurt the most.

Treat her right however, and return her love in equal measure, and you will bring out all her best qualities. She'll stand by your side if you commit murder; she'll nurse you through illness devotedly, indeed follow you to the grave. Ms Emotional is quite capable of fading away when the man she loves dies – genuinely dying of a broken heart herself.

When Ms Emotional will stray

Ordinarily, infidelity would never cross the mind of the pure Emotional woman. She gives her body entirely to the man to whom she has given her heart. She only wakes up to the attractions of other men when her relationship has gone so wrong that there is very little feeling left. She'll rarely have an affair for the sake of sex or even to find the love that is missing in her marriage. She will usually do so only when she is fully intending to leave her husband.

There are some exceptions. The unhappily married Emotional woman, whose commitment to the happiness and security of her children makes her reluctant to leave their father, might become involved with another man. The woman who fears losing her own secure home, even if she has no children, can do the same. But this is never casually done. In her heart her lover is her 'husband'. The secretive side of her nature can mean she is quite adept at covering her tracks, but her emotional honesty will cause her to suffer for it. If she tends towards feeling guilty anyway the situation will be intolerably burdensome for her. She will find her real husband's sexual attentions unbearable, and will do everything she can to avoid them.

More unusually, there is a certain kind of Emotional woman who has split in an almost masculine way her desire nature from her love nature. She is usually the kind of woman mentioned earlier, whose formative experiences have given her a distaste for sex and a horror of her own strong desires, or have caused her to find brutal and unloving sex more arousing than anything else. In these cases she may fall deeply in love with a man for whom she feels little sexually – indeed, thinking of him in sexual terms can seem an offence against the love she feels for him. Sometimes she is then driven to 'fall' as she sees it – having brief and occasionally unpleasant sexual encounters that confirm all her distorted misgivings about sexual matters. Unsurprisingly, her self-esteem is usually very low, and she can be tortured with fear about what would happen if her partner ever found out.

Ms Emotional and sexual problems

The emotions that power Ms Emotional's sex drive can, in other circumstances, sap it. She needs to be feeling loving or, at the very least, powerfully emotionally connected to her man to feel desirous and enjoy sex. Without these feelings sex can seem insipid, or crude. Sometimes she doesn't quite understand why she has ceased to respond to a man who is still the perfectly good lover that he always was, and the less she knows herself the more likely her body is to do her protesting for her. The headache she complains of is a real one.

When her sex drive is affected by problems surfacing in her relationship there is only one remedy: the problems must be tackled first before her desire returns. Trying to cope by attempting to improve the sex itself is like treating a broken leg by buying new shoes. When love as she defines it has gone from her relationship she might cling to it for other reasons, but she will rarely be able to feel sexual with the man again.

On the other hand, there is usually a natural ebb and flow to her desires. She might have cyclical moods, and times when she regularly feels most sexual. Even when she is not so predictable, she is even more sensitive than most women to outside influences. If she is under pressure at work, tense generally, or worried about matters outside her relationship, the impact will be felt within it. Many other women and men experience this too, but the all-consuming nature of her emotional states means that she finds it less easy to switch off from pressures that others can, at times, leave outside their front door. The answer to this is patience on her partner's side. Pressing her to have sex when she is unhappy can create a problem needlessly between them. Instead she needs some quiet understanding, and much unsexual physical reassurance.

A more complex problem can be caused by an ambivalent attitude to her own sexuality. She has usually absorbed her parents' attitude to sex and taken it as gospel. When these ideas are repressive they can conflict with her desires. It is always difficult for her to deal with a disparity between what she is supposed to believe and what she feels. If she is highly sexed she can make strenuous attempts to control her sexuality, and find it difficult to enjoy sex or let go with her partner. Women of other Sexual Styles with a similar problem can often work through it with the help of a counsellor or a sex therapist, or even an understanding and much loved partner, but she finds this harder than most. Sometimes the way she is best able to deal with it is to 'become' someone else during sex — using fantasy and role-play to distance her sexual persona from the day-to-day person she feels most comfortable being.

Sometimes her partner tolerates her lack of desire for sex for his own reasons — he might be getting the sex he needs elsewhere. Even so, she usually needs to find an outlet for these repressed energies. If she turns her back on sex completely it helps her to find another physical expression — dancing, swimming, exercise. Or else she needs to turn the force of her passion on to a cause — a charity, a political party, a religious philosophy — so that she can sublimate her sexuality in a way that gives her great emotional satisfaction and puts her own troubles into perspective.

The Emotional Man

'I hate and love. You may ask why I do so. I do not know, but I feel it and am in torment.'

Catullus, Roman poet

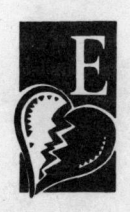

The Emotional Man

Sensitive is the catchword that describes the Emotional man, but what does it mean? Is it that empathetic sensitivity that means he's alert to your feelings, or is his sensitivity confined to himself, nursing every slight or hurt? Does it mean he's capable of great love or that he can't stand pain or rejection? Does it make him a poet or a counsellor? A priest or an alcoholic? Mr Emotional can be any of these and more. That's the trouble with trying to classify him. Emotions are varied and complex, positive and negative, and Emotional men can be very different from each other.

Not that the Emotional man has an exclusive on deep feelings. Where he differs from other men, however, is that everything he does is shaped and powered by his intense and profound emotional state. It doesn't matter how clever, talented or intellectual he is, when he is in the grip of strong feelings he acts without regard to conscious thought. Or rather, his thought processes can be radically affected and altered by the emotion he is experiencing. Often he is unconscious of this. He is not aware that rage has influenced his logical thinking or that misery is clouding his judgement. Where other men will think, 'I must calm down', or can detach themselves for periods of time from their moods, he, instead, is swept along regardless. The emotions flood his system, insidiously transforming how he thinks. Cut him open, and the words 'anger', 'guilt', 'love' or 'grief' will be written on every cell.

It's the same in his sex life. Mr Emotional makes his choice of partner based on gut responses. He can usually operate sexually when he's not deeply moved, but there is something superficial in this for him. Until he meets a woman who manages to touch him in his most sensitive spot – the seat of his emotions – he can rate sex little higher than a game of squash or a burger. When his emotions are engaged, however, sex becomes an altogether more elevated experience. It is important to distinguish between his reactions and that of Mr Romantic. In the Romantic man's case what is touched is light-headed wondrous excitement: classic 'love' feelings. For the Emotional man it could just as easily be hate, fear or abject dependence. The sensations of physical sex pale into insignificance compared to the way he is profoundly shaken by how he is made to feel. When love fails for Mr Romantic he can soon be off looking for the next woman. Mr Emotional feels the disappointment more profoundly and personally. He can take years to recover.

Perhaps that's why he is such a magnet to many women. Byron's words: 'Man's love is of man's life a thing apart,/'Tis woman's whole existence', are often true, and galling to women. The Emotional man, however, can be different. Sensing that he has the capacity to love with the same single-mindedness that they do is often what draws women to him. It's partly, also, because he arouses the maternal instinct in women: when he suffers they want to make it all better. Other men can be perplexed by his ability to attract women without saying or doing anything at all. Mr Emotional spent the evening glowering into his drink, and *they* flocked to *him*.

But women need to be wary of him. Just because he is capable of deep feelings doesn't mean that they are necessarily constructive. Emotional men are at the mercy of the fluctuations of their moods, but there is usually one distinguishing emotion that dominates all others.

The primal nature of his driving emotions is the clue. The fact that they go beyond words is because the pattern was often laid down in earliest childhood before his brain had developed the sophistication to process rationally, when he was all feeling. All of us are imprinted deeply with the experiences of our early life, but Emotional men and women are least able to rise above these or change the programming. The Emotional man is stamped with the hallmark of the most intense and prevailing emotion that characterised his childhood.

When he experienced his family as deeply loving and caring, his own capacity for great love flowers. But if he felt neglected or put down this can become warped. Depending on the individual's environment, the emotion that colours his personality into adulthood could be anger, guilt, revenge, sadness, and so on. He feels other things, of course, but not so profoundly. The over-riding emotion, when triggered, is what makes him feel 'himself'. The woman who draws out this fundamental emotional state, good or bad, is the one he bonds to, sometimes forever.

The actor Richard Burton is a good example of this, particularly in his relationship with Elizabeth Taylor. Burton was born in 1925 and brought up in a Welsh mining village, one of 11 children. When he was two, his mother died after giving birth to her last child. Until then, Burton had been a clingy baby who would cry and scream when his mother was out of his sight. That this loss affected him for the rest of his life is evident. As his brother, Graham Jenkins, reported in his book *Richard Burton: My Brother*, Burton once explained that he drank so heavily to 'drown fear' and the fear was of loss: 'To have everything is to lose everything. The dread of losing is the greatest dread of all.' After his mother's death, he went to live with his sister, Cis, whom he adored, and her husband.

Burton was a womaniser, before and during his first marriage to Sybil, whom he married when he was 24. He loved Sybil, but not in the same way that he loved Elizabeth Taylor, whom he met in 1962, when he played Antony to her Cleopatra in the movie. 'I would say my love for Sybil was more a love of a man for his daughter ... Before Elizabeth I had no idea what total love was ... I was shocked.' Even more tellingly, in his autobiographical story, *A Christmas Story* written during his relationship with Taylor, he writes about a character based on his sister, Cis: 'It wasn't until 30 years later, when I saw her in another woman, that I realised I had been searching for her all my life.' The Emotional man often gives his heart to the woman who reminds him of the most significant woman in his childhood.

Burton's marriage to Taylor was marked by great passion, tremendous rows and reconciliations, and out-of-control drinking. They married in 1964, divorced nearly ten years later, remarried, and then divorced again very quickly. The relationship was finally over when he married his third wife, Susan, in 1976. Burton went on to marry a fourth time, shortly before he died, but Taylor continued to obsess him until the end. In a conversation with Graham, towards the end of his life, Graham asked if he missed Taylor. Burton replied: 'Of course. All the time ... We've never really spilt up and we never will. We're always there when we need each other.'

Yet, despite this great love, Burton had seemed driven to ruin their relationship, as sometimes happens with Emotionals. His drinking escalated and he was unfaithful, although 'only physically'. He was powered by a sexual appetite that often disgusted him. He believed in monogamy, but couldn't sustain it. In an interview he once said: 'I am not excusing myself. I am very puritanical about sex outside marriage. I don't believe it doesn't matter if you are unfaithful. It's torture because you betray both yourself and her.'

Just as damaging, was his Emotional propensity to bring on himself what he most feared: the alienation and loss of people closest to him. In certain moods, often when he was drunk, he was devastatingly cruel to Taylor, and to anyone he loved or who loved him. He once wrote to Graham, in apology after one of these occasions: 'My chief and most vicious faculty when I lose my balance on the tight-rope is to attack with malicious venom the people I love most.'

Lord Harlech, chairman of Harlech Television in which Burton was a shareholder, once said: 'His approach to everything is wholly emotional.' Like some other Emotionals, he seemed compelled to bring about what he feared most: to have everything he desired, and then to lose it.

Burton is the darker version of the Emotional man. Mr Emotional's feeling nature can also be his gift. The more aware Emotional man is not only acutely in touch with his own feelings, but he has the ability to comprehend the emotional states of others, often on the slightest evidence. While many men need to be told that you are sad, angry, or whatever, the Emotional man can feel it in his bones. If he is well-intentioned he can use this knowledge in healing ways. Not that he will try to talk you out of it — he knows that doesn't work — but simply by being understanding and sympathetic he can make it possible for you to bear your inner turbulence, knowing that it is accepted and acknowledged. The Emotional man who has no control over this channel to another's deepest feelings can be swamped by the intrusion of emotions that are not his own. His capacity for compassion is paralysed by his sensibilities, and he suffers helplessly alongside. A more robust Emotional man will feel his heart bleed, but not to the extent that he is immobilised.

When he is motivated by more destructive impulses, however, he can use this sensitivity as a weapon. His uncanny talent for intuitively understanding what makes others tick can impel him to press emotional buttons to cause suffering. He delves to find the most sensitive point in others and then attacks it. Like much of what drives the Emotional man, this impulse is largely unconscious. He doesn't set out to hurt, but he is propelled towards what he understands as the essential meaning of life — strong feelings. Everything else is something of a charade from his point of view. Living, as he does, in a welter of passion, he needs to connect with others in the same way, even if it means strife and unpleasantness.

The more selfish Emotional man only sees matters through the lens of his own current feelings. He knows he's hurt; he knows he's angry. That's what counts. When he is too taken up with his own emotions he loses the ability to empathise with others. What he feels is so powerful that he can't comprehend that someone else has feelings that could be just as important. This is the man most likely to wreak havoc in the lives of people close to him.

Heathcliff, the creation of Emily Brontë in her novel *Wuthering Heights*, is the Emotional man at his most elemental. Adopted into the Earnshaw family as a young orphan, Heathcliff shows a great capacity to love, although wild and untamed. His deepest feelings are stirred by the man who adopted him, and by the child Cathy. This love for Cathy shapes his entire life, enduring when he is away from her for years, and long after her death. It is open to speculation what he would have become if his childhood experiences had been happy. As it was, after his adoptive father's death he was treated harshly by Cathy's brother, humiliated, beaten and degraded. Cathy, too, betrayed their love when, as a teenager, she was drawn to the glamour and the riches of a well-brought-up neighbour. The rest of Heathcliff's life is powered by the desire for revenge and the pain of his thwarted love. He goes away, educates himself and becomes rich. If he had been of another Sexual Style this process would have tempered his feelings. Instead it merely gives him the ammunition to indulge them. He returns to wreck systematically the lives of everyone he deems responsible for his pain, including marrying the sister of Cathy's husband and treating her abominably, and even using his own son as an instrument of revenge. He continues to love Cathy long after her death and, maddened by his agony, 18 years later starves himself to death. As a child, talking of the revenge he wants to wreak on Cathy's brother, he says: 'I don't care how long I wait, if I can only do it, at last. I hope he will not die before I do!'

All Emotional men have the capacity to look below the surface of life to what drives other human beings. Words and actions are not taken at their face value. The more balanced Emotional man can use this instinctive grasp of motive to develop a subtle understanding of human nature. When this is harnessed to intellect the result can be great art. It can also lead to paranoia if he assumes that his own dark drives are typical.

You should never underestimate his capacity to feel. This is not the man with whom to play emotional games for the fun of it. You can wound him forever, or unleash passions that can't be talked away or laughed off.

Identifying Mr Emotional

Don't be fooled into thinking that the man whose eyes filled with tears during *Gone With The Wind* is Mr Emotional. It's most probably Mr Romantic, whose sensibilities are much more sentimental and near the surface; his tears soon dry. When Mr Emotional is moved it is at such a profound level that it is impossible for him to shake off. While other people can be saddened by, say, a documentary about human suffering or an environmental disaster, they might not even remember to send a donation when cheered by the situation comedy that follows. In some cases that same documentary can change an Emotional man's life. People who dedicate their lives to causes are often Emotionals, because the feelings unleashed never lose their strength. That is the root of both his troubles and his greatness. No strong emotion is ever diluted for him. 'Revenge is a dish best eaten cold' is the motto of the Emotional man. The rage might have cooled, but is replaced by an icy burn that is equally powerful: he is prepared to bide his time. Equally, strong love, once evoked, maintains its strength. The raw power of emotion never loses its edge for him.

You can spot him most easily by what he doesn't say, more than by what he does. Yes, he can make conversation when he is on an even emotional keel. His Emotional nature doesn't stop him developing a keen intellect or a good sense of humour. But when his emotional state is powerfully intrusive he can be rendered almost wordless. In the grip of strong feelings he is unable to identify with the superficiality of social life, which seems far less real than his emotional state. Whereas others can 'make an effort' if they are depressed, sad, or otherwise feeling a strong undertow of emotion, and thereby somewhat dissipate it, the Emotional man is swamped and isolated by what is going on inside him. Even when he is happy, he is more likely to sit around with a smile on his face than to translate his feelings into social bonhomie. Not that he is ever happy-go-lucky. Even strongly positive emotions are too profound to be light-hearted. Indeed, his is the Sexual Style most likely to suffer from angst or depression, even when nothing in his life appears to be causing it. And don't expect him to be able to explain why. With the exception of those with a strong dose of another Sexual Style, most Emotional men separate talking and feeling. The use of words is for social or professional matters and is quite inadequate for describing or quantifying what is happening in their hearts and souls.

For these reasons he is not at his best in company. When he is very alert to the emotions of others he can be disturbed by what he is picking up in a large gathering. When he is more self-obsessed he can't be bothered with the small-talk that detracts from the more compelling voice of his inner life. The niceties of behaviour often pass him by as well. He can't see the point in being polite for the sake of it. Often he is disconcertingly honest. 'Tact' can seem a synonym for 'lying'. On the other hand, the Emotional man whose experiences have made him cynical can become cleverly devious as a form of self-protection.

At his most classic he could be described as the strong, silent type. Silent, true, but the strength can be deceptive. It is the strength of *feeling* rather than of action or self-control. He usually has 'presence' however: the ability to make himself felt even when he is not saying anything. This is different from the presence of Mr Romantic, or Mr Imaginative — who are noticed by others because of what they say and do, or the image they project. Mr Emotional, by contrast, just 'is'. His strong feeling gives out an unmissable vibration, even if you don't know what it's about. When he speaks it's because he has something to say, and people usually listen.

On the whole clothes will be unimportant to him. They are what you put on to protect yourself from the elements, and because convention demands it. He is the man least likely to be concerned about what he wears, and will quite happily allow a woman to take charge of his wardrobe. If he tends to depression he will put on the same clothes day after day — not as a statement but because he really couldn't care less. Even when he is much happier he is extremely unlikely to notice or consider fashion. It's an example of the kind of superficiality he most despises. What he wears is usually what first came to hand, and unless he is in a profession that demands a degree of sartorial elegance he only shops for clothes when the ones he already has are wearing out.

The Emotional man is happiest in a profession that uses his feeling nature, rather than one that requires him to deny it. The more compassionate type will be drawn to the caring professions in some capacity, such as doctor, counsellor or priest. He can be excellent at this when he is able to use his abilities to help without becoming too emotionally involved. Some Emotional men, however, feed off the intensity of another's feelings. Then an unhealthy situation can develop in which he is dependent on the person he is supposed to be helping, and much is stirred up without being healed.

Actually, there are very few fields of work in which he cannot find an outlet for his instinctive grasp of human responses.

Anything that brings him together with others, either as colleagues or clients, allows him to use this faculty. The genius that marks out certain businessmen, bankers, lawyers, accountants, and so on, is that their technical expertise is underpinned by their ability to interpret people's moods, and perhaps use this knowledge manipulatively. This applies even more directly to advertising and PR. If he has developed a good channel between heart and brain he can be a writer whose work reflects an understanding of the human condition. He can get inside the skin of his characters and knows what it feels like to be them. The same with certain actors. If he has artistic talent, however, he is more likely to express it through music or painting, which speak directly to the emotions without the barrier of words.

The Emotional man who has grown up distrustful can also be finely attuned to darker emotional currents. He can use this positively in any line of work that demands knowledge of the underbelly of life, such as detective work or even psychology. When it is not part of his job, his suspicious nature is less useful. He can believe he is being plotted against, so makes pre-emptive strikes on people who might be totally innocent. This causes him to be a difficult employer, or an employee who finds himself isolated or unpromotable whatever his talents. Indeed, the need for power can be a driving force for the Emotional man. If he can't gain power in his profession he might try to wield it in his private life.

He needs to feel emotionally involved in whatever work he does. This often makes him an obsessive or a workaholic. He doesn't like doing something just for the money. When his emotions are not engaged he can despise what he does – and himself for doing it. At his best, this gives him an enviable integrity. He trusts what he feels, and won't be swayed by what others say or do.

When he is deeply involved in his work, and perhaps deeply involved also with his partner or family, then he may have few outside interests. He can, however, be drawn to pursuits that calm him — private pastimes, such as fishing, or anything that gets him away on his own, or spending time listening to music. He likes animals too. Not just because he is comforted by stroking them, like Mr Sensual, but because he can also endow them with emotions and sensibilities that match his own. Battling with the elements can also appeal — sailing, rock climbing, and so on. The forces of nature fascinate him and can take him out of himself.

The Emotional whose daily life is less involving may fill the void with interests that obsess him. Perhaps he makes intricate models, or collects toy soldiers. Usually you can see beyond the apparent pleasure to the emotion that drives it. He might be retreating to the safety of childhood, for instance, or recapturing happy times spent with his parents, or exercising a need for control that was thwarted when he was younger.

His attitude to food and drink also has its roots in his emotional nature. Sometimes he only likes the dishes and flavours of his childhood, not so much for the taste but because they represent the known and secure. If food equalled love when he was growing up then he might be unable to connect with the sensations of appetite and fullness, and eat mainly for comfort or to assuage sadness. Sometimes he has a disdain for eating, and is scornful of those to whom it means a lot. He can't be emotionally neutral about any aspect of his life and this can make him passionate about food — but rarely for epicurean reasons. At one extreme this can lead to eating disorders, as he expresses his pain or self-disgust by starving or bingeing — or if food meant love in the past he rejects love by rejecting food. A more positive manifestation is when he becomes a vegetarian, or will only buy organic and free-range produce. This goes beyond regard for his own health to a concern for the suffering of animals, or a rage against the pollution of natural resources.

It's the same with what he drinks. He might be emotionally attached to having hot milk at bedtime, like his mother used to give him, or a whisky after work because it reminds him of his father. When he finds the turbulence of his emotions hard to bear he might use drink as an anaesthetic. Similarly he can turn to drugs. Therapy to deal with this won't work unless it tackles the underlying problem of how he is to deal with his difficult emotions in the future.

The Emotional man is rarely gregarious, and hasn't got much time for superficial friendships. He tends to have few friends, but those he does have mean a lot to him. They are usually old friends – not, like Mr Sensual, because he is comfortable in their presence, but because they touch emotional chords in him. He's just as likely to continue to see the bully who made his schooldays a misery, if he admired him intensely, as he is the friend with whom he had more pleasant times. His loyalty, once given, tends to be unwavering when he feels profoundly, and he will usually forgive lapses of behaviour in those to whom he feels emotionally connected. When anyone else crosses him, however, he can take disproportionate revenge. His deep friendships are marked by an understanding that goes beyond words, which is one reason he finds it hard to make friends in later life. Sometimes his only real friends are women with whom he has been involved, because the emotional connection is deeper than any he can make with companions.

Sometimes he finds people generally a disappointment. He won't have much time for other people when this is so. His emotional nature then tends to be satisfied in less personal ways – through religion, a political philosophy or campaigning. This kind of Emotional man can even put his life in danger to serve humanity at large, yet not notice the sufferings of the people closest to him.

The unattached Emotional man

Adolescence can be a particularly turbulent time for the Emotional boy. All boys find the hormone-induced ups and downs difficult to take but he is usually buffeted by these more than most. While other boys find that they are driven by a sexual appetite that makes most girls appear attractive, the Emotional boy is likely to find that his newly awakened sexuality makes him more aware than ever of his deeper feelings, which tend to be aroused by one particular girl. Whether this relationship becomes sexual or not depends on lots of things, such as his upbringing (and hers), whether she returns his feelings, and how connected his sex drive is to his emotional pattern. However there is usually something about her that strikes the emotional keynote of his childhood. Everyone is driven to make relationships which, to some extent, echo the emotional themes of their childhood, often as a way of working through them and transforming them. He, on the other hand, seems to need to re-experience them just as they are, without changes. If his mother was rejecting, therefore, he might fixate on an aloof, rejecting girl, and the fact that he can't win her fires his feelings rather than cools them. With happier childhood experiences he can forge an early relationship with a maturity in its emotional depth that can make it last a long time.

If he has a naturally high sex drive, and the right woman doesn't come along, he can be fairly cold-hearted in his sexual dealings. He can't value someone who doesn't stir him emotionally, and therefore feels little compunction about treating her badly. Actually, what seems like cruelty is often emotional honesty: he can't pretend to something he doesn't feel. Usually, however, his emotional antenna is so sensitive to what he needs that he is drawn to someone who assumes importance to him sooner rather than later. As nursery and infant teachers will agree, some little children bond unusually strongly. He can have been deeply love-struck as early as four, five or six, and carry the impression of his equally young love as a blueprint throughout his life. Even when this is not so, there's often something reminiscent of his mother, for good or bad, in the women to whom he feels drawn. In a few cases he bonds more closely to other boys. When he is heterosexual, he can go on to make relationships and even marry, but the women are never as important to him as his male friends.

Flirting is not his strong point at the best of times. If he is any good at it at all it is when he couldn't care less about the outcome: when he is only concerned to 'pull'. When he meets an emotional soulmate, however, these tricks desert him. He speaks, if at all, with his eyes. It's a miracle that the most purely Emotional man ever gets together with the woman he wants. Sometimes he has known her for a long time, and has been able to check out his instincts against reality; they make a relationship first, and the sex follows. It can be more instant — but instinct tells him that behind the lust lies something more intense.

On the whole it doesn't suit him to be a Lothario. He's only interested in sleeping around when he can't find the woman who closely fits the missing jigsaw piece of his emotional needs. But when his essential nature is diluted with a fair dose of the Imaginative, Romantic or Sensual, he can be diverted by women who only partially fit into his emotional make-up. Sometimes, unfortunately, he is too often misled by these other drives to settle down: something in him remains profoundly disappointed or untouched. 'Unfortunately' because the Emotional man who can't find his heart's match feels incomplete. When he can't experience a fundamental emotional interaction he can feel unbearably lonely. That's why, when he does manage to find it, he can be extremely tenacious.

If you are the woman who profoundly suits him on an emotional level you will activate the obsessive qualities that bind him to you no matter what. He'll notice other attractive women, but he is unlikely to want to pursue them while you hold him in an emotional thrall. Unless there have been perverting experiences in his early life his sexual drives will be focused on the person who moves him most deeply.

Prince Charles, an Emotional man, exhibits this tenacity. The press has made bewildered noises about his attachment to Camilla Parker-Bowles, with whom he fell in love before he married Diana, and with whom he admitted to be having an affair once his marriage went wrong. How could he reject the beautiful Diana for a woman of around his own age, with a face more lived-in than beautiful? Easily, is the answer for the Emotional man. Beauty of face and form could not be less important to him when he has found his emotional soulmate. The Emotional man is helplessly enslaved by strong love, and he cherishes the unique loved one who meets his deepest needs.

Not surprisingly, Emotional men can be very jealous. Usually this is a fairly normal reaction to circumstances, but he is more acutely aware than most men of undercurrents that can activate his jealousy. Some Emotional men, however, have jealousy as their driving emotion, usually because they were very insecure as children. These men can be tortured by dark imaginings of infidelity even when there is no cause.

The Emotional man who finds relationships most difficult is the one who has experienced more suffering than joy in his childhood. Imprinted, as he always is, by his earliest strong emotions, he doesn't feel comfortable with happiness, contentment, or trust. In these cases he is drawn to difficult women — and if they aren't difficult, his own unconscious need to create discord can lead him to behave in ways that blight even a promising relationship. If his most formative emotional experience has been disappointment or rejection, he is impelled to push every emotional button in the woman who loves him until he finds the one that causes her to behave in the way he most fears. Then he is unhappy in a way he understands, and as he always expected to be.

I know a man I shall call Tom, who considers himself unlucky. He has been in love four or five times, and after a brief honeymoon period the relationship becomes unbearably hate-filled and destructive. He thinks it's the fault of the women, and, indeed, they do behave badly. But he starts it — by behaving in ways that madden them. I've known a couple of his loves — pleasant women, who before and since have had decent, normal relationships. None of Tom's affairs ended well, and the distraught women usually leave him in a way that causes him pain and humiliation. It's no coincidence that his mother died before he was three. The anger and pain he felt on being 'left' by her has been transferred to all women, and he is driven to make them act out his expectations that all women hurt you and leave you.

Even when he is not so destructive to himself and others, Mr Emotional is usually moved to turn up the emotional temperature in a relationship. Unlike Mr Sensual, with whom he is sometimes confused, it doesn't suit him if the relationship settles down into a pleasant jog-along routine. He needs to feel the presence of his woman intensely — either in a closely loving relationship, if that is his strongest emotional need, or in a more tortured partnership, if this suits him better.

What attracts him to a woman superficially depends on other aspects of his personality. It could be beauty, intellect, maternal qualities, high-spiritedness, sexuality, and so on. But with him, this is always the *route* to his heart. Once his feelings are engaged none of this matters any more. He won't 'see' her with his eyes or his mind if she continues to have a hold on his heart. If he is moved mainly by pity or compassion he can prefer women who are ugly, sick, or disadvantaged in some way. Ultimately everything the rest of the world values pales into insignificance once the catch to his emotions has been sprung.

Sex and Mr Emotional

It can take the Emotional man time to understand how his emotional nature affects his sexuality. Perhaps he followed the crowd and slept around fairly indiscriminately. Sooner or later, however, he discovers that this doesn't suit him. As one Emotional man said: 'I need the time to make an emotional, not just a physical connection.' At some point he finds that a deep involvement opens up a new world of sensuality — making the less emotional contacts seem pointless. When he knows this about himself he will often pass up purely physical temptation. He then finds it difficult to comprehend how other men can sleep with someone 'just for fun'. Fun, in fact, rarely enters into the experience for him, attached as his sexuality is to emotions that are profound and not light-hearted. The best sex for the Emotional man is with someone who moves him deeply. Then it is much more than their bodies connecting. Sex isn't so important for itself but as a symbolic enactment of his feelings. It can be easier for him to 'show' his feelings than to 'tell' them.

Some Emotional men are highly sexed: physically they need to make love often, but they can be troubled if they have to make do with lovers who mean little to them. There is something inauthentic about the experience and sometimes it seems like a betrayal — of himself, or of the woman he has yet to meet who has a claim on his heart. The highly sexed type sometimes finds the woman who has the key to his heart through sex. What started off as a brief encounter becomes transformed when sex with her is so profoundly right that it opens up his feeling nature.

On the other hand, the Emotional man who has a low sex drive is perfectly capable of holding out for the right woman. Even when he has found her he doesn't necessarily need to express his feelings through sex very often, and won't feel deprived so long as the emotional tenor of the relationship suits him. On the whole, though, Mr Emotional can find that sex gets better the longer the relationship lasts. When he has a deep need to feel secure, the commitment of a long-term relationship enhances his pleasure in love-making.

While his feelings can intensify the sexual experience for him, they can also interfere with his sex drive. Only Mr Romantic is as affected as he is by mood, though for different reasons. Mr Romantic likes to be excited − excited-angry, excited-ecstatic, excited-special. These high-octane feelings are often transitory, and when they disappear, so does his lust. Mr Emotional, instead, needs to be moved in less exciting but more profound ways. He can ache with a compassionate love that makes him a sensitive and concerned lover. On the other hand, when he is swept up in one of his periodic passions it can switch off his lustful feelings like a tap. If he is upset by his lover, for instance, he is not going to be turned on in bed. While other men often use sex as a way of making up after a row, if he is hurt he is more likely to turn away from his woman, and punish her by not touching her.

It is not uncommon for power play to be an erotic factor in his sex life. He can like to feel he is 'taking' his woman, or alternatively enjoy feeling dominated by her. While many men enjoy these sexual games, when it is important to Mr Emotional it is not a game. Indeed, he won't tire of love-making that always follows the same pattern, finding it more difficult to be turned on without the feelings unleashed by an unequal power balance. In extreme cases this becomes more obviously sadomasochistic, with unvarying rituals that include pain and fear. Dressing up, which can be titillating for Mr Romantic and Mr Imaginative, can assume even greater importance for him. His lover as the schoolgirl or the stern nurse accentuates the power play, as it does if he is dressed as the baby or the Nazi. Similarly, this kind of Emotional man can find talking dirty a turn-on. This often harks back to his sexual awakening in boyhood, when crudeness was extremely exciting, and it re-evokes what he felt then.

The Emotional Man

This type of sex can be abhorrent to another kind of Emotional man. But even the gently compassionate Emotional can be affected by a more disguised form of power. For instance, one relationship counsellor talked of a man who needed to 'rescue' women. He fell in love with distressed or neurotic women – and married two of them. In his case, his rescuing was so efficient that they became stronger and happier and better balanced. When this happened he lost all sexual interest in them. They no longer needed looking after; they were healthy enough for an equal relationship. The loss of his benign power sapped his sex drive and it couldn't be rekindled.

The best sex for Mr Emotional will always touch an emotional nerve. He can be as alert as Mr Sensual to smells and texture, but in his case this is not a general sensual sensitivity, but is confined to particular sensations that elicit powerful memories for him. The perfume his mother wore, for instance, might contain an erotic charge for him, or he might be fixated on more basic body smells, connected as they are in his unconscious to a babyhood delight in his physical functions. Or the smell associated with his first sexual experience – creosote in the garden shed, or the soapy smell of his girlfriend, for instance – can continue to be erotic throughout his life. He can like textures that remind him of his baby blanket, or even prefer rubber because it evokes his undersheet or the nipple of his baby bottle. Water, slippery creams, oil – sensations that take him back to the pleasures of being cared for as a baby – can be equally erotic. Most of the time he is unaware of where his preferences came from. He just knows that certain experiences open him up emotionally, and increase the significance and the pleasure of sex.

Some Emotional men are freer when it comes to experimenting with different ways to make love. But it is not for the sake of change. Usually this is important for him because he sees it as a way of pushing back the bounds of what he and his lover feel for each other, or because it symbolises what they are prepared to do to show what they feel – not just for the sake of the different sensations.

He can sometimes find sharing fantasies deeply satisfying, especially those that strongly create an emotional mood. At times this can be more compelling than the sex that follows, but it can certainly enhance his delight in the sensations of physical sex. Often though, he likes to keep his sexual thoughts private; they are too strong and disturbing to share, and he fears the effect they might have on his woman. The man who feels most himself when his withers are wrung, however, can sometimes derive a contrary pleasure from a partner whose fantasies make him jealous. The jealousy is supportable because it is succeeded by love-making that confirms she is his.

Scene-setting can be as important to him as it is to Mr Romantic. The right choice of music, especially, can be as powerful as foreplay. The wrong atmosphere, on the other hand, can turn him off. If his nerves are jangled or he is caught up in emotional turmoil, he finds it all but impossible to connect with his physical body.

Some Emotional men find pornography a useful route to arousal. If he is like this, it is rarely straightforward nudity or even hard-core 'normal' sex scenes that turn him on. It is usually porn that creates the emotional mood that most arouses him. If he has mixed up needs about power and domination that aren't being met he might only find satisfaction through literature and films that deal with these issues. Sometimes his interest is narrowed down to huge breasts or very large women, evoking terrifying – or comforting – mother figures. Very occasionally he might prefer pornography featuring children. When this is the case he was usually inappropriately exposed to sexual activity young, or was abused, and the turbulence of terror, shame and excitement becomes a factor in his sexual responses into adulthood.

Like men of all Sexual Styles, he is more likely to split off his sexuality from his other needs than is his female counterpart.

This is most likely to be so when the image of womanliness that moves him most profoundly is non-sexual. In this case he might keep many of his urgent sexual needs secret, or find that when he loves a woman his feelings go beyond sex, or he feels, in common with Mr Romantic, that she will be sullied by having to fall in with his sexual demands.

All being well, however, the two dovetail. When he gives his heart he can be a delightful partner. Like Mr Sensual he has the potential to be physically demonstrative if he is feeling loving, even when sex is far from his mind. Unlike Mr Sensual, however, whose thoughts can quickly turn to sex, he will often be satisfied by non-sexual embraces that show love and concern. When he has sex with the woman he loves he will often maintain that the quality of orgasm is quite different, and certainly more intense, than anything he has experienced in less emotionally engaging relationships.

The Emotional man and marriage

When he finds the right woman, Mr Emotional can be a loyal husband. He likes to be emotionally rooted, and he doesn't give his heart easily. The more intense Emotional man finds opening up in a new relationship quite difficult, and even the emotionally spontaneous man can find endings almost too hard to bear. It's quite in character, therefore, for him to prefer to settle down than to live with emotional uncertainty.

The gentler Mr Emotional can also be a fairly easy husband. Sometimes what he craves most is a secure, welcoming maternal atmosphere. Unlike Mr Sensual, who likes stability for its own sake and can put up with a fair amount of discomfort to that end, Mr Emotional needs to feel his marital home is truly 'home'. The more intense Emotional man can be harder to live with. If he is powered by stronger, difficult emotions, then his wife can find herself barraged with jealousy, rage, gloom, as he creates these and other less comfortable atmospheres. It doesn't mean he doesn't love her, nor that he is not, in his own way, 'happy' – but that he is simply being himself.

A problem can arise because of his difficulty in expressing himself when he is experiencing strong feelings. However articulate he is the rest of the time, he often becomes silent when under duress. It's not so bad if he is feeling very loving, as he will usually contrive to make it plain in one way or another. But if he is hurt, or very angry he can often only seethe. He expects you to know what he is going through – or thinks you do and are simply ignoring it – but if you are busy or otherwise switched off from him you can miss the cues. If it's important to him he won't forget. He might reproach you, bitterly, later – sometimes years later: he can be quite eloquent once the first impact of the emotion has passed. Sometimes, indeed, he will exact a revenge long after you have forgotten what caused his anguish. In extreme cases his unhappiness leads to violence, as his frustration at not being to express what he feels erupts into action.

But all of this makes him a compelling partner. No woman who lives with him can underestimate her importance in his life. Sometimes this is a childlike dependency. He can, literally, die of a broken heart if the woman he loves dies or leaves him. Even if he is violent, his wife will often try to explain to bemused onlookers that she knows he loves her and needs her. This love will usually extend to children they have together. He can be a highly involved father – sometimes a 'new man' – although the more childlike Emotional man can find himself competing with his children for his wife's affection. In certain cases, indeed, he will take against one of his children. He is rarely 'fond': he loves or hates, even when it is his own flesh.

For this reason his original family often plays a major role in his life, even after he is married. Sometimes he never quite separates from them, and even when they make him angry or upset, he needs a continuing connection with them. He won't take kindly to *you* criticising them, even if he does so himself.

When he loves them, you'll have to learn to love them too — or else. In certain cases he hates them, and all that they stand for. This is easier in one way, because he won't need to see them, but his hurt and rage never quite abate, and can surface throughout his life, even after they are long dead.

The Emotional man who makes the best husband is the one who cares as much for his wife's emotional state as he does for his own. In these circumstances he can be a true best friend as well as a lover. When he strikes a good balance between his concern for his own and his wife's feelings, and she is able to do the same for him, they can make a marriage that is the envy of other people. As Stendhal said: 'I was small before I loved ... Half — and the most beautiful half — of life is hidden from the man who has not loved passionately.'

When Mr Emotional will stray

All being well, Mr Emotional is not the type to be unfaithful easily. When he weighs up the pleasures of sexual attraction against the possible emotional damage it can cause he will often think better of it. This is especially so if he suffers from guilt. The potential pain to himself is then equally inhibiting.

This kind of Emotional man is most likely to stray when his relationship has ceased to make him feel deeply. Like the 'rescuer' whose sex drive went when his women didn't need him so urgently, a change in circumstances or in his partner can change the essential emotional atmosphere of the relationship. He will then be vulnerable to another woman who makes him feel alive by touching him on an emotional level. In this case he will usually leave for his lover, although it can cause him great anguish.

Less often he can use sex to revenge himself on his woman for slighting him, whether this is imagined or real. Then, it's not the sex itself that is so important but the effect it has on his partner, and he can make sure she knows about it, one way or another. In this instance he is less likely to leave her – though she may leave him – and he may not care anything for the woman he slept with.

The Emotional type most likely to be unfaithful on a regular basis is the one who finds his own sexual needs distasteful or shameful. If he has split them off from his more tender emotions he might not want to share them with the woman he loves. This is the man most likely to have a weekly appointment with Miss Whiplash, or have an accommodating mistress with whom he can satiate his more unusual sexual tastes.

Usually, however, taking another sexual partner is a big statement for him, and he is unlikely to do so lightly. The more paranoid Emotional can cover his traces quite well, as he is used to hiding the truth for fear of becoming vulnerable. On the whole, though, what he does or feels is usually written all over him. His partner might not immediately know what he has been up to, but she will find it hard to miss the signs that something has happened.

Mr Emotional and sexual problems

All men are likely to suffer from bouts of impotence from time to time, and for the Emotional man this is likely to be connected to strong feelings that sap his sex drive. This is only a problem if he doesn't understand why it has happened to him – then the difficulty can be prolonged by needless anxiety. Once he becomes aware that his libido is intimately interwoven with his emotional state he can accept that he won't be able to perform when he is upset or disturbed. Sometimes he needs to have it pointed out to him that his grief for the death of his father, for instance, or the fact that he has been made redundant, is the cause of what he sees as sexual failure.

When he is sexually switched off from his partner for a long time, it is usually far more than a passing mood, especially if his sex drive is normal to high. This tends to mean that there is a more important emotional mismatch between them. Sometimes he has become involved with someone else, who now claims his loyalty. But even when there is no one else on the scene, if his feeling nature is disappointed it affects his sexual responses. Sex therapy based on the physical is unlikely to do much for this, whereas anything that helps him and his partner tackle the underlying emotional problems has far more chance of success. Although he can find talking about these matters hard, an empathetic counsellor who can draw him out and help him identify what is wrong can make a great difference.

There is a more difficult problem for the Emotional man who has married or settled down with a woman when the focus of his emotional attention is elsewhere. Usually this kind of man is most profoundly moved in the abstract – by work or by a cause, or by religion. In these cases sex is purely an appetite for him, and has no power to engage him profoundly. When the appetite goes he can live quite happily without sex. In these cases there is little to be done, because he is not prepared to do anything about it. For this man sex is relegated to an unimportant corner of his life, along with the other things he considers shallow elements of daily existence, such as eating, dressing and superficial chit-chat. Love me, he says, love my passion – and don't bother me with minor complaints.

The Emotional man who feels that aspects of his sexuality are unacceptable can find that his desire to make love to his partner wanes as he tries to suppress his urges. Sometimes using fantasy helps here: by creating an erotic emotional climate with words he can find that physical satisfaction follows. It also enables him to test out his partner's reactions in a less threatening way. The best outcome in these cases is when he discovers that some of what he has been hiding is perfectly acceptable to his partner, and they are able to integrate some satisfying variations into their love-making. When this happens, the Emotional man can find that their relationship becomes even more profound.

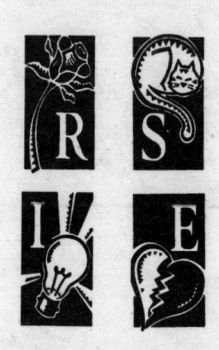

The Emotional Combinations

The Emotional Combinations

This section looks at Emotionals who have a strong subsidiary Sexual Style. It should be read in conjunction with the main Emotional chapter, and you should also look at the sections on sex and love for the secondary Style, or Styles. Each person will manifest their sexual combination in a unique way but, if you have identified your Sexual Style correctly, the broad themes will apply.

The EMOTIONAL-Sensual (E-S)

This is one of the most loyal of all the Sexual Styles. It is loyalty born of genuine, unwavering commitment. When Sensual is added to the Emotional nature, the great need to merge with another at a deep emotional level is reinforced by the Sensual need for security. The E-S wants to express feelings through sex and physical closeness, rather than words, creating a profound and enduring bond.

This closeness does not have to be comfortable. The unpredictable aspect of Emotionals is which of the many and varying emotions defines their feeling nature. Early experiences can predispose them to have a seemingly inexplicable need for an emotional connection that is wounding. It is a paradox that some Emotionals can be 'happy' when they are at their most unhappy: certainly their commitment is unaffected. The Sensual preference for certainty over insecurity increases the E-S's natural tendency to be faithful and dedicated when feeling strongly. An E-S with a happier emotional background can make a life-long relationship that appears as pleasurable to outsiders as it does to the people involved.

This combination is also extremely intense. It makes for people who are instinctive – led by their impulses, emotional or physical. However intelligent they are, however intellectual in their working lives, their strongest motivations come from what they feel, in all senses of the word.

One such person was Sidney Webb, who, among other things, was the founder of London School of Economics, a working-class socialist who became a government minister. He was a contemporary of George Bernard Shaw, who called him the 'ablest man in England'. In a letter to a friend, Webb once made a comment that could stand as a slogan for E-Ss: 'Man is still 9/10 an irrational animal – how little influence intellect has, compared with that exercised by emotions.' He was referring to himself, and in particular was lamenting his lack of success with women, which was blighting his life, and making other considerations seem insipid.

Webb met Beatrice Potter when he was 30, and fell deeply in love with her. He was in despair because he knew he was small and ugly, while she was beautiful, upper-class and rich. Nevertheless, he had to let her know what he felt. She, mainly Imaginative, told him that they could be friends, but the friendship should not be 'blurred by the predominance of lower feeling'. As an E-S he had a different perception of the value of such feelings: 'You blasphemed horribly against what is highest and holiest in human relations,' he wrote. In the same letter he revealed another E-S trait: when it comes to intimate matters words are inadequate, and can desert them at key moments. 'I could not speak my mind last night,' he wrote, 'but this agony is unendurable.' He wanted her to know the 'throb of life'; said he couldn't stop loving her even if she wouldn't return his 'hurricane of feeling'.

The Imaginative in Beatrice found Webb's feelings as repellent as his physique. Even so, he deluged her with passionate letters. At one point he wrote obliquely about his sexuality: 'I wonder whether a woman ever adequately realises the dreadful "tearing" nature of a man's real love ... I have a strong nature.' Eventually, after more than two years, Imaginative Beatrice was won over by Webb's intellect and reforming principles. She agreed to marry him, and he sat for a photographic portrait for her. She told him sharply that she didn't want a full-length picture as, 'It is the head only I am marrying.'

The Webbs remained happily married for over 50 years, until Beatrice's death in 1943. This was despite the fact that she found his sexual attentions distasteful. As an Emotional first and Sensual second, Webb tolerated it when they stopped having sex. Most importantly he had found his great love and Emotional soulmate.

Physical sex is important for E-Ss, but only with someone they love. If sex is denied them, they can also derive great emotional satisfaction from other aspects of their sensuality: the physical involvement with the here and now. An E-S who has been deeply hurt can sometimes pour the greater part of his or her emotions and sensuality into something other than a human being.

Lucy Irvine is an E-S of this kind. She wrote *Castaway*, based on her year surviving on the desert island of Tuin in 1981. She fell in love with Tuin in a passionate, almost sexual way, evident in her diaries. She wrote: 'The island had me like a lover ... invading me physically and mentally, claiming all my attention. I had to explore, to wander, to be naked and timeless and warm.' She stroked every rock, tree and shrub, giving herself up to every sensation. 'I will lie upside down and the sun will come right up underneath my breasts and between my toes ... I am going to commit adultery with a sunbeam ... They enter directly from above when the sun is perpendicular to the earth. You cannot deny the sun. His seduction is absolute: invasion, conquest, occupation ... it is Tuin that has entered my body.'

Lucy shared the desert island with Gerald Kingsland, whom she called 'G'. They had had to marry before the authorities would allow them to stay there alone, and G expected her to have sex with him. For most of the time she wouldn't. 'Sex was something too valuable to be misused.' With the strong Sensual component in her nature, Lucy had enjoyed sex in the past, and had lost her virginity before she was 16. When she eventually submitted to G to keep the peace, she wrote of her disappointment with the experience: 'I only wished I had never experienced the aching joy of my own body answering another's ... If only I had never known what it was to soar, to arch and ache and wing.'

Lucy expressed her sensuality in homely ways: trying to make gourmet meals from limited ingredients; and, '[G] commented that he had never met anyone who wanted to please him so much. He was referring to small everyday things, how I made every effort to ensure that his tea was not smoky, or cut him a pillow if he came with me on a walk and needed to rest *en route*, and the way I reminded him to wear his hat out fishing because I knew too much sun made him nauseous.'

In her autobiography, *Runaway*, it becomes clear why Lucy was better able to express her E-S nature with an island than a person. Passionately fixated on her friendly but cool father, her greatest love affair was with a very similar man who broke her heart. She was also violently raped when hitch-hiking in Greece. When Emotionals are too damaged, the fear of becoming involved with people outweighs the desperate yearning to be in a significant, exclusive relationship. But the emotions – and the sensuality, in the case of an E-S – must find an outlet.

More usually, of course, E-Ss derive greatest satisfaction from a close and loving relationship with good sex. Should the emotional bond weaken, however, the sex will cease to have the same satisfactory significance.

The EMOTIONAL-Imaginative (E-I)

This Sexual Style needs powerful emotions to be aroused by a partner, and these are often evoked by a stimulating mental rapport or a mutual need to offer support by talking matters through. Sex may or may not be important in the relationship — but it is certainly a less real way for the E-I to display his or her feelings. Talking together feels, ultimately, more intimate than love-making, which can be a subsidiary, if pleasurable, aspect of the relationship. Alternatively, talking *about* sex, or sharing fantasies, or being experimental together are ways that this Style marries together the aspects of his or her nature: sex then contributes to the emotional bond.

Emotionals have a need to be passionately committed in every aspect of their lives. When Imaginative is also part of their natures, they need their intellect to be involved with their emotional concerns. This often means that they make their most enduring relationships with people who share their visions and ideals.

This was the case with Marie Curie, who was jointly awarded the Nobel Prize for Physics with her husband, Pierre, in 1903, for the discovery of radioactivity.

Although Marie was Polish, they met in Paris, where she was studying at the Sorbonne. Pierre was a professor of Physics and Chemistry. When they met he was 35 and she was 27, a very pretty woman who had been disappointed in love when she was a teenager, and had been interested in nothing but science since. He had never been in love. He had not met his intellectual equal before, and he had once mourned to his diary: 'Women of genius are rare.'

Their first meeting set the stamp on their relationship: 'A conversation began between us and became friendly,' Marie wrote later. 'Its object was some questions of science upon which I was happy to ask his opinion.' Their wedding was a quick civil ceremony with no exchange of rings or celebration afterwards; the honeymoon a bicycle ride through the French countryside. They spent the time talking about Pierre's current obsession – his work on crystals. When they set up home together they refused all offers of furniture except for a bed, a large table and two chairs in which they would sit each evening facing each other working.

There was undoubtedly passion in their marriage – Pierre's letters particularly suggest their relationship was strongly physical – but the greatest bond between them was a mutual respect for each other's brilliance and a fascination for ground-breaking scientific research. They had two daughters, whom they loved. Every other detail of normal married life was unimportant to them. They cared nothing for money or any creature comforts, including food and clothes – only the excitement of their working partnership. When Marie's work on isolating radium began to show exceptional promise, Pierre gave up his own research to join her. They worked side by side for four years in a shed that was stifling in summer and icy in winter. 'It was in this miserable old shed that the best and happiest years of our life were spent, entirely consecrated to work.'

Pierre was killed in a road accident in 1906. They had been married for nearly 11 years and Marie was 38. For weeks she wrote obsessively to him: the only way she knew how to handle her grief. That this intellectual meeting of minds had produced a great love is quite evident: 'In the street I walk as if hypnotised, without attending to anything. I shall not kill myself. But among all these vehicles is there not one to make me share the fate of my beloved? ... My Pierre, I think of you without end, my head is bursting with it and my reason troubled. I do not understand that I am to live henceforth without seeing you, without smiling at the sweet companion of my life ... Yesterday at the cemetery I did not succeed in understanding the words "Pierre Curie" engraved on the stone. The beauty of the countryside hurt me, and I put down my veil.'

The E-I is often the least clingy of Emotionals. So long as they know they have a strong relationship they can tolerate some separateness. Their bond is nourished by sharing the interesting aspects of their life apart and talking them through. But the restlessness of the Imaginative can, in some E-Is, dilute the constancy of the Emotional. To put it another way, when their interest in a partner becomes less compelling it can sometimes weaken the emotional bond. It can also lead them on a search (Imaginative) for the great union they require (Emotional). The writer, Saul Bellow, who won the Nobel Prize for Literature in 1976, is one of these. His E-I nature is apparent in his work, as well as his relationships. Martin Amis nicknamed him 'Soul Bellow' in recognition of the emotional quality of his writing. In an interview he gave when he was 80 he said: 'The unexamined life is not worth living ... Writing continues to fix your mind and your heart on perennial truths and, if it's not about that, I've just wasted my time.'

Bellow had been married five times. As an Emotional he seemed impelled to act out the emotional drama of his childhood, consciously or not. He said he saw his father as 'an angel of strength, beauty and punishment'. There is nothing about love, kindness or softer feelings in this, and it is not surprising that, of his first four wives, he said: 'I chose flinty hearts — let's put it that way. I was a missionary more than a husband.'

In common with all Emotionals he was able to put up with difficult and apparently unrewarding relationships because they fitted like jigsaw pieces into his Emotional expectations: 'I think nothing but karma can explain the ridiculous and self-mutilating things that I did in the course of my life. I lived for many years with a woman who didn't really care in the slightest for me. How did I get into that and what sort of blindness was it that made it possible?' The Emotional longing for a deep soul union was there, too. 'You have a feeling that this is a woman who will meet you halfway or more and you can really have an exchange of souls with her and so on, and then you discover she has no such things in mind — at least not for you. The fact that I married women rather than having affairs with them meant that I had in mind a permanent solution to life's most important questions. I was in earnest and kept on being in earnest, believing that you could soften even the flintiest of hearts.' One of his relationships lasted nearly 20 years, another 13. Even so, the Imaginative in him was the driving force to continue the search to resolve the childhood pattern he was reproducing with his wives. In his last marriage, to Janis, aged 36 at the time of the interview, he seemed to have found the compassion and the soft heart he was looking for, as she nursed him devotedly through a difficult illness.

When the E-I finds the emotional soulmate the intellectual considerations matter less. Even the most exciting and mentally stimulating companion will not gain the E-I's affections, however, unless the deeper emotional chord is struck.

The EMOTIONAL-Romantic (E-R)

Whenever Emotional meets Romantic in combination there is a quality of passionate openness in emotional expression. These are the Emotionals most likely to let the world know what they feel, be it love, anger or resentment. In love relationships, the channel to their deepest feelings is opened by a glamorous figure they can admire intensely, or a relationship with someone who puts them on a pedestal. These refined, other-worldly feelings can sometimes make the physical expression of love through sex seem coarse. For this reason, this is the Style that can form an attachment that is never consummated or reciprocated. It can also result in a person whose Romantic expectations are constantly spoilt by darker Emotional impulses. In rare cases they revenge themselves on members of the opposite sex by putting out romantic lures and then taking the initiative to break the captive's heart before their own is broken. More often, however, it means that for the E-R significant and enduring emotions are evoked by a relationship that seems special in some way, or that has fairy-tale connotations.

There is usually a crucial element of power play in the relationships Emotionals make. In some cases it is wholly benign: the 'powerful' partner draws great satisfaction from cherishing and looking after the weaker one. With E-Rs this power balance is often expressed in an excess of admiration. Either the adored or the adoring, the E-R knows that one of them holds the key to the other's happiness or despair. Inevitably this sometimes results in painful dependency. In these cases E-Rs can tolerate behaviour that other people might find difficult to handle. When their Emotional pattern is to derive deep, if uncomfortable, satisfaction from emotional pain, the very difficulties can enhance the commitment.

Katherine Hepburn was an example of a female E-R. One commentator succinctly dismissed her three main romantic involvements with terse judgements: the psychopath (Howard Hughes), the bully (John Ford) and the hopeless drunk (Spencer Tracy). Whenever a person has a history of damaging involvements they are usually Emotionals who are magnetically attracted to people who inflict the pain they hate yet crave.

Hepburn chased all three of these men, none of whom could, or would, marry her. Her affairs with them had to be secret. Romantics often find that difficulties about meeting and physical distance keep romantic feelings simmering, and for an E-R this can strengthen the bond.

Hepburn's relationship with Tracy lasted 25 years until he died in 1967. Their first meeting set the tone of their relationship. They were introduced by Joseph Mankiewicz. Hepburn sized up this new man and said: 'Mr Tracy, I think you're a little short for me.' 'Don't worry,' laughed Mankiewicz, 'he'll cut you down to size.' Afterwards Tracy said: 'I don't want to get mixed up in anything with this woman.'

Despite the fact that Spencer Tracy treated her with irritable contempt much of the time, Hepburn would do anything for him, and admired him intensely. 'Isn't he great?' she would say; or, 'He's formidable!' or, 'He's an actor's actor.' The treatment meted out to her only served to increase her devotion. It is an interesting insight into her feelings about herself that she used to shower as often as six times a day.

Beauty and aesthetic considerations are often important to the E-R. When this person's emotional needs are healthier and happier he or she can form a lasting attachment that is serene and loving, and with an elegance of lifestyle and manners that is enviable. The Romantic element can also lighten the Emotional's propensity to become engulfed in fears or dark moods from time to time. The excitement of infatuation can burn off sombreness, though it may still be lurking. The words in Irving Berlin's song capture the essence of the the E-R: 'There may be trouble ahead,/But while there's moonlight and music and love and romance/Let's face the music and dance.'

The Romantic element, however, can make this Emotional less steadfast in relationships, though more devoted and committed than the reverse Style, the ROMANTIC-Emotional. When mutual, or one-way, admiration is essential to meet their deeper emotional requirements, then the loss of this can make them feel so desperate that they have to leave the relationship.

Rudolph Valentino, one of the first great lovers of the screen, was an E-R. He was born in Italy in 1895, and went to America aged 18 to make his career. He could operate perfectly well sexually, but sex was not a motivating force for him, neither was it important in his love-life. Indeed, one of his first jobs, aged 20, was as professional companion, or 'walker' for rich women, and he soon found it more financially lucrative to be a fully-fledged gigolo, offering sexual services, which he called 'love-breaks'. Emotionally, however, he was drawn to dominant, controlling women. He seemed to prefer these relationships not to be sexual, but to evoke an enduring admiration and respect: 'A man may admire a woman without desiring her. He may respect the brilliance of her mind – even the beauty of her body.'

Not much is known about Valentino's relationship with his mother, but it is significant that he married his first wife shortly after his mother died – and within days of meeting her. She was a lesbian, and an aspiring starlet, and she quickly left him to return to her girlfriend. When he had his first big break in the movies soon after, she filed a divorce suit against him for desertion and demanded maintenance. Meanwhile he had fallen in love with the set designer Natacha Rambova: 'I saw before me no ordinary woman, but rather the reincarnation of some mighty goddess of the past.' Their relationship was virtually sexless. He revered her, and she took him under her wing, like a mother. Indeed, she took control of his career, and helped steer him to even greater success, fighting studios on his behalf. Significantly, Valentino wore a platinum slave bracelet that she had designed for him.

Rambova's interference in Valentino's career made him unpopular with the studios. As his star rose, his unquestioning admiration for her also began to slip. She was outraged when he signed a contract with United Artists that had a clause stipulating that she was no longer to have any official connection with his movies. It was a tacit admission that, for him, she had fallen from her pedestal, and so no longer had her great emotional hold over him. They were divorced in 1926, when he was 30, and he died of a ruptured appendix less than a year later.

As an Emotional first, if Valentino had lived he would likely have formed a more lasting relationship in time. If romance should evaporate, E-Rs will often find that the relationship has taken root in their hearts, and that there are now more important reasons for staying together. When the feelings aroused are sufficiently deep the attachment can continue. There might be great regret for the passing of the more exciting qualities in the relationship, but E-Rs often find that, even so, their commitment holds firm.

Combinations of three or four

It is rare to have a genuinely equal balance of Sexual Styles. One will be dominant — in these cases Emotional — and the remaining two or three are also unlikely to be found in equal measure. In most cases one of them will combine most strongly with the main Emotional Style (in the ways described above) and the third and possibly fourth will add colour and subtlety, but little more. Most usually, aspects of the weaker Styles will be noticeable in other aspects of your personality — your attitude to clothes, career, loved ones other than partners, and so on. The following descriptions are therefore only broad guidelines to the possible ways the Styles can coexist.

The EMOTIONAL-Sensual-Imaginative (E-S-I)

Deep feelings are aroused in this Emotional type by relationships that are physically and intellectually satisfying. The Emotional-Sensual is usually a very constant combination, unless this person has had difficulties in the past which have distorted the capacity to make lasting relationships. Adding Imaginative to the mix militates against the deep quiet contentment that Emotionals can derive from partnerships. They need to be more compellingly interested, to have more variety in their lives (often sexually as well), and for communication that is verbal as well as instinctive. When this Emotional has been damaged, however, the injection of Imaginative can increase the desire to flee from close involvements that can cause pain.

On the other hand, the Imaginative element can also make them more comprehensible to their partners. Instead of keeping their feelings to themselves, they are more able to express what they are privately experiencing. Indeed, they may have a need to talk things through. Sometimes in this combination sexual variety (Imaginative) and intensity (Sensual) are the route to the E-S-I's most important feelings. With a partner whose predilections match they feel they have come home.

Usually when E-S-Is find a partner with whom they are sexually and intellectually compatible, they take them into their hearts. The transforming nature of the bond this compatibility generates can lead to profound emotions that can endure even after the other elements have long since weakened. These E-S-Is then feel fully committed to partners who have become less compellingly interesting, and with whom sex, perhaps, has ceased to be so satisfying — although the relationship will feel less rewarding. If the deeper emotions are not touched, however, then sex and good conversation are not enough to make this person feel that the relationship is worthwhile.

The EMOTIONAL-Sensual-Romantic (E-S-R)

The feeling nature of this Sexual Style responds best to physical passion within a romanticised relationship. Whenever Romantic combines with Emotional there is more ready access to feelings, or they are more obvious to others. With an addition of Sensual this person has a need to show love through sex.

Because there is a Romantic demand for admiration to be present in the relationship, or for more obvious displays of love, however, the E-S-R can be more unpredictable than the pure EMOTIONAL-Sensual. Even strong sexual desire can be sublimated when the emotional atmosphere of the relationship ceases to be so romantically gratifying.

The E-S-R tends to gloominess. Sensuals have a leaning towards depression, and Romantic demands are the most ephemeral and unstable elements in any relationship. As the E-S-R has a longing for romance in some form, when this requirement is not met life can seem somewhat barren. The deep feeling nature of the Emotional takes this very hard.

Emotionals always find the end of a relationship traumatic, and can take a long time to recover from the feelings of failure and loneliness this prompts. But if the Romantic element is strong in the E-S-R's nature then there is a compelling desire to find the partner who will activate these necessary feelings, and the search will be on.

At best, however, E-S-Rs can be sensual and delightful companions, who feel profoundly committed to partners who bring some glamour and an earthy interest in sex to the relationship. If the sex wanes and the romance goes, inevitably the E-S-R will feel disappointed or depressed, but the relationship can still survive if this person continues to feel emotionally moved by the partner. These are people who are usually happiest in the first years of a relationship, but who have the grit to see it out despite disappointment or unhappiness.

The EMOTIONAL-Imaginative-Romantic (E-I-R)

Passionate attachments can be formed by this style, even when the physical side is insubstantial, so long as there is interest, excitement and the heightened emotions of new love. But these very elements make this the least predictable of Emotionals. The E-I-Rs are people whose own impulses cause them to suffer. The intense Emotional need to bond is here complicated by the capricious demands of the Imaginative-Romantic combination whose requirements in tandem attract this Emotional to relationships that are inherently volatile.

Sometimes this combination derives profoundest satisfaction from a 'relationship' that is quite distant or never consummated. Lively interaction, compelling conversations, and the intoxication of 'what could be' fantasy answers a deep need in them, which fixates them on this elusive person. For this type, a conventional relationship can never be quite so satisfying.

Usually, however, the E-I-R will be attracted to good-looking and interesting people, who enjoy fun and open communication, and with whom they can have a proper relationship. Over time, the relationship will only last, however, if more profound emotions have been touched — and in that case the excitement and intoxicating feelings can disappear without affecting the importance of the relationship. Nevertheless the silent empathy which is usually so satisfying to the Emotional is less fulfilling for the E-I-R, who can feel lonely when the more thrilling elements of the relationship have disappeared. If the loneliness is acute, then the Romantic and Imaginative in their natures will make them feel it is necessary to find someone new. As Emotionals, however, they are more likely to stay in a relationship that has ceased to be fully satisfying because of their deeper need to be in an exclusive relationship.

The EMOTIONAL-Sensual-Imaginative-Romantic (E-S-I-R)

Emotionals need above all a soulmate with whom they can spend the rest of their lives. Not surprisingly they long for a relationship that has the elements that can satisfy them profoundly at all levels — intellectual, sexual and romantic. In reality, as with most people, once in a partnership they find that some elements are more important to them and, indeed, they don't notice, or don't mind, the lack of others.

At the extreme, this Emotional is so choosy that he or she never ventures into the arena of relationships at all. Usually it is a person who has experienced great pain or rejection in early life, and rather than risk being deeply hurt by becoming involved with the wrong person, these E-S-I-Rs prefer the satisfying (to them) pain of loneliness rather than compromise their ideals. The obsessive, which always lurks in the Emotional nature, is expressed in a lofty dismissal of fallible humanity. This person, instead, will bury him or herself in an all-consuming passion for work or an abstract cause.

Like the Sensual who is highly demanding about partners, however, E-S-I-Rs are more likely than most to make a lasting relationship which seems to meet all their requirements. The Emotionals' steadfastness when feeling deeply allows these people to tolerate periodic disappointments in areas of the relationship. Over time they can look back and see that they truly have 'had it all'. Even when this is not so, however, Emotionals who find a partner who seems to offer all the elements at the beginning of a relationship can find their hearts open to a great love. In this case, the emotional impact is so great that it can outlast disillusionment in almost every area, so long as the partner continues to make this Emotional type feel deeply.

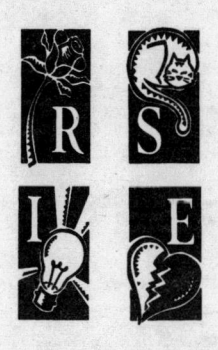

Sexual Styles in Relationships

Sexual Styles in Relationships

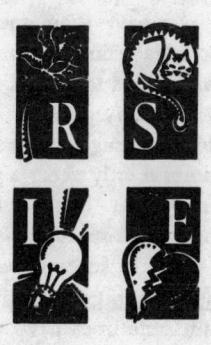

This section looks at the relationships that the various Sexual Styles make with each other. Once you have identified your dominant Style, and your partner's, you can read on to find out what makes the relationship work best, and what the potential difficulties might be. If you have a strong subsidiary Style, it is worth looking at the relationships for that one too, so that you can complete a more rounded picture.

Remember that it is your *Sexual* Style that determines the pleasures and dissatisfactions in your relationship. While you may have elements of the other Styles in your personality, it is the one that most closely reflects your attitude to love, sex, and long-term partnerships that will ultimately have an impact on the relationships you make. While these guidelines can tell you a lot about flings, short relationships, and the early days of love, they are most reliable for relationships that last many years. Your Sexual Style becomes most apparent when you have experienced the ups and downs of relationship life: faced problems and life-changing experiences together. It will then become clearer what the most pressing needs that you have are, in emotional and sexual terms. These will determine how you feel about your partnership, and whether you want, or are able, to continue living together. As you will see, all these relationship combinations have their good points – and their drawbacks. There is no 'ideal' combination that is problem-free. It is the nature of relationships to have difficulties, particularly relationships that last for many years.

Each section includes some suggestions for negotiating Stylistic differences. Sometimes it only needs a proper understanding of what makes your partner tick to find a way through difficulties that seemed insurmountable. The give and take that all relationships need to succeed becomes more possible when there is a mutual recognition of differing needs, and the resolution of these can sometimes pave the way for a deeper and more enduring love.

The Romantic Man and Woman

'I knew it was love, and I felt it was glory.'

Lord Byron

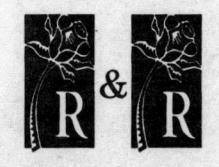

The Romantic Man
and Woman

They know they were made for each other, sometimes from the moment they meet. One of the reasons Romantics trust in love at first sight is because the visual is so important to them. Seeing a beautiful person across a crowded room awakens awe as much as lust. Actually, although Romantics prize beauty, their definition of it can also be quite wide. An exceptionally stylish person; someone with chic; presence; the aura of greatness; the glamour of fame; exceptional charisma — all of these touch the Romantic's impressionable heart.

Romantics know themselves to be blessed by the gods, and although there is a gracious element of *noblesse oblige* in their characters, they don't really want to spend too much time with lesser mortals. The Romantic at a party searches the room for kindred spirits: other special, superior beings who stand out. The Romantic flirts quite charmingly and intensely with everyone, but will also be looking over each person's shoulder for the better option — or the shining stranger. The Romantic trusts the instinct that signals the presence of this dream creature. 'I felt him standing behind me before I'd even seen him'; 'When I heard her name — even before we met — I knew she was the one.' The Romantic's antennae are always at full stretch, quivering to catch an answering vibration from another Romantic.

When the attraction is mutual the courtship is magic. No one is more spell-binding than the Romantic who is in love and who wants to be loved in return. The Romantic man and woman seek to entrance each other, using every formidable wile in their repertoire. Everyone enjoys being in love, but it is when Romantics feel most themselves. They glow; they are quicker, lighter, nicer, cleverer, better-looking and at their most alluring. They love themselves like this, and they love the people who make them feel like it. They love life illuminated in this way and their happiness attracts others to them.

The beginning

Young Romantics in love can live on air, and their dreams. They derive a great, if narcissistic, pleasure from each other's company. They see an ideal, perfect person, and in that person's eyes is a flattering reflection of themselves, equally perfect. What more do they need? They certainly don't need other people, nor money, nor even any other excitement beyond what they find in each other. Nothing else *is* so exciting. Should they go out in company they find it hard to pay attention to anyone else. They are the couple canoodling in a corner, or laughing at each other's jokes, or talking together as spiritedly and intensely as if they had just met.

They are happiest when it is just the two of them. They spend long, lazy evenings together, making love, or talking by the fire – deeply delighted by the simplest pleasures. These are pleasures that all new lovers cherish – often poignantly, because they feel it is a golden moment in time, which will eventually become just a distant, treasured memory. Not so the Romantics. They are agreed that their love is transcendent, that it will continue to be special and glorious. It makes them feel powerful. They talk about what they will do and achieve. They can enjoy the cheap wine and the inexpensive takeaway, because they know that before long it will be transformed into champagne and caviar.

This love feels grand and generous, because all they demand

is each other's presence. The Romantic woman doesn't need flowers and scent, she just wants his love and his attention. The Romantic man asks nothing of her except to be what she is and to show that she adores him for himself. The fly in the ointment is their jealousy. When they are apart they find it hard to believe that someone else is not going to try to deprive them of their prize. Who wouldn't want this sensational person? Even when they are together they find it hard to bear their Romantic partners bestowing attention on anyone else, even a friend of the same sex. Sometimes this jealousy translates into emotional scenes, accompanied by trembling anger or tears. But these serve to fuel their love rather than dampen it. It shows how much they matter to each other, and the making up is very sweet.

Settling down

When love of this order strikes them they will usually make a commitment very quickly. This is the couple who can agree to marry within weeks — or even days — of first meeting. They believe that the strength of their feelings is a sign of permanence. Even if they don't marry immediately, or at all, they know themselves to be a united couple. It takes hardly any time for them to drop 'I' from their vocabulary and replace it with 'we'.

Now comes the hard part. Those feelings don't last — or, at least, they change. Speeded up responses slow down; they become more used to each other; they start to see faults in this wonderful person and are faced with the unpleasant knowledge that their lover doesn't think they are perfect any more either. How long it takes for this to happen varies from couple to couple and from Romantic to Romantic. Sometimes it can be many months — even years, especially if they haven't been together as much as they would wish.

This is a critical stage for any Romantic couple, and how they handle it determines whether this relationship can last or will end abruptly. To give them their due, they have been duped into believing that romance can last by their favourite films, books and songs. They didn't take much persuading however. The beginning of love is beautiful and exciting for everyone, but for Romantics the message that it can last is particularly seductive because it is what they want to believe.

There are many disappointments connected to the passing of the first flush of romance. One of these is that for the romantic temperature in a relationship to remain compellingly high efforts have to be made to keep it that way. Now it *does* matter whether the Romantic man brings little presents, writes ardent postcards or proves himself to be not just a dreamer but an action man. The Romantic woman, too, can't just get by on being delightful: she must show her admiration more clearly, curb any little irritating habits, be careful not to shine too brightly in case she outshines him.

Previously their relationship felt so wonderfully intimate simply because they were together, lovingly, so much. In fact, there was often precious little intimacy in the real meaning of the word. They both saw what they wanted to see, and hid what they didn't want to have discovered. They don't really know each other that well. What they have connected to is the image – and although image is very important to the Romantic, it is far from being the whole person, or even the truth. Sometimes in the chilly dawn following the honeymoon one or both of them finds that the strong feelings have mysteriously evaporated. When this is the case they feel appalled consternation, and can exit from the relationship with the cool efficiency more associated with the Imaginative.

I heard of a couple like this from a counsellor. It took six years for Celia and Edward to arrive at this point of disaffection – and then it was as if those six years of married life had never happened. Their marriage was flamboyantly romantic. When they were apart they spoke several times on the telephone every day. They would leave each other love-notes, hidden in briefcases and coat pockets. They bought each other little presents. Celia would rush home from work before Edward to prepare stunningly elegant dinners and would change for the evening into something glamorous and sexy. One day Edward announced that he had met someone else – and he moved out within an hour. Shortly afterwards he sent Celia two copies of a solicitor's letter listing their possessions with suggestions on how they should be divided. He asked her to sign both copies and return one to him. In one of their last conversations before Edward moved out he had told Celia that she was the sexiest woman alive and that he couldn't imagine life without her.

Celia saw the counsellor on her own, attempting to make sense of what had happened. She began to see that once the genuine romance had gone out of their relationship they had begun to pretend. Rather than face the disappointment they felt when the glorious feelings had gone, or use the new phase to build a more maturely loving relationship, they had tried to prolong the romance. Celia played at being the sexy, happy, perfect woman, when inside she felt inadequate, and scared that if she dropped the act he wouldn't love her any more. She deduced it must have been the same for Edward. He played the ardent suitor because it was what he wanted to be. When he re-experienced the feelings with a new woman he didn't have to pretend anymore. Celia had to face the fact that they never really knew each other and that the love between them had been superficial, a mirage.

Fortunately it doesn't have to be as grave as this for the Romantic couple. There is nothing wrong with them wanting to prolong the romance – indeed, for them to be happy it is best if they do. But if they concentrate on this to the exclusion of the less exciting but more enduring elements of love then they create an illusion rather than a relationship.

The greatest challenge in the Romantic partnership is to balance the romantic excitement with a developing intimacy. It is a delicate balancing act. Romantics don't like too much intimacy in the way that other Styles might define it – certainly not the 'warts and all' aspect, which comes with being open and honest, and knowing your partner as thoroughly as you know yourself. Ms Romantic doesn't want to have to be faced with Mr Romantic's fears and weaknesses or lack of talent, for instance. To love him as she needs often involves pretending that these aspects don't exist. Mr Romantic doesn't want to have to recognise that his Romantic woman has disagreeable qualities as well as charm, or that she has pressing needs that conflict with his own. Neither do either of them like facing up to their own less lovely sides. The insecurity that lurks in the recesses of the Romantic makes it uncomfortable for them to acknowledge anything they suspect would make them unlovable. With another Romantic, indeed, they may be right. Their similarity in this respect reinforces their natural inclination towards a certain amount of secrecy and denial. It is often, indeed, why Romantics bloom in relationships with a less perfect match of temperament. Sensuals and Emotionals, for instance, can see the faults and love the Romantic anyway. This balancing act is made more difficult because although they long for constant togetherness when they are in love, this love is actually prolonged when there is more distance between them. More experienced Romantics know this. 'It's terrible – I can only see my girlfriend one night a week!' a Romantic man complained to me. When I asked why, he said: 'If I see her more often it won't be so special.' He had had a difficult day, and was in a bad mood. 'Anyway,' he reflected, 'I don't want her to see me like this. She wouldn't be very pleased. It's better for both of us if I'm feeling happy and full of energy.'

The best chance that this couple has of letting each other into their own private worlds, and learning to accept and love each other's foibles comes early on in the relationship. In the glow of intoxication, even undesirable aspects in each other's natures appear endearing and acceptance is easier. When the excited high of first love wears off, therefore, there is still the disappointment but also a closeness that gives the relationship more staying power.

Another uniting factor is the home and lifestyle they create together. When love is no longer the be-all and end-all, Romantics find that they are more fastidious and acquisitive than they had suspected of themselves. They need elegance, quality, and beauty all around them. They want the best clothes, the best food, the finest wines. They want other people to be able to *see* how special, important and valuable they are. This is a great leap from the days when 'things' and other people didn't matter; when Ms Romantic could make herself look glamorous in thrift-shop clothes, and Mr Romantic was happy to make one beer last for the entire evening while he talked about the next acting role he was up for, or the poems he wrote in the small hours, or the radical changes he would make in his company when he became managing director.

Romantics who can achieve their goals and make the money that buys them the accoutrements of success can make more stable relationships. Too much struggle, particularly when their relationship has become less exciting and compelling, kills their finer feelings. On the other hand, romantic energies that are no longer diverted towards each other can be reinvested in practical ways. Romantics look for romance in every area of life, and consequently they often find it. They can feel somewhat compensated for the loss of heightened love feelings by a beautiful home and family, or a glittering career.

Daily life

Next to being madly in love, Romantics want excitement, fun, and pleasure. There is a drive to be happy in their natures, and two Romantics together reinforce this in each other. No couple is better able to make the mundane special, or to discover excitement in the most ordinary occurrences. The most contented Romantic couple, therefore, routinely put effort and thought into how they can enjoy themselves and by doing so they prolong the liveliness in the relationship that is so important to them. At home, they amuse and interest each other with diverting conversation. They like this spirited side of themselves, and enjoy displaying it. Well-disposed Romantics can be as charming and winning towards each other as they are with strangers. They save witty anecdotes to tell each other; take note of a fascinating news item to discuss. They also make efforts to create a special atmosphere in the home — particularly the Romantic woman: lovely flowers, good music, well-prepared food. This couple is unlikely to sit in front of the television with a tray on their knees.

They also both need something to look forward to. Happy Romantics make plans together: where they are going to go during the week; what they are going to do for their holidays. A corner of their lives must have magic in it, and anticipation often provides it.

All this is when things are going well, however. When they are not, the atmosphere can be just as intense, but more acrimonious. A peaceful evening is a boring evening as far as Romantics are concerned, and they'd rather argue than feel ignored. Indeed, there must be some sort of passion in their relationship for them to believe it is worth sustaining. At least when they are in the middle of a tempestuous row they are having some impact on each other. Some Romantic couples, indeed, have long-lasting relationships that are very stormy. The fearful elation and the adrenalin rush it creates is quite addictive. It is also close physiologically to happier passion and so can lead naturally into love-making of the kind that Romantics like best — arising spontaneously from strong feelings. These stormy episodes are less wearing emotionally to Romantics than they are to other people. Their ability to let out their strong emotions as they feel them often means that they pass without ill-effect. Romantics, anyway, don't want to dwell on anger or misery. They want to be happy again, and they look for something that will make them so.

More dangerous than conflict is a daily routine that leaves them estranged. Romantics actively enjoy time alone when the reunions are happy and loving or even negatively highly-charged — but not when they are detached. This can happen when the Romantic man looks for his thrills outside the home. It doesn't mean that he has affairs, necessarily, but that he derives the romance he needs from his work, or he seeks fun and adventure in other activities. While Ms Romantic will always look to her relationship first for romance, and will try to keep it romantic, Mr Romantic is often motivated to search more widely. Neither does he usually want to make an effort. If what he needs is not immediately available he'd prefer to find it ready-made than work on it. The problems are self-evident. The Romantic man so disposed is more likely to prefer to find another woman with whom he can fall effortlessly in love. The Romantic woman may do the same. If she's too neglected, indeed, a love-affair is the best way she knows to restore her self-esteem.

Communication between the Romantic couple

The Romantic couple are best at communicating happy and loving feelings to each other — better in fact than anyone else. Love makes them articulate; they like to share happiness, and enjoy themselves even more when they are doing so, and talking about it.

Communication is more of a problem for them when they are feeling unhappy generally, and certainly when their relationship is not going well. Everyone finds this difficult, but for them, it is harder than most. They don't like to examine unhappiness, they prefer to chase it away. Talking about it can seem frightening, useless or self-indulgent.

It is particularly hard when one of them is suffering and the other isn't. One reason is that Romantics find other people's misery somewhat irritating. They do their best to cheer someone up, but if their best is not good enough they can feel offended as well as alarmed. Another reason is that Romantics find it hard to empathise with another person's feelings when they are very different from their own. A happy Romantic quite literally can't understand why everyone else isn't feeling as happy as she or he is. Secretly, Romantics believe that no one feels as strongly as they do – even another Romantic – and that no one's feelings are quite so important. The happy Romantic can't conceive that his or her partner's feelings wouldn't go away if enough effort were made; the unhappy Romantic feels that no one else has known such intense suffering. This is not a good recipe for sharing and dealing with the feelings together.

It is even harder when their partners and their relationship are the causes of the problem. A Romantic who doesn't feel loved enough doesn't have the incentive to talk about it. Pride is one reason. Another is that having to ask for what he or she needs spoils the spontaneity that Romantics value so highly. A further reason is that a very disappointed Romantic is tempted to find what is missing with another person.

Whether the Romantic couple tackle this fundamental problem or not depends almost exclusively on how motivated they are. A young Romantic couple who believe in the existence of a perfect relationship are likely to decide that something is seriously wrong when difficulties arise. A more mature Romantic couple may still *want* to believe that a relationship without problems exists, but experience has taught them that this is not so. One failed relationship too many can bring them to the point where they are prepared to try to find solutions. Romantics who don't do this are likely to end up alone. In *The Relate Guide to Starting Again* I wrote about Karen, a Romantic woman. She had been married three times to Romantic men, and in each case she had a child by them. All these marriages broke up within a year of the baby being born. She came for counselling because she was in a fourth relationship that was in the process of collapsing.

The counsellor discovered that Karen's relationships with the men had started by being intense and exclusive. They had been totally wrapped up in each other and felt that nothing – and no one – else mattered. In each case this changed when Karen had a baby. For a while *this* was her most important relationship. The men couldn't take the 'betrayal', and left. She had not had a child by her current lover, but the honeymoon period had passed and he now resented any attention she paid to her children. Actually, Karen revealed to the counsellor, she too felt that something had gone drastically wrong when she no longer felt that the man was number one in her life. The counsellor had hoped that if Karen could understand that a relationship could be satisfying even when it wasn't emotionally exclusive, she would have a better chance of making a lasting relationship in the future. As it was, after the 'honeymoon' period of counselling was over Karen announced that she wouldn't be coming any more. Her live-in lover left her at the same time. At the end of counselling Karen still hoped that she would eventually meet the man with whom she could say, 'we are everything to each other'.

Karen's resistance to counselling shows just how difficult it can be for Romantics to deal with these issues. If they don't cope with difficulties it drives them apart, yet when they try to find solutions they can find that the uncomfortable process makes them both less loving. Again, this is why Romantics can often make relationships that are more rewarding in the long-term with partners of a different Sexual Style.

Unless they also have a strong dose of Sensual, Emotional or even Imaginative in their natures, too much intimate examination of themselves and their relationship is not going to be as helpful for them as it is for other people. Although this goes against the spirit of counselling, in which I truly believe, they are sometimes better pursuing other tactics. Their best chance is to put their main efforts into strengthening what they perceive to be good about the relationship. The more that they can enjoy and share, the better. When Romantics have more in common than their Sexual Style, indeed, their relationship can be happy and worthwhile even if it is low on intimacy. Accentuating the positive can make the occasional difficult interludes less distressing. Fortunately, this suits their temperaments well. If any people can build a relationship that relies on fun and enjoyment, this couple can.

Sex in the Romantic partnership

As you would expect, the Romantic couple need sex to be romantic too. They want to ache with lust, so that they are swept up into love-making that is too passionate to resist. They know exactly what this feels like, because they experienced it at the beginning of their relationship. All being well, they had the most beautiful sexual experiences of their lives when they were first madly in love, and they long to recreate those rapturous feelings of spiralling excitement, spontaneity and glorious abandonment.

But they can't. Like everything that they treasure most about love and relationships this aspect changes too. It's impossible to feel sick with desire for the person you sleep next to every night and see every day of your life. Neither are Romantics especially interested in ways of making sex better and more interesting, or in starting love-making from 'cold' – bringing on desire by caressing each other and awakening sexy feelings through touch. They want the feelings first. And when the first passionate phase of the relationship is passed these feelings are often aroused in other ways – through anger and reconciliation perhaps, or, dangerously, through making each other jealous. Sometimes these feelings can be artificially manufactured through seeing a passionate or romantic movie, play or opera together. They are both very sentimental and susceptible to having their emotions touched by drama, and the tide of tenderness or excitement can carry them through to the bedroom.

Because sex follows strong feelings, however, the strength of their sex drives is almost irrelevant to the amount of sex they have. A sexy Romantic woman will avoid sex with her Romantic partner if they are having problems, while still wishing that she could be satisfied. A Romantic man who needs a lot of sex might still have sex with Ms Romantic, even if he is disappointed with her, but he will consider it a second-rate experience and not trouble himself to take much time over it. Either will be vulnerable to the sexual attentions of someone new – particularly if they are feeling unloved, undervalued, or missing the excitement of infatuated love.

Nevertheless, because they feel the same about what makes sex good, love-making can be very fulfilling for them. They like the build-up. Going out for a romantic meal, when they are both dressed up and on their best behaviour can be erotic for them; equally so can an amble together, holding hands and talking. Gentle lighting, soft or emotional music, loving chit-chat – all this can put them in the right mood. They like their partners to be clean and look good, and they are fastidious themselves. The Romantic woman quite understands that her partner may not fancy her if she is wearing any old thing, and her hair and her teeth are unbrushed. She'll lounge around in something that makes her look good – elegant or sexy; check that her make-up is OK, discreetly dab on some of his favourite scent. Mr Romantic will shower before he makes any advances, shave off his five o'clock shadow, spray on some aftershave and check whether his breath is smelling. Actually, both of them feel more in the mood for sex when they can look in the mirror and say: 'You look wonderful!'

On the whole, Romantics like to be 'good' at sex, and set out to please as much as to be pleased. Sophisticated and sexually interested Romantics of either sex can be superb lovers, even more concerned about giving pleasure than they are in taking it for themselves. Whether sex is important to them or not, however, they like it to be somewhat elegant and not too animal. They like their partners to look good, and to look good themselves, while they are making love.

The exception to this happens when the Romantic man has separated his sexual feelings from love, which is sometimes the case. This type of man often finds nothing beautiful in sex, and prefers not to have to sully his love for his partner in this way more than he has to. He is unlikely to have developed his sexual repertoire for this reason, and either tries to subdue his sexual urges or is occasionally unfaithful with women he cannot respect. Surprisingly enough, this often suits Ms Romantic, even if she needs more sex herself. If she has to make the choice she would always prefer to be cherished and made to feel loved than to have her desires satisfied. This kind of Romantic man is often the most ardently and openly romantic of them all, and shows his love in the ways that gladden the heart of the Romantic woman.

Ms Romantic who, for her own reasons, finds sex distasteful can also appeal to the Romantic man. It suits his sense of how men and women should be when he is the most desirous partner. He feels strong and virile. His romantic feelings are often excited by some reluctance from his woman, and so long as she doesn't make him feel coarse or unattractive he can often put up with less sex than he needs. Romantics can live quite happily in virtually sexless relationships, so long as they are admiring and loving.

The difficulty for both of them is the value they place on physical appearance. They find it hard to feel desire for a partner who is looking less good or is in poor physical shape. The Romantic woman can rationalise this better than the Romantic man. So long as he smells and feels nice, she is prepared to shut her eyes and go along with it – especially if he makes her feel beautiful and desired. The Romantic man can be more particular. If his woman no longer looks attractive to him he can feel that it is his right to look elsewhere. The Romantic man tends to see himself as young whatever his age, and can feel that he needs a partner to match. Nonetheless, the Romantic woman is the most artful of all the Sexual styles when it comes to keeping her looks, and appearing youthfully alluring whatever her age. She doesn't mind if it means hard work or expense either. She does it as much for herself as for her lover. Her standards are so high that if she is satisfied with her own reflection in the mirror, it's a fairly safe bet that he will be more than satisfied as well.

Long-term prospects

On the face of it, the long-term prospects of a Romantic union are not especially good. Feeling happy and in love is so important to them, and yet so hard to sustain. They 'only' want to be happy, they say. Is that too much to ask? Nevertheless, Romantic partnerships can and do stand the test of time, so long as other elements are there.

As has been seen, Romantics are more committed to staying together when they have enough money and success to create the life of which they have dreamed. They like to feel superior; humility is an uncomfortable emotion for them. That is why it is so important for Romantics to create a glamorous and enviable lifestyle, and why they may be prepared to put up with some disappointments rather than lose it. Both the man and the woman of this Style can draw comfort from a marriage and a situation that is enviable to outsiders, even if the reality is not quite what it seems. Ms Romantic will forgive Mr Romantic a lot if he is successful, and seen to be so; Mr Romantic can feel the same — and he also continues to value his Romantic woman if she looks good and dresses better than other women in their circle. There is always the possibility that one of them will fall in love with someone else and therefore give up what they prize so highly, but they are less likely to be looking to do so if they have realised their dreams together.

For Mr and Ms Romantic need to realise their dreams. There comes a time for both of them when excited speculation about the future must bear fruit. Ms Romantic, especially, usually needs to feel that her Romantic man is fulfilling his promise. She is often as attracted by his potential greatness as she is by his devastating sex appeal. Some Romantic women like to be on a pedestal themselves, and to attract subservient admirers. When Ms Romantic is drawn to Mr Romantic, however, she is often looking for someone who can live out her dreams for her. Whether she is successful or ambitious herself or not, she prefers to be able to admire her man. If Mr Romantic proves to have been all talk with little follow-through it is hard for her to believe that their love is worthwhile. This kind of Romantic woman is prepared to put up with a certain amount of hardship – even be the main financial support – so long as she is convinced that it is temporary. As a way of life it has less appeal – she needs, above all, to feel feminine. She doesn't want to have to nurture like a mother or provide like a man. Eventually she has to be cared for and indulged.

Mr Romantic can have a similar tendency. Some Romantic men want to be allowed to be the little boy for life, or to fixate on a powerful, iconic woman whom they can look up to and adore. This kind of Romantic man is less likely to fall for a Romantic woman. When Mr Romantic is drawn to Ms Romantic it is because he is looking for the incarnation of femininity – and, by his definition, it means that he must be the object of her worship. Or, to put it another way, with her esteem and devotion he can rise to great heights for both their sakes. In this case he wants her to be beautiful, special and loving, but not a threat. When he does what he sets out to do, this can be very satisfying for them both. But if she needs more for herself it can prove difficult.

A couple I know lived this pattern. Andy fell in love with

Nadine, a proud, stunning-looking single mother, whose other Romantic relationships had proved short-lived and disastrous. She was, in some ways, the trophy wife that most Romantic men want – she was chic and exotic and had great wit and charm. She was also damaged by disappointed love, and consequently fearful and insecure. She made Andy feel strong, masculine and pleased with himself. Her bad experiences of love had also put her off sex. Andy did not have a particularly strong sex drive, and, anyway, Romantic men sometimes find that their love increases when desire is not easily satisfied. He was happy to be fairly undemanding sexually because romantically it was so right. In common with many Romantic men Andy was also jealous and possessive. Nadine was most able to be open-hearted with other women and, indeed, often had sexless crushes on them. Andy resented these women friends more than he minded men who paid court to Nadine – sexually he felt safe because her interest in sex was so low. This marriage lasted happily for five years, but then it started to go wrong.

Nadine had never fallen wildly in love with Andy, but she did admire him. She made the compromise that some Romantic women do: she traded love for elegant security and the opportunity to look up to a successful man. Andy was a highly-paid, creative man. He rescued her from financial distress and gave her opulent comfort. Nadine flowered in these circumstances. Creative herself, she began to develop her talents. Andy encouraged her initially, and then began to feel discontented. She was locking herself away in her study when she should have been looking after him. Worse, she started to become successful as well. Even more disturbingly, she began to show renewed interest in sex, and he started to feel undermined by her enthusiasm and receptivity. Andy couldn't take these changes. His Romantic soul was touched by his image of Nadine as the broken, sexually frightened beauty – it was not much to do with Nadine the human being. He began to make difficulties about her working, was rude to her female friends, told her that she was unbalanced sexually. Nadine had been attracted to Andy because he had been the strong father; now he was behaving like a petulant boy. She could no longer admire him. He had made her feel valued, but now he was making her insecure. It is not surprising that she took the Romantic escape route – she fell madly in love with someone else and left Andy.

The catchphrase of Romantic men and women could easily be the lines in the poem by W B Yeats: 'I have spread my dreams under your feet;/Tread softly because you tread on my dreams.' No Romantic can bear to have dreams trampled upon, be they about love, work or life in general. Romantics who want to make their relationships last need to bear in mind that their Romantic partner's dreams are as important as their own.

A force for stability, at least for some years, is that Romantics who are disappointed in their own dreams can project them onto their children. The Romantic man sees his son captaining a national team, his daughter winning beauty crowns; the Romantic woman knows that all her children will be beautiful, talented and successful. United in their hopes, they can sometimes sink their life savings and dedicate all their free time to giving their children all the opportunities they need to do well. It is a compelling shared interest that also removes the spotlight from their own relationship and how they are getting on.

The Romantic partnership can last many years – or for life, although many fall by the wayside. When it is going well, however, it is better than good – it is glorious. Romantics believe that it is 'better to have loved and lost than never to have *loved* at all'. Romantic love obeys different rules from other kinds of love. Its strength, beauty and passion can't be judged in the light of whether it succeeded in the long term. If it was everything that both of them wanted at the time, then it was worth it, no matter how long it lasted. Romantics will agree on that.

The Sensual Man and Woman

'The deep, deep peace of the double-bed after the hurly-burly of the chaise-longue.'

Mrs Patrick Campbell

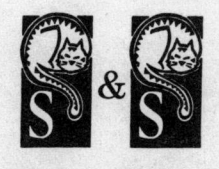

The Sensual Man and Woman

Two well-matched Sensuals have a natural capacity to make the most enduring and *contented* relationship of any combination of Sexual Styles. They match in the way that makes living together so pleasant — because both of them derive such enormous pleasure from the small and realisable things in life: a good meal, comfort, cosiness, affectionate tactility and, of course, sex.

It's sex, not surprisingly, that brings them together in the first place. They lust before they love, usually, and the *coup de foudre* in their case is often a longing to get their hands on each other. Even when they can't — or sensible caution stops them doing this immediately — the longing will be what they are most aware of and what makes their attraction to each other more compelling than anything else.

It's not just the lust that makes them compatible, however, and their compatibility goes beyond a shared need for sexual satisfaction. Indeed, some Sensuals do not have a great need for sex, and sometimes their differing views in terms of how much sex is important is quite marked. Much more reliable in the long term is that they have a similar need for constancy in relationships, and for an emotional atmosphere that is warm but calm, without too many upsets. This temperamental match means they are prepared to work quite hard at keeping the peace, or, at any rate, putting into proportion the kinds of upsets that trouble other couples. They ask themselves, does it *really* matter in the scale of things? They are prepared to be extremely forbearing, or even wilfully obtuse in the interests of a quiet life, and they love and value each other for doing the same.

Mr and Ms Sensual are also united in gentle pleasure-seeking that is connected to instant gratification: they want their creature comforts, and they want them *now*. They have the great, shared ability to derive satisfaction from the simplest things in life, and together they can create a sybaritic paradise that increases their love and devotion, and which makes staying together the dearest wish of them both.

The beginning

This is the couple who spend most of the time at the start of a relationship in bed. Ideally, they will have their favourite food and drink waiting on the bedside table to enjoy in between bouts of love-making — although passionate lust plus the intoxication of new love tends to make them lose their appetites, at least temporarily. Nevertheless, the famous eating scene in *Tom Jones* must be one of the best celluloid depiction of two Sensuals, as the couple greedily devour a huge feast with their hands, their eyes fastened on each other, becoming more aroused by the minute as they do so.

The hungry feasting on each other's bodies, however, is the best way that Sensuals know to check out their feelings. For a relationship to last happily, they must delight in each other's bodies even if, eventually, they develop a routine in which sex plays a more minor role. Talking about themselves — the way most couples explore their love, and intensify their feelings — has a subsidiary and less crucial significance to this pair. They do it of course, before love-making — or preferably after — but what matters most is the love-making in between.

What they are also seeking to determine, whether they realise it or not, is how *comfortable* they make each other feel — something that can be even more vital, or at least equally important, as it is to discover how much they can excite and satisfy each other. This is not so true of a couple of inexperienced Sensuals, who can be so bowled over by sexual discovery that it is all that matters to them. More mature Sensuals, who have been around, however, have usually known plenty of exciting and satisfying love-making that has eventually palled without the X-factor of this soothing sense of ease with each other. Indeed, in their thrilling interaction with other Sexual Styles this has often been missing. Excitement, thrills, and intoxication need to be underpinned by this less dynamic but more enduring sense of 'coming home'.

Settling down

No other Style combination enjoys the experience of making their relationship permanent and building a home together as much as this pair do. Once Sensuals fall in love, settling down is what they want to do. Two of them together derive deep satisfaction and pleasure from the sheer ordinariness of the process. There is bliss, and excitement, in spending the day stripping wallpaper in a room that is empty except for cartons of takeaway food and a mattress in the corner.

Other couples can also find this kind of activity extremely pleasurable when they are in the romantic first phase of settling down together. For Sensuals, however, it is almost romantic in itself – and making their home better, more comfortable, and more suited to their needs continues to be a pleasure for them – even when they are doing it years down the line, and they are adapting it to be more convenient for their changing capabilities.

Their home is their castle – a fortress, even. The Sensual couple may not move often – they love what is known and settled too much – but they will spend as much time and money as they have on making where they live warm, comfortable and welcoming. When they are forced to move – to upgrade or find more space, indeed, it will often be to a suitable house nearby. Change is unsettling for them and they are comforted by familiar streets, shops and faces. They are often broken-hearted when their neighbours move and they have to contend with new people – even if they had little to do with the people next door, or didn't madly like them. They knew where they were with them – and knowing where they are is what Sensuals need to be content. In actual fact they become fond of anything and anyone that is familiar. Habits and routine delight them for just this reason as well. They put their best efforts into refining and shaping the minutiae of their daily life so that it becomes deeply satisfying.

This gift for enjoying what others might think dull is one of the most important ingredients in the continuing success of their relationship. For instance, they derive maximum entertainment from eating and food generally – something you can do every day, more than once a day – and find as much enjoyment in it each time. They often both like cooking, although the more conventional Mr Sensual might think that it's not his job. Even he, however, is likely to have a speciality that he shows off on occasions – it could be barbecuing, or an individual way with eggs, or a cake that his grandmother taught him to cook, and which he has been making ever since. Many Sensual men are much more sophisticated in the kitchen, and more concerned to roll up their sleeves and cook regularly. Happy Sensual couples often cook together. They give each other cookery books as gifts and keep their eyes open for exotic ingredients they can try out. An evening spent preparing food, and then savouring each mouthful when it is ready can be bliss to them.

Equally satisfying can be a shared interest in gardening. Sensuals tend to have green fingers, and even when they are not naturally talented at it they'll make the effort to learn. Poring over seed catalogues together, and then pottering amicably about their patch, one digging, the other weeding, is what they call satisfying intimacy.

They also like doing nothing at all. Few people can feel so content at the end of an evening merely watching television, scarcely exchanging a word. Usually they'll sit side by side, or close enough to touch. Often they'll be even more intimate: they'll cuddle, or she'll lie with her head in his lap, or sit on his knee. Growing children can be quite scornful or embarrassed by this silliness, and wish for their parents to be more 'grown up'. In truth, it can sometimes be a bit of a relief to them as well. Sensual parents need to be hugging and fussing over someone, and their children can find themselves subjected to more cuddles and kisses than they think is entirely appropriate as they become bigger. At least when their parents are involved with each other they can escape these sometimes suffocating and unwelcome attentions.

These are ways that happy, loving Sensual couples might choose to spend their time. Others can be much less content with each other, more unfriendly, and much more separate in their habits and pleasures. Mr Sensual, for instance, might be more focused on his work and his responsibilities. Home is where he expects to switch off and be looked after while he indulges his private pleasure in reading or listening to music. Ms Sensual concentrates her affections on the children and her home. Indeed, they can both be even more puritan and much less fun-loving. They do what they do out of duty (and Sensuals are extremely dutiful) rather than because it gives them pleasure. Even the cooking, the gardening and the decorating are done with stalwart efficiency rather than loving excitement. But it is precisely this dutifulness that can make this relationship just as strong as the more agreeable Sensual partnership. Commitment is important to them, as is stability. They might be less happy, but they are realists and don't expect to be happy all the time. Indeed, the Sensual who is less tuned into pleasure is probably the most constant of this Style – he or she is less likely to notice or mind too much when it is missing, and therefore won't see any point in looking around for something better or even in improving matters within the relationship. Two of these Sensuals together can have a fairly uncomfortable, arid-seeming life together, but dismiss its inadequacies as 'normal'. Occasionally, these very committed couples have affairs, particularly Mr Sensual. But these are very much 'on the side'. These affairs compensate for what might be missing in the relationship (especially if it is also the satisfying sex) but they do not threaten his relationship with Ms Sensual in any other way.

Even happier Sensuals are in danger of letting their relationship slide so deep into habit or sloth that they find, some years later, that what they do is not so much fun or so satisfying any more. The trouble is that they reinforce each other's natural tendency to do what they have always done, be distrustful of the untried, or choose inaction over activity because they just can't be bothered. Harmonious companionability turns into the silence of nothing to say. They go out for a meal 'for a change', and while other couples chatter around them they pass only the occasional comment about the food. Nothing new has happened in their life for so long that they can't think of anything to talk about. Even so, while a relationship like this can make other couples unhappy or at the very least impatient, the Sensual couple are less demanding of each other. Even the predictable boredom has its compensations: steadiness, the security of the known. They can derive the small dose of excitement they need in other ways – from work, friends, other members of their family.

All the same, it's a shame if they let their relationship get to this stage, and many Sensuals are more vigilant about avoiding it. They can usually find more to share and talk about to rescue themselves from complete inertia – and both will feel better if they try.

Mr and Ms Sensual often play 'mothers and fathers' after many years together – not just to their children, but to each other. Both in their own way like to have life under control. Mr

Sensual sees himself as a provider, and has a sneaking suspicion that if he doesn't tell everyone what to do they won't be able to manage. He can be quite strict with Ms Sensual, laying down the law about where they live and when they must move, how things should be in the home, what they should spend their money on, where they will go for their holidays, and exactly what they will do when they get there, and so on. Ms Sensual controls in her own, usually motherly, way. She monitors what Mr Sensual eats and drinks, makes sure he is warm enough, checks on the state of his health and fitness, and will keep on at him if he's not doing quite as she thinks best. They can irritate each other at times by these controlling ways, but so long as they are generally happy together they also see them for what they are — signs of love and concern. Mr Sensual might roll his eyes to heaven as Ms Sensual stops him on the way out of the door to straighten his tie and settle his collar, but he also feels warm inside. Ms Sensual can feel exasperated that Mr Sensual is dragging his feet about whether they can afford the new extension that she has set her heart on, but it also makes her feel safe that he is being careful and wouldn't do anything to jeopardise the security of their home and lifestyle. Privately, they both know who is *really* in charge. Mr Sensual thinks that he is. Ms Sensual believes that she influences what is most important. This is a very satisfactory state of affairs for both of them.

This parental behaviour towards their partners is precisely what can make things difficult for Sensuals matched with another Sexual Style — particularly sexually. This is most marked in the case of Ms Sensual. Other men often can't see her as so desirable if she becomes a mother to them. Women of other Sexual Styles might appreciate Mr Sensual's paternal strictness in one way, but they can also perceive it as unromantic and stifling and therefore find his sexual attentions unwelcome. With each other, however, there is no such problem. Their sex life tends to run parallel to their domestic life — their desire is not so intimately connected to their day-to-day interaction. Sex is somewhat separate, and mainly to do with their physical chemistry, not so much their feelings or their ideas about each other. They may, even, call each other 'mother' or 'father' — but that doesn't stop themselves thinking of each other as 'lover' once they are between the sheets.

Daily life

Quiet routine is the mainstay of the Sensuals' daily life together. The more sexy couple will set their alarm early so that they can have a cuddle or make love before the day begins — they want to do it, but they don't want it to make them late. It's a good start to the day, and neither of them is likely to be fussy about how sweet they smell or how good they look. A night spent closely snuggled together is all the foreplay the more highly-sexed couple needs. The best way that they can reaffirm their intimacy is by further love-making at night.

Both of them are likely to be very industrious, so they appreciate even more their time off together. Evenings tend to be spent in homely ways — and at home. The more self-aware couple make sure that they go out fairly regularly as well — but not too often. They like their excitement well-spaced, and it acts chiefly as a contrast to the deeper pleasure of being comfortable, relaxed and quiet at home. They prefer, indeed, to have their excitement *at* home. They are often excellent hosts, who enjoy entertaining. They enjoy the planning and preparation of these events, and even the clearing up, as much as they do the occasion itself, and they will put themselves out endlessly. You've barely crossed the threshold and they are begging you to put something in your mouth — a cup of coffee, a glass of wine, some nibbles. There's usually a delicious aroma emanating from the kitchen. They are very solicitous about their guests' comfort. They'll check that you're warm enough, or not too hot, make you put a cushion behind your head, beg you to think again and be sure that you couldn't manage just a *tiny* bit more pudding. They can be very witty and articulate people, but often they feel that their main contribution as hosts is to offer the arena, the comfort and the sustenance, and to let the excitement and the conversation take care of itself. Ms Sensual sits smiling happily at the way the plates are being wiped clean by her guests. Mr Sensual busies himself opening bottles and keeping the glasses topped up. They like it if the evening takes off and becomes rowdy and interesting, but they are equally happy with a bunch of old friends who simply exchange memories and anecdotes in a friendly, cosy way. When their friends return the compliment they are more likely to talk about the food on the way home than they are the scintillating political discussion.

Most of the time they are content not to see other people too often. The prospect of a video and a meal on their laps is more entrancing. When they have children, much of their effort and time is spent concentrating on them. Two Sensuals with a young baby will normally love all the physical tending that is involved. Mr Sensual often finds an unknown side of himself opening up when he becomes a father. He doesn't like all of that 'new man' stuff about letting his feelings out and becoming in touch with his feminine side, but he's surprised at how delightful it is to bathe a soft, slippery little creature, and even changing and cleaning up a baby has its pleasures. He finds that he's as good at the bedtime rituals as he is at the rough-housing: rocking and soothing – even discovering that he remembers all the words of the lullabies his mother used to sing him.

Mr and Ms Sensual are also closely involved with their older children. This is slightly more difficult for all concerned. The Sensuals are alarmed at the independence that adolescents require. All the normal parental worries and considerations are intensified for them. They worry about their children's safety when they are not there right under their noses. They want to control what their children eat, wear, study, who they date and what they are going to do when they are grown up. This is the couple who can't sleep until all their brood is safely in bed with the front door securely locked. Or they pace the floor, ready to telephone the police, their children's friends – anybody – when one of the 'little ones' is half an hour late.

This couple find it difficult when the children leave, particularly when much of their loving attention has been concentrated on them to the detriment of the relationship. Other couples, too, find this stage difficult, and many split up when the children are no longer there to keep them together. But the natural caution of the Sensuals stops them doing anything rash. Once they've overcome the worst of the transition, indeed, their relationship can blossom again. They can give more time to sex, for instance – something that might have been impossible for years. Their ability to draw pleasure as well as comfort from the simple things in life also sees them through. The retired Sensual couple obtain great satisfaction from the fact that they can now devote themselves to the home. Wait long enough and there may well be grandchildren to become involved with and fuss over. Meanwhile, a furry animal or two also helps Mr and Ms Sensual resettle while they wait.

Communication between the Sensual couple

Mr and Ms Sensual can't understand the emphasis placed on communication in a relationship. Even when they are by nature intelligent and talkative people, this aspect is the least important to them on a deeply personal level – indeed, it's not what they think of as intimacy, and they might have their best and most interesting conversations with other people. However clever or intellectual they are, indeed, talking involves effort, and putting themselves out – effort, they feel that is better conserved, and should be rationed.

They are happiest when they agree about things. And when they find that they do agree, there is not a pressing need to go on talking about them. Disagreements are unsettling to them, and consequently they prefer to avoid them. Rather than battle with words, their preferred method of handling any conflict is to pretend it doesn't exist. Mr Sensual tends to do what he wants to do, and what he thinks is best anyway. Ms Sensual does the same, but with a greater degree of subtlety. She may well try to manoeuvre him into thinking something was his idea, or bide her time and bring it up later.

This works perfectly adequately for them over the minor issues in life, but is far less satisfactory when there is something more important – or there are graver problems in their relationship. When this is the case they are likely to fret quietly, or to sulk. Mr Sensual might go in for some intermittent forceful bullying. Ms Sensual might become depressed and turn for comfort to food. None of these methods solve anything, and can turn a potentially happy relationship into something resembling an armed truce or worse. Very angry or upset Sensuals can have sensational blow-ups of great ferocity or a sudden uncontrolled tantrum, because they have not practised relieving their feelings at an earlier, more manageable stage. These spats frighten them both, and they are usually extremely sorry afterwards. What they do is vow that it won't happen again – but instead of finding a different way of dealing with these difficult feelings or problems they repeat the same pattern. They control their emotions as long as they can, until they can't any longer.

The pity is that they are better placed than most couples to cope with these issues in a more helpful way. They respond well to the idea of practical solutions, and they are also realistic about love. This means that they are able to tolerate conversations in which one of them expresses disappointment or pain, especially if he or she makes a reasoned argument for changes to improve matters. Because conflict is the last thing they want, indeed, both are motivated to make changes to keep their relationship comfortable.

When counsellors have told me about working with couples

like this, what has struck me most forcibly is that counselling works best for them when it helps them make practical – almost physical – changes in the way that they relate to each other. For many people the most important part of counselling is the revelation and understanding of emotions, their own and each other's. When this is the case there is a natural improvement in the relationship, so long as good feelings are also present. This is never enough for Sensuals. Their emotional life is just not important enough to them, and understanding their partner's emotions leaves them concerned but helpless. For their relationship to improve, they have to put in place different ways of behaving – experience how much better this makes them feel, and continue from there.

One striking case that I wrote about in *The Relate Guide to Better Relationships* involved a couple called Alison and Mike. They came with a truly tragic story. Their second child had been born with a heart defect and died shortly after birth. During the child's illness and death Mike had had an affair with Alison's best friend. Their relationship was hanging on by a thread. Alison was grief stricken and also terribly angry; Mike was also grieving and consumed with guilt – partly to do with the affair and partly because he felt that – somehow – he should have been able to stop his child from dying. He thought he should have been strong enough. He felt, as Sensuals do, that he could control things, but that he had failed. The counselling taught them a lot about 'why'. Neither, in the Sensual way, was good at expressing feelings. Alison did this by mothering Mike, but now she needed some mothering herself. Mike had needed to blot out his own terribly strong feelings and had chosen the easy Sensual way – sex; sex with the grieving Alison, of course, had been out of the question.

These realisations were useful – indeed Alison was able to forgive Mike, and he was able to forgive himself – but this didn't help them move on. Slightly more helpful was the talking programme the counsellor instituted. This involved them taking it in turns to talk about themselves and their feelings. It was slightly artificial, and rather difficult for them: every day they took half an hour each to say precisely what was on their minds, while the other listened without speaking. Both came to be able to recognise and express the weaker and more fearful sides of their natures, which, in the Sensual way, they had always ignored. But the most helpful of all was when the counsellor asked them to 'meet each other's needs to increase intimacy'.

This time they were to take it in turns, daily, to ask the other to do something for them or with them that they would like. After a couple of false starts, they were able to do so. What they asked for were the small-scale pleasures that Sensuals like: Mike wanted Alison to massage his aching shoulders after he had been digging in the garden; Alison wanted them to do something together with their surviving child on Saturday, and so on. By the end of the counselling the counsellor said that their marriage was in better shape than it had ever been, and that what they had learned would make it even better as the years went on. 'The changes they made seem simple but can be quite difficult. They worked really hard because they wanted their relationship to last and they both changed. Many couples aren't ready to put in the effort.' Of course they worked hard, and of course they wanted their relationship to last – they were Sensuals. It is this ability to work at relationships that makes the effort of learning to communicate so rewarding to the Sensual couple.

Another intriguing case involved a young couple who were very embattled, yet also wanted to stay together. None of the talking helped, and they simply weren't interested in understanding why they were at odds. Almost in desperation, the counsellor helped them renegotiate every aspect of their daily lives, from the moment they got up in the morning. They used to row about who should rise first, and the counsellor suggested that they should synchronise this exactly – both putting a foot to the ground at the same time. Strangely enough this worked excellently for them. They agreed who should do what for the children. One took the cereal from the shelf, the other brought the milk from the refrigerator, and so on. This made them so much happier that they contracted everything they did throughout the day in a similar way. By the time they left counselling this had become a habit that had revolutionised their life together.

These methods of 'communication' can strike other Sexual Styles as extremely odd. Indeed, they seem odd to Sensuals who have not tried them. But they work, and they don't need a counsellor to preside over them. Sensuals who are happy in their daily routine are happy with life, and therefore their relationships feel much more pleasant. Sensuals who are able to ask for and receive what they would like from their partners, so long as it is not something disturbing for their partners to do, find that intimacy increases. As a couple they might be very similar, but they still have different needs. Sensuals can tend towards selfish indulgence of their own needs. A programme of asking and receiving is one way to curb their selfishness, and yet increase their general happiness. Actually, all Sexual Style combinations could benefit from a degree of this kind of negotiation, but the Sensual couple who live most intensely in the present, minute to minute, will find it the most beneficial of all.

Sex in the Sensual partnership

Sex can be the most fulfilling and intimate part of this couple's relationship. Both of them find expressing deeply loving feelings much easier this way than any other – and they can still derive immense satisfaction from their sex life when their love has become merely companionable and not so strong. One of the best things they have going for them, indeed, is that they can continue to find each other attractive throughout their relationship. They don't need beauty, elegance or physical perfection. They want a pleasurable, tactile experience – a body that they know and love, that smells naturally delicious to them and feels nice. It takes a lot for a physically well-matched Sensual couple to lose all sexual interest in each other.

Two experienced Sensuals, who have learnt what they need sexually to be satisfied, are well placed to develop a gratifying and rewarding love life. The happiest Sensuals are those who make the effort to give plenty of time to love-making. Mr Sensual will often find rushed and perfunctory love-making perfectly adequate, but he can fully enjoy a more prolonged and considered session, and is usually willing to do anything that makes love-making more satisfying for him and for his partner. Ms Sensual, with her more complex female needs, will always need more time – especially after the early days of heightened lust when all her responses were so exquisitely tuned up. If her needs are ignored, however, even the most highly-sexed Sensual woman will lose interest in sex, sometimes turn off altogether – which leaves her vulnerable to the attractions of a sexually compelling man who is ready and willing to give her the attention she is missing.

The less experienced Sensual couple might never have got the sex quite right – particularly for Ms Sensual. They might be disappointed but not know that anything is wrong, or, if they do, what they can do about it. Re-reading the Sensual Man and the Sensual Woman chapters can give some clues. All Sensual couples, however experienced, can benefit from pure sexual time out. Booking a holiday alone, or even a night away together, or even at home (when any children are looked after somewhere else) is important for them. They should use this time to hole up and experiment with ways of touching that are delightful to them. They should be prepared to show their partners what they have discovered about their sexuality for themselves – and let each other know when they are giving each other pleasure in the right way. Some good food and their favourite alcohol can smooth over any embarrassing moments. Considering that good sex can be so important to these people, they are often surprisingly shy at talking about it or letting go of any inhibitions.

The most pressing problem this couple is likely to encounter is a difference in their sexual appetites. When one of them needs more sex than the other then it has to be handled in a way that suits them both. When it is the Sensual woman who needs less sex than the man, this is sometimes easiest. Sensual women can be more prepared than most to go along with love-making when they are not particularly aroused themselves. Intimate touching is always a pleasure to them – and so long as their partners are not totally wrapped up in their own urgent needs they can enjoy a less exciting but nonetheless pleasurable sexual encounter. If the Sensual woman's feelings are not taken into consideration on too many occasions, however, and she stops connecting sex play with satisfaction, she can feel short-changed. On the whole, she wants to be able to give herself up to sex and enjoy every minute, and she wants to feel that he is as concerned with her pleasure as he is with his own. Frequent hasty sex for his sake alone can lead him to take less care of her needs, which must be respected if she is to enjoy herself fully. In this case, the Sensual man can find it worthwhile to have sex less often than he feels he needs in the interests of making it special for both of them when it does happen.

It is more difficult – as, indeed, it always is – when the woman wants sex more frequently than the man. A Sensual man, however sophisticated, believes that sex starts and ends with his erection – until he is taught otherwise. When his woman makes it plain that she needs more sex than he does, he can feel as threatened as do men of other Sexual Styles. The clever and patient Sensual woman has a few tricks up her sleeve when it comes to knowing how to turn him on – and indeed, the Sensual man is more susceptible than an Emotional, Imaginative or Romantic man to being turned on when his mind is on other matters. Nevertheless, in common with other men, the Sensual man baulks at feeling pressured, or in having his manhood questioned by a woman who thinks his sex drive should be higher than it is. It is often best for Ms Sensual to bide her time, and wait for a moment when he, too, is desirous. Making the most of these occasions to ensure that the love-making is as prolonged and as voluptuous as she could want can make up for the lack of frequency.

The trouble is that whether their sex drive is high or low, Mr and Ms Sensual equate sex with love. They find it hard to go on feeling loving, in fact, when their relationship is virtually sexless. Being touched lovingly, with expert knowledge, and with concern to satisfy, makes them feel more loved than almost anything else they can possibly do for each other.

It makes a profound difference for both of them when they can realise the pleasures to be gained from non-sexual touching. Ms Sensual is usually more alert to this than Mr Sensual is — focused as he is on his penis and the pleasure to be had from it. In fact, spending time in gentle, aimless, affectionate petting can be as satisfying, in a different way, as sexual intercourse. Enjoying themselves cuddling and kissing, as perhaps they did in the early courting days, makes up for love-making being less frequent. The bonus is that it makes them feel loving and relaxed as well — and, as Sensuals, this means that they are likely to be in the mood for love-making more often. Ms Sensual, particularly, likes to be shown that she is loved in this affectionate way, with an absence of sexual pressure. Both of them respond to knowing that their bodies are loved and needed, sexually or not, and physical closeness always results in a flowering of their loving feelings, and therefore an increase in the general level of satisfaction in their relationship.

Long-term prospects

This couple would rather stay together than part. They are prepared to work to make their relationship good. They are fairly undemanding about what *makes* a relationship good. They have all the ingredients, in fact, to live together as happily as is realistic, for as long as possible.

Nevertheless, some of these relationships do founder. They break up in the end, because of the inherent laziness of Sensuals. They *are* prepared to work at a relationship, but on the whole they'd rather not. Neither do they challenge each other to make it work, as often happens when they are paired with one of the other Sexual Styles. In a climate, indeed, when as many relationships do break up as survive, even the Sensuals heed the seductive message that it might be much *easier* to find a new partner and re-experience the effortless joys of love in the early stages before there is any work involved.

But Sensuals are happier with relationships that last, and they also derive profounder contentment with one that has been through the ups and downs of life and proved its strength. They are too realistic to trust easily, but when they know that they can trust they feel an immense and grateful satisfaction. The Sensuals are possessive people, and the ugly side of this becomes apparent when they don't feel secure in their partner's love. Mr Sensual becomes domineering and controlling; Ms Sensual becomes jealous and depressed. With each other, over time, however, they have no need of these tactics because they are relaxed and assured in each other's love.

As has been seen, the Sensual couple can sometimes make an enduring relationship that is unloving, uncomfortable and unhappy. Equally, with slightly more effort, and the blessing of a naturally equable temperament, they can be the oldest hedonists in town – thoroughly enjoying themselves and each other, and able to teach the younger ones a thing or two about sex and love that is worth learning.

The Imaginative Man and Woman

'There's a cool web of language winds us in,
Retreat from too much joy or too much fear.'

Robert Graves

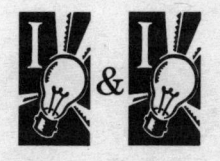

The Imaginative Man and Woman

When Ms Imaginative meets Mr Imaginative there is an instant rapport. Even if there is no spark of physical attraction, they will feel they have met a potential friend, and be delighted. Good looks will catch their attention – but when they don't look away again it is because of the harder to define 'chemistry'. In their case this chemistry is an unconscious recognition of qualities that are most appealing to them.

The sexually curious Imaginative will pick up the signals that here is another person who has the same uncomplicated approach to sex. It is not about 'love me', or 'make me whole', but 'let's have fun'. The twinkle they see in each other's eyes is a tonic. They don't mind going to bed with someone who is looking for more from sex, but they are happier with a person who feels the same as they do.

When the attraction goes deeper they are excited by each other's mental alertness and curiosity. They see a reflection of their own intense interest in conversation, novelty, and a meeting of minds. When two Imaginatives meet and are attracted they will be enveloped in a fog of words. Hardly able to contain their delight long enough to listen, they will signal their enthusiasm by a dialogue that is almost sexual in its intensity.

Actually, they do listen, even when they are talking at the same time. The mental quickness of Imaginatives allows them to take in what someone else is saying while in the middle of speaking themselves. Even when they are mainly concerned to show off their verbal dexterity they love people who are equally good at expressing themselves, and will be charmed rather than annoyed by the interruptions.

How could they fail to be charmed? They recognise instinctively that this person has the same values that they do. They share the same open attitude to the pleasures of new experiences, adventure, dialogue, and the excitement inherent in ideas, principles and the 'big picture'. Not only that, but the same things disturb them: boredom, routine, messy emotions, and conflict that is irrational and poorly argued. The Imaginative is looking for a mental soulmate, a playmate, and someone who will continue to be interesting. These attributes can last long after the unpredictable, feeling-driven aspects of love and sex have turned into something else. Mr and Ms Imaginative believe that they have found just the partner they've been looking for.

The beginning

When two Imaginatives are attracted to each other consummation usually follows quickly. They tend to be uninhibited about sex and want to satisfy their curiosity as soon as possible. When they are both very keen on sex the beginning of their relationship can be intensely passionate. This is the couple who will make love anywhere, any time, whatever the difficulties, given the slightest opportunity. They find the novelty extremely erotic, and can't keep their hands off each other.

Sex will never be quite so erotic between them again. The newness, the mutual exploration, the eagerness to try different things — all these have built-in obsolescence. 'Newness' by definition is transient. Mutual exploration reaches its limit. Trying different things, initially spontaneous, eventually involves more hard work and thought. If they have little Sensual in their natures they will come to find that the most exciting part for them has been the thrill of the novelty and variety, more than the actual physical sensations. Even if one or both are fairly Sensual too, the eroticism diminishes when the sense of adventure goes.

Not all Imaginatives are so interested in sex, although while they are newly in love lust will be amplified. If one or both of them rates sex low, the initial passion will be more about the Imaginative's favourite pastime: getting to know the inner workings of a loved one's mind. Usually they will also become fellow adventurers in a whirl of social and intellectual activity: seeing things, doing things, spending half the night afterwards dissecting and analysing their experiences and planning future projects. Sometimes one is the guide and the other is the pupil: Imaginatives can love both teaching and learning. Indeed, even the 'teacher' recognises that there can be a lot to be learnt from the open, fresh and questing mind of an acolyte.

Even while there is intoxication and overwhelming lust, the Imaginative in love retains a clear-headed appreciation of what else the relationship has to offer. It's fairly easy for both the Imaginative man and the Imaginative woman to exit from a relationship with rapidity and with an untouched heart. But meeting a fascinating, like-minded Imaginative makes men or women of this Sexual Style more motivated to continue the union and make it permanent.

Settling down

Don't mention the phrase 'settling down' to the Imaginative couple — they think it is a rather sad concept. When their whirlwind relationship has proved itself by standing the test of time, they *will* settle down, but if they are going to continue to be happy it mustn't *feel* settled. One Imaginative couple I know have been formally engaged for six years, and have lived together ever since. But taking that final step into marriage is something they are not quite ready for, and perhaps never will be.

Sexual Styles

So long as they can spark each other off mentally and their life together is interesting and challenging, most of the things that other couples care about seem irrelevant. Their relationship can be central and compelling and full of love without any conventional trappings. Over time, sex doesn't have to be good, they can even tolerate infidelity; money and prestige don't matter in themselves. But when the spark and the adventure go, so does the main basis for love.

For people whose Sexual Style is more Imaginative than anything else the best relationship they can have as a couple is a never-ending dialogue that ranges across every issue large and small. A shared sense of adventure also unites them. The happiest Imaginative couple have a life that is busy and involving, with many different activities, a constant stream of friends, new and old, and holidays that are interesting and unusual. All Imaginatives, indeed, need to be refreshed by variety, and find each other more interesting when their lives generally are entertaining.

They are usually an example of the thoroughly modern couple. Imaginatives, unlike other Sexual Styles, don't need too much togetherness and don't have the same anxiety about their partners leading fairly separate lives. When their interests coincide they will do a lot together. But if they have different tastes or preoccupations they feel it makes sense to pursue them independently. Amy and Alex are a strongly united Imaginative couple who are very much in love. They have lived together for eight years, but in practice spend very little time together. Amy likes going to clubs, seeing new bands and other acts, chatting with friends, dancing, and having a laugh. Alex prefers quieter social occasions, talking intensively about important things. Three or four nights a week they go in opposite directions in search of a good time. Their holiday likes and dislikes are different, too. Amy likes educational holidays, where you learn to paint, cook, meditate, and so on. Alex likes walking holidays, in which he explores a different area each time along with a small group of like-minded friends. They do holiday together occasionally, but usually prefer to do so apart.

What does unite Amy and Alex — and is important for the success of the relationship of any Imaginative couple — is that while they are not especially interested in doing the same things or seeing the same people, they *are* extremely interested to hear about each other's different experiences. Their parallel tracks eventually converge in intense and exciting conversations that are almost like courting rituals, in which they aim to delight and fascinate each other with well-polished anecdotes and observations. These times are when they feel most in love, and when love feels deep and uniting. The Imaginative couple that doesn't do this, indeed, is in danger of drifting apart. When they are no longer interested in what each other has to say their hearts become disengaged as well.

The main danger for the Imaginative couple is that neither of them feels comfortable with the darker side of emotions. They too can feel depressed when something goes wrong, or they are ill. Anxiety comes and goes, as does anger, fear, sadness, and other feelings connected to the obstacles inherent in life. The Imaginative, on the whole, tries to deal with the upwelling of difficult emotions in two main ways: by finding a solution, or by ignoring them — sometimes both.

For instance, one of them is feeling inexplicably sad about something. He or she talks about it, comes up with a series of solutions, but the feelings remain. So what he or she then does is try to work the feelings off through a flurry of activity, or by burying him or herself in work, or reading — something either interesting or intellectual, until somehow or other the feelings pass. These coping mechanisms can be extremely useful at times, but can also cause them to miss the significance of a message from their subconscious — a message which, because it is wordless, they cannot understand.

The problem inherent in this is more acute when one of them is suffering but not the other. Imaginatives find other people's intrusive emotions even more irritating than their own. Ms Imaginative is grieving for the recent death of her mother. She is disturbed by the strength of her feelings, and by the fact that they seem to hit her out of the blue whenever she thinks she's dealt with them. Mr Imaginative is extremely sorry for her. He wants her to 'get over it' for both their sakes. They talk about it and she seems better. But the next day or the next week she's suffering again. Mr Imaginative might be patient, compassionate and caring for a few months, but sooner rather than later he feels aggrieved. Why can't she pull herself together? Their conversations go round in circles. Whether he says so or not, he is becoming bored and exasperated. A gulf of misunderstanding and fear opens up between them. Sometimes, indeed, it creates a rift that they never get round to mending, even after the crisis has past. Instead, when Ms Imaginative is ready to face the world again she looks for her comforts and needs outside the relationship in the Imaginative way – through other activities and other people. She, too, was profoundly shaken by the fact that she couldn't 'pull herself together' and sometimes she sees it as *his* failure too, because he couldn't help her.

This example illustrates that Imaginatives often respond to the aftermath of emotional pain by trying to organise their lives so that they will not have to feel it again. Being less dependent on other people is one of the ways they do so. While their opposites, the Emotionals, embrace pain – sometimes even seek it – Imaginatives prefer to flee from it. This is one of the aspects that can create a basic instability in Imaginative relationships. When too much emotion threatens what they find important, their instinct is to solve the problem by removing themselves from it. This sometimes means, of course, leaving the person and the relationship that is causing such chaos and disruption.

Perhaps it is Mr Imaginative who has the emotional problem. He is made redundant, and experiences a vertiginous drop in self-esteem. Ms Imaginative tries to make it all better by coming up with schemes and action-plans, and telling him how wonderful he really is. This doesn't work; he just doesn't seem to be able to tap into his usual get-up-and-go. He doesn't know why, and she doesn't know why. It's so *illogical*. Mr Imaginative reacts by escaping from the problem in the Imaginative way — filling his life with activities to take his mind off it, going out, seeing friends. This keeps him functioning, but it doesn't help his self-esteem, or bring him nearer to solving the problem. Ms Imaginative is exasperated, and starts to lose respect for him. Respect is an essential word in the Imaginative love-vocabulary, for the Imaginative needs to feel respect for someone in order to want to talk to them or share things with them.

Respect, as Imaginatives define it, however, is intimately connected to interest. Emotions are bothersome rather than interesting. Mr and Ms Imaginative can form long-lasting relationships on the basis of respect inspired by interest. They can be mentally very different in their views and opinions, but equally invigorated by verbal duelling. They might disagree on almost every point of discussion, but find the very controversy exhilarating — indeed even sexually exciting. The broadly Imaginative person does not find disputes as distressing as other people do, so long as they are rationally argued. Equally the respect between them might rely on general agreement about specific issues — they respect the mirroring of their own beliefs. It can be just as exciting for Imaginatives to have a less equal relationship, in which one leads intellectually and the other follows. Or perhaps they learn from each other. Imaginatives from different cultures or with a large age-gap can fit into this category — turned-on and fascinated by the window into their partners' worlds.

Daily life

Once they have thrown off the torpor of sleep, the well-matched Imaginative couple are immediately engaged in conversation at the start of the day. They might describe their dreams and analyse them, or, if not, they'll talk about their day ahead over breakfast. A silent morning between two Imaginatives, for whatever reason, gives the day a bad start. For them, even a few minutes of proper conversation reaffirms their intimacy as much as, for other couples, love-making or a kiss and a hug can do.

They like, if possible, to arrange their week in such a way that they can look forward to its different possibilities. They won't feel happy unless at least one evening includes an interesting outing, or meeting with other people so that they can enlarge their horizons through conversation. It is even better if there are more such occasions in the diary.

If this couple have to stay in because of financial or practical constraints (such as children) they won't just want to watch, mindlessly, whatever comes on the television, but will search the programme schedule for something interesting. They might talk throughout it, or about it afterwards – they are best able to process information if they have been able to discuss it and put their own words to it. Thus, even watching television can make them feel loving and happy together. Two Imaginatives spending an evening silently are a couple who no longer feel loving and probably feel hostile – but who don't want to address their feelings by mentioning them aloud. In contrast, Emotionals and Sensuals can be supremely happy in what seems on the face of it an identical situation. Their contentment often goes beyond words, and certainly doesn't rely on them.

Many Imaginatives have other ways to keep themselves happy. They might have an absorbing hobby, or an interest in study or reading, which doesn't require the participation of their partners. In these cases they can spend their leisure time privately involved in their own worlds. When both of them have engaging but solo interests then silence is, for once, golden. A problem arises, however, when one of them has fewer inner resources, and draws most satisfaction from interaction with other people and outside interests. In these cases, when one Imaginative partner is happily involved in introspective activities the other becomes peevish – constantly interrupting in a disruptive way so as to generate the kind of attention he or she needs. Although they are both Imaginatives, their requirements are different. A mutual loss of respect follows, with all the attendant difficulties.

All being well, however, their needs dovetail – at least most of the time. They are usually top of everyone's party list, because their presence lights up a gathering. They find it incomprehensible that other couples stick together at a social occasion. They will usually only begin and end the evening in each other's company. In between they will be working the room, talking to as many different people as they can – or to one particularly fascinating specimen. Parties gratify them on two levels: they can indulge their interest in other people, and increase their enjoyment by talking it through together later.

Communication between the Imaginative couple

At its best, communication zings and flows between the Imaginative couple. They are united by their shared desire to be interested on a mental level, whether they are intellectual or not, and by their need to sort out what they think, rather than be guided by their feelings and instincts. With an Imaginative partner they can be themselves; it is easier for them to respond to and understand people who operate in the same way that they do, and who have the same priorities. There is less room for misunderstanding or for a seemingly inexplicable breakdown in what appeared to be a good relationship. When problems occur this couple is likely to experience them in a similar way, and have a better chance to work on them to find a mutually satisfying conclusion. They talk it all through. They come up with practical solutions. In the process they respect each other's coolness under fire and clear, innovative thought processes.

This is, of course, when problems are logistical, without a heavy emotional price-tag. As has been seen, they fall down when the problems are based in the quagmire of emotions, or when there seems to be no action or talking that dissolves the difficult feelings underneath. They use their usual strategies, but they don't work. Imaginatives with little Emotional or Sensual in their natures find that serious problems of this kind often signpost the end of a relationship, or at least their commitment to it.

Their difficulty with emotions can go further than this. The quote at the beginning of this chapter needs examination. Yes, Imaginatives do retreat from fear (or anger or depression) or anything else that swamps and interferes with the part of themselves they value most highly – their deductive faculties. If they possibly can they distance themselves from it by talking it away.

But joy? It's not so much that Imaginatives retreat from joy, although even pleasurable but strong emotions can scramble their brains a bit, which they don't like. It's more that in the midst of an experience the Imaginative knows better what he or she thinks than what he or she feels. An Imaginative having an intensely interesting experience – talking to someone, seeing an exhibition, an adventurous journey – is aware of the mental excitement more than the feelings aroused. Only if they have a good dose of Sensual – which glories in the sensations of the here and now – do they feel the emotions. Joy is often experienced in retrospect (even, sometimes, sexual pleasure) when thinking it through at leisure, or, more importantly, talking about it. 'Emotion recollected in tranquillity' is the best and most understandable emotion Imaginatives know. That's why they have such a pressing need to talk through their experiences: it is the closest they get to emotional understanding. Without talking about what they have seen or done, in a strange way it doesn't seem to have existed. When there is an intellectual disparity in the Imaginative partnership and they don't understand what each other is trying to say, therefore, both can feel unbearably lonely.

Intimacy for Imaginatives is intellectual. They can love each other deeply without understanding each other emotionally. They prefer to ask 'what do you think?' rather than 'what do you feel?'. Emotions are less interesting, or rather scary. When their intellectual needs are met, so are their emotional needs — but when something goes wrong with the intellectual connection intimacy dies, and they have not equipped themselves to deal with the consequences.

In the interest of seeing their partnership through bad times, therefore, the Imaginative couple has to make an effort to deal with this weak point. This is made harder by the fact that neither of them has a talent for it. Precisely the events that can unite couples of other Sexual Styles can drive them apart. But because Imaginatives respond particularly well to counselling — which involves the talking-cure they most understand and respect — they can help themselves through difficulties as a couple by signing up for some professional help. It is also useful for when one is suffering more than the other. This person can find the emotional support, and the clarification that is needed, from someone who is skilled but not intimately involved.

Mr and Ms Imaginative are also receptive to books on relationships which can guide couples through how to communicate in emotional minefields. Most of the heart-warming feedback I've had about my own series of Relate books has come from Imaginative couples. I've heard about relationships radically transformed through working with these books. The couples have been motivated to solve their problems in their own preferred way — by talking — once the guidelines have been made clear, and the logic is apparent to them.

Apart from this, however, Mr and Ms Imaginative are well-equipped to construct a good channel of communication because they enjoy it so much. They both like being 'talked out of' moods, or being lured into forgetting about them by something interesting to do. The wealth of goodwill they can build up when everything is going well between them will stand them in good stead when they hit one of the sticky patches that afflict all long-term relationships.

Sex in the Imaginative partnership

Imaginatives divide into those who find sex riveting, with all its combinations and possibilities, and those for whom sex is something of an irrelevance, of limited interest. In between are the Imaginatives who start off fascinated, curious, and extremely willing to try everything sexually, and then lose interest some years down the line. Sexual harmony, as ever, depends on whether Mr and Ms Imaginative in this relationship think the same about sex. So long as they do – whether they are frenetically sexually active or virtually dormant – they will be happy.

A sexually-interested Imaginative couple will approach sex with a spirit of adventure. When they have a similar need for variety and novelty they can construct a passionately interesting sex life. Even when they do, however, and even when they find their sex life delightful and involving, it is rarely the main focus of their loving feelings for each other. When it is, the relationship can be immensely satisfying while it lasts, but it will run its course sooner rather than later. Once they have experimented to their satisfaction, have gone as far as they want to in discovering different ways to excite each other, they will usually decide it's time to find someone new. When they reach this stage at the same time they will often part as friends, with little bad feeling and much fondness. Sometimes one of them remains sexually interested in the other for longer, and will feel more regret. But even this person will find that the sadness does not go too deep if a lively sex life has been the chief binding factor. Only an Imaginative with strong elements of another Sexual Style will find the feelings involved in sex powerful enough to touch deeper emotional levels.

In a long-term relationship, the Imaginative with a powerful sex drive finds the limitations of a one-to-one sexual relationship restrictive. Mr and Ms Imaginative of this type need plenty of sexual variety to keep them turned on — as the individual chapters devoted to them show. This is the couple who will scour sex manuals, magazines, and blue films for ideas to keep the sexual temperature turned up. The scouring process is, in itself, arousing for them. Locking into ready-made fantasies can be just what they need to give their own sex life a fillip, even if what they then go on to do in their love-making is more conventional. This is the couple most likely to venture into the dangerous area of wife-swapping, three-in-a-bed, and other permutations that excite them but keep their sexual adventurings 'in the family'.

A less dangerous solution for them is an exquisitely long-drawn-out build-up to sex. They decide they are going to make love later; they talk about it, and what they will do; they arouse each other with fantasies or sexually explicit language; perhaps they play games that involve putting off the moment of consummation until they are maddened with lust. All this is better, for them, than physical foreplay and can be deeply satisfying. Alternatively, even 'old married couples' of this Imaginative type can enjoy sexual situations that are bizarre or which are semi-public and have an aura of danger: such as a quick, fraught copulation amongst the coats upstairs at a party. It's certainly the kiss of death to the sex life of the lustful Imaginative couple when routine pervades their lives on any level.

The Imaginative couple at the other end of the scale — for whom sex is rather unimportant — can sometimes live quite happily with little or no sexual contact. In their case, however, sexual activity often directly arises out of the intense intimacy that comes from a meeting of minds. When their mental wheels are turning in concert they feel more alive, and consequently closer and more sexually motivated. The Imaginative couple who find sex only slightly amusing — or even decidedly uninteresting — can feel that their mental intimacy is almost sexual in itself, and they don't need to make love to increase it. If they don't have any Sensual in their natures, and their natural sex drives are low, sex can seem to be one of life's little sidelines with limited appeal.

The in-betweens – the Imaginative couple that starts off enthusiastically investigating the highways and byways of sex, but when curiosity is satisfied turn their attention to matters that seem more interesting – can enjoy the fact that they shared a sexual past, but not regret it vanishing. So long as they continue to captivate each other on other levels their relationship can be as intense, alive and loving as couples for whom love-making is more central.

It is always a problem in a relationship when sexual needs or desire levels conflict. The more cerebral Imaginative with the lustful partner can find that they battle about the frequency – or even the fact – of sex. The Imaginative with little Sensual in his or her Sexual Style, finds it hard to understand why other people put so much emphasis on it.

Whatever the reason, and whether it is the Imaginative man or the Imaginative woman who places most importance on sex, if they are not getting what they need inside a relationship, they will have few scruples about finding it outside. The Imaginative, being emotionally unmoved by sex, places little importance on it, even when it is an urgent 'itch'. Imaginative couples can still be supremely happy together, even if one or both of them is chronically unfaithful, so long as their relationships include the elements of mental intimacy and general interest that they find more bonding and compelling.

Long-term prospects

An Imaginative marriage, or long-term commitment that retains these elements, can last for a long time, even forever. Sometimes it can last without them. Because Imaginative men and women do not feel a pressing need to be deeply engaged emotionally, they can continue coolly in an enduring relationship because it suits them on a practical level, even when all interest has gone.

Mr Imaginative, indeed, can be fairly content to stay with Ms Imaginative even if he finds her boring and has lost respect for her, so long as he can compensate by finding the missing elements – sexual, intellectual, or in terms of variety – elsewhere. Ms Imaginative is capable of this too – but being a woman she finds it less satisfying. On the whole she needs to have a partner who is satisfying on an Imaginative level to be truly happy.

An example is Ellen. It took her nearly 20 years of marriage to Max to lose her faith in the relationship. For most of those 20 years their marriage had suited them both very well. There had been a strong physical attraction between them when they met – they were strikingly attractive – but it was the mental cut and thrust that had been the strongest pull. Ellen thought Max was brilliant. It didn't matter that at 30 he had never held down a job, or that after their marriage he went into a boring and underpaid career. She was dazzled by the way his mind worked, his theories, his politics, his voracious interest in world affairs and in reading all the latest challenging books. Max found Ellen's raw, untutored but original intelligence fascinating. She was younger and took on his opinions wholesale. He loved being her mentor.

Soon after their first child was born Max virtually stopped making love to Ellen and embarked on a series of affairs. These were short-lived, and none of them meant anything to him. Typical of the Imaginative he felt compelled to seek new sexual experiences. His loss of interest in Ellen was nothing personal – she was still a beautiful, sexy woman, more so than the other women. He just could no longer be excited by a woman whose body he knew so well.

Ellen was initially devastated when he stopped wanting to make love to her. When she found out about his first affair she was very upset. But, as an Imaginative herself, she was able more quickly than other women to distance herself from what was happening. All that was best in their relationship was still alive. She didn't like it, but it didn't alter her feelings for him. A few years later she embarked on affairs herself and, like Max, was able to disengage herself emotionally from her lovers. They provided sex, but otherwise she was uninterested in them. She dictated the terms of the affair, and when she became bored she dropped her lover for a new one. Max knew, but pretended not to. 'What does it mean when a man has saggy balls?' Ellen once asked, after an encounter with a new lover. A man of another Sexual Style would have reacted suspiciously or angrily. Max accepted the question at face value and said mildly, 'I don't know. Perhaps it's to do with age.'

Home was a battleground, but not because of the affairs. They never spent an evening in companionable silence, or a quiet mealtime making desultory conversation. They were always embroiled in passionate debate. Often there were furious arguments, and Ellen sometimes went wild with temper. In common with other Imaginatives, they were not good at dealing with feelings – that upwelling of emotion that isn't logical or manageable. Ellen's way was to attack, blow her top, scream, break things. Max's way was to goad Ellen into this kind of behaviour, so that she ended up expressing his anger and pain while he could look on loftily, with a patronising sense of being in control. This kind of habitual interaction could have blown apart couples of other Sexual Styles but, as with other Imaginatives, their emotional exchanges left almost no scars. They were as explosive as fireworks with as little to show for it afterwards. Next day they behaved as if nothing had happened. Actually, they quite enjoyed it.

What they enjoyed even more were the holidays they took as a family. They never had much money, but they scraped enough for the fares to exotic locations and then roughed it. They travelled around in the cheapest way, camped or stayed in flea-ridden hotels, bought food from markets or ate in the cheapest cafes. The months prior to going away were spent poring over maps and guidebooks and planning what they would do.

So why, after 20 years, had Ellen had enough?

For three years Max had been working in another city. He'd landed a highly paid job and they had plenty of money for the first time. Holidays were no longer exciting extended treks, but short luxury breaks. Max couldn't be away from the office for too long. The new job also meant that they only saw each other at the weekends. Max arrived, exhausted, on Friday night and left shortly after Sunday lunch. Instead of thrilling debates and cataclysmic rows they caught up with practical matters and news of the children. Max was often too tired even for this. Anyway, now that he had a more interesting job he was less concerned with reading and the issues that had previously fascinated him, or in talking them through with Ellen. On the occasions they did argue, usually on a Sunday, there was no next day to be normal together and talk of other things, just a tense, five-day wait for the cycle to begin again.

Ellen knew that something had been lost, though she wasn't sure what. The truth was that the intimacy and passion in their relationship had been mainly to do with their vibrant intellectual connection. Without it Ellen felt isolated. Deep down, what she really wanted was the fireworks back. Max wasn't as perturbed by any of this as Ellen – he was getting the intellectual stimulation he needed through work, and, as an Imaginative man, this was enough for him. When Ellen stormed about their relationship he didn't realise it was more serious than her other bursts of temper. He was shocked and perplexed when she eventually left him.

The Imaginative couple can also find that some difficulties arise over starting a family. These articulate, rational people, are very concerned to find the 'right' time to do so. In the age of effective contraception, they can find it as difficult as anyone to pinpoint this mythical perfect moment, and may procrastinate so long that Ms Imaginative's fertile time is over. Ms Imaginative finds it more difficult than most women to understand her own broodiness and urge to have a baby, if it conflicts with her intellectual evaluation of the appropriateness of doing so. She doesn't value these primitive instincts, and neither does her Imaginative husband. Whether she 'makes a mistake' and has a baby, or chooses her moment with care, Ms Imaginative can also be shocked by the way that she becomes plunged into hormonal chaos after the baby is born. For the first time she might be struggling with depression that is endogenous, and can't be rationalised. She can also find a baby — the most illogical of creatures — difficult to understand and control. Mr Imaginative, standing by and watching helplessly, can be both overwhelmed by his own unwelcome emotions and severely critical of his Imaginative wife's inability to deal with the newcomer in a reasonable and civilised fashion.

Even when they are both perfectly delighted with their new family, a chasm can open up between them. Ms Imaginative, at least for a period, becomes more emotional and less rationally focused. If she stays at home with the baby she becomes, sad to say, rather boring in Mr Imaginative's eyes. She can, for a time, find the things that interest her partner rather boring too — or else she demands that he fills the Imaginative vacuum in her life by telling her things, exciting her mentally, living life for both of them. If he finds this one-way interaction irritating then the mental closeness they had built up over the years can evaporate, sometimes forever.

But having a baby changes every relationship — it's how the couple deal with it, and what happens afterwards, that counts. This is not the first or last incident in the lives of the Imaginative couple that will find them at odds, at least temporarily. So long as they keep in mind what brought them together — and what they still have in common — they have the potential to build a relationship that continues to be vital, interesting and stimulating through the years.

The Emotional Man and Woman

'Love alters not with his brief hours and weeks,
But bears it out even to the edge of doom.'

William Shakespeare

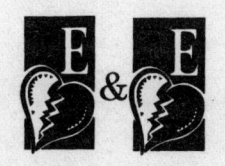

The Emotional Man and Woman

Every Emotional needs a life-long partner, so it is not surprising that when two Emotionals meet and fall in love they can't bear to let each other go. Emotionals are intense people, no matter how cool or frivolous they might appear on the surface, and this intensity allied to strong feelings for another person translates into an obsessive tenaciousness in relationships.

Emotionals are looking for someone who touches on their deepest, strongest feelings. With a certain emotional temperament, indeed, they can find love in pain, in anger, in rejection or in tyranny. In other cases, they have a deep need to serve, to nurture, to adore or to follow. Sometimes they are fearful and feel most complete with someone who shares and understands their fears. Usually, when their hearts are captured by another Emotional it is because their needs mirror each other's. They can be very similar or, more likely, apparently quite different — but their differences are shaped to match like jigsaw pieces, so that the server or the follower joins with the tyrant, for instance. This fitting together so exactly gives even more staying power to the relationship.

All this is in the future however. When they are attracted to each other the emotional interaction that will shape their partnership is not clear to either of them. They'll feel it though, as a faint echo, like a psychic intuition that they have always known this person — that they have, indeed, found the one they have always been seeking, knowingly or not. Sometimes, as in all initial attractions, this undercurrent translates as lust. They are drawn to each other with a compulsion that is sometimes hard for them to understand in any other way. On occasions this attraction is instantaneous, for other couples it grows over time getting to know each other. Some Emotionals are quite impulsive, but they are often slow to give their affections. When they love they tend to do so unreservedly, but their great emotional sensitivity means they can fear being hurt. Loving and losing is unutterably painful for them. Many prefer ultimately to be bonded in a relationship that is unhappy than to experience the greater unhappiness of parting with a partner. They prefer, of course, to love happily – to heal whatever unhappiness they carry inside. Whatever happens once this relationship develops, however, one of the great attractions of another Emotional is that this person too is unwilling to break up a partnership easily. Love might be painful, it will certainly have its difficulties, but with another Emotional it will at least be enduring – and with its continuance can come deep satisfaction, and sometimes peace.

The beginning

It is much harder to characterise any aspect of a relationship between two Emotionals than it is other combinations of Sexual Styles. That is because 'emotion' as a catch-all term covers such a breadth of different feelings. One thing is sure, however – when they fall in love it will be very intense, life-changing even. They can be filled with all the happy frivolity of new love, but it will be much more than that. They embrace this intoxication wholeheartedly, and are tremendously invigorated by the happiness – particularly the kind of Emotionals who are more used to heavier, gloomier emotions. All Emotionals want to be happy, even if some of them are driven to create atmospheres that are quite the opposite. When they are romantically in love it is one of the few times that they are blessed with an effortless happiness that is quite exhilarating.

Sex will be very important to them. Some highly-sexed Emotionals quickly consummate their relationships, most, highly-sexed or not, are more cautious, particularly the women. Whichever, making love marks an important transition for them – more so than for any of the other Sexual Styles. It's not so important how satisfying the sex itself is. It doesn't even matter if either of them finds the significance of the move into intimacy so overwhelming that sex is difficult, impossible, or uncomfortable. What matters is that they have exposed themselves to each other in more ways than the obvious. Even if they are sexually experienced and have made love many times before with other people, indeed, sex feels quite different with the person they believe is the soulmate for whom they have been waiting. An Emotional who has been fairly casual about sex in the past has usually found something rather distasteful about it. Unless he or she is very damaged by previous experiences, however, this loving sexual exchange feels dramatically better and different – and can transform for ever his or her ideas about sex.

Settling down

Two Emotionals can live together in quiet accord, or can shake the walls of their house with passionate rows. One thing is sure, once they have decided that they have found the person they want to be with they feel completely committed, and will usually marry.

The 'fit' of these two people means that the atmosphere of their relationship is settled very early on, and the way they interact can remain unchanged throughout their life together. They have chosen each other because of the way they are made to feel – and this feeling is central to the continuance of their union. Romantics often tend to classify themselves as Emotionals, because they can express their feelings uninhibitedly. They, too, choose each other for the way they are made to feel – but by this they mean the heightened emotions of romantic love. When this passes the relationship often founders. But although Emotionals enjoy the early 'in love' days, it is rarely this exhilaration that is as important to them as the feelings that are lurking underneath. Once the relationship has settled down these surface and become more obvious.

It is hard for people who do not have a strong Emotional component in their natures to understand why less happy and sometimes unhealthy emotions can keep this couple entwined. Indeed, it is hard for Emotionals themselves to understand. Consequently, it is difficult to explain as well. But the fact is that whenever these people don't feel deeply they don't see the point: in work, in relationships – in any activity that does not move them. Their intellect and their physical responses can be lively and in good working order, but these concerns have little power to motivate them. All that matters – what drives them – is powerful emotional reaction. Even when they are unhappy or depressed, they are grappling with real life as they understand it. Strong emotions focus them, willingly or not. When these strong emotions are evoked by another person, therefore, their attention is held. They may not like it, but they know what they are doing, and they feel alive.

This is why it is important for the Emotional couple to feed their own and each other's feelings in such a way as to keep them compelling. If they don't do this, or the interaction between them changes to encompass emotions not so strong, the bond unravels. Gentle contentment, for instance, can make them restless. What, they ask themselves, am I doing with this person? It does not feel so important any more. Even peaceable Emotionals living together are tied by something much stronger than quiet harmony. Usually they are united in their fear of the world, and only feel safe when they are together.

All this explains why they are impelled to push each other's emotional buttons to keep the feelings fresh, insistent, and sometimes scaldingly hot — wittingly or not, and usually unconsciously. And no one is more skilful at knowing precisely what he or she has to do to make this happen. Emotionals have an instinctive genius for understanding what makes another person tick, and what will make them flare up, or behave in certain ways. Because it is instinctive, however, they often don't even know that they are doing it.

How they 'settle down', therefore, depends on what emotions are important and compelling to them, and what they need to derive from each other. Often it is a supremely satisfying sense of being needed or cared for. One of them can be a compassionate, caring person who derives most satisfaction from nurturing another. This person's Emotional soulmate is someone who finds life very difficult and challenging. Together they make up a warm partnership, which works best when the *status quo* doesn't change. The fearful partner continues to feel insecure, except in the presence of the strong and caring spouse, who has every opportunity to prove the depths of his or her love and concern. Even this couple, however, has too much invested in the comfort of this interaction to relinquish it very easily. Somehow or other, the very concern the nurturer shows makes the other person more fearful. Not having to learn coping strategies means that the ability atrophies further. Indeed, the fearful person knows subconsciously that love is dependent on this dependency, and feels almost obliged to play up his or her inadequacies.

The union can be more obviously unhealthy, however. Ms Emotional, programmed, perhaps to feel fear and self-loathing, matches up with a sadistic Mr Emotional who needs the electric charge of cruelty to feel powerful or even to mask his own feelings of fear and self-loathing, which are less comfortable for him. She hates his treatment — so why is it that somehow or other she behaves in ways to activate his rage? Or why, if he should be weakened in some way does she take over the sadistic role in the partnership? Or why, indeed, when she finds the strength to leave him, does she end up with someone who behaves in similar ways? Actually, the emotions generated by a power struggle are always intense, which is why it is usually a factor in a long-term Emotional relationship. The person wielding the power generates a current of internal excitement, and the person subject to dominance experiences a fear that is painful, but enlivening.

Sometimes it is them against the world. Clara and Simon, a couple I know slightly, have been married for nearly 50 years and have been united by a low-level paranoia. In common with some other Emotionals, they are well aware of their own dark impulses, and believe these are shared by everyone else. Much of their married life has involved mutually satisfying conversations about other people's motives — how they were envied, plotted against or actively harmed. Much of this is typical Emotional speculation — there is no hard evidence, simply 'feelings', 'intuition', reading motive into apparently harmless words or actions. They didn't dare trust anyone else, so they became even more essential to each other. For many years Simon worked in a cut-throat industry, and Clara stayed at home, doing the occasional work for pin-money. Simon took on the hostile world for both of them, and shielded Clara from the worst of it. In the past, Simon had the occasional affair with a colleague, which even Emotional men are wont to do when they are young and lusty — but he never trusted these women and what they wanted from him. He thought they were offering sex as a strategic, professional move, and while he took what they offered, he despised them for it. Clara knew about these affairs, and the knowledge kept her frightened of losing Simon, and intensified her need to keep him. Simon trusted Clara because she was dependent on him, and also upon his large salary. When he retired, however, there was a threatened change in their relationship. Clara had become involved in charitable works, and sat on a number of committees. Now she was out of the house more than he was, and his distrustfulness grew to alarming proportions. She seemed to be made happy by her full, interesting and valuable life in the outside world. Would she stay with him – or need him in the same way? Could he bear her acceptance of the world that they had both decided was hostile?

What happened was that Simon undermined Clara's satisfaction with her new life, and she let him. He told her that all this activity was making her ill – and, indeed, she became ill. He told her that the committees only wanted her because of their money, and she believed him. Her ill-health, and her suspicions led her to give up her charitable work. When last heard of they were in retreat – enclosed in their own safe world, hardly seeing other people, convinced that it was the only real safety they could possibly know.

With no other partner – with the possible exception of the Sensual – could Emotionals be so free to let their prevailing emotions dominate their lives. There is security in this, but also, sometimes unhappiness and fear. Emotionals might be challenged with a partner of another Sexual Style, but they can be lifted out of themselves and begin to understand another way of living and behaving. With another Emotional, however, they sacrifice this possibility in return for the certainty of long-term stability, and also the comfort of feeling what they have come to believe is the reality of life, however uncomfortable it is to experience.

Daily life

When their emotional relationship feels as profoundly right as this, it is understandable that they don't really feel that they need people other than their partners. More than this: they only feel completely themselves and comfortable with their partners – other people act as a backdrop, an interesting counterpoint, but are not truly 'real'.

It's not surprising, therefore, that their daily life centres on the home. They might be busy, active people, with involving careers, but home is where they recharge their batteries and act in accordance with their feelings, rather than as they are supposed to behave. Even when they are fully committed to their work, and it is supremely important to them, at work they must be professional, considered, considerate — and, if they are not, there are consequences. Only with their partners can they give full rein to the person they want to be — and the emotions that power them. For this reason, they might be averse to entertaining. They'd rather ration the amount they see other people, and may feel that they are intruders in the home. Other Emotionals can be more sociable, but use people to reflect back at them the state of their relationship. The martyr will want to show how he or she suffers; the couple who fight about sex can drop explicit or coded comments about this at inappropriate times in company.

Family life is equally important to them. They will be intensely involved with their children — particularly Ms Emotional, and often the Emotional man as well. Sometimes, unfortunately, their children become part of the battleground. Either can feel threatened by the other's attachment to the children, particularly Mr Emotional. Sometimes, however, Emotionals who sense that they need to be uniquely focused on each other never have children at all. There might be a fertility problem, but even if there isn't somehow or other they avoid it — either by putting it off until it is too late, or by developing a 'sexual' problem which is, in reality, an expression of this emotional need.

Every day will see some sort of re-enactment of the emotions that tie them together. It's essential to the deepening of their bond. The happier and more stable Emotionals will make continuing efforts to please and satisfy each other. The Emotionals who are united by a more complex and difficult attachment will have their daily dose of conflict — or whatever else it is they need. Because this is so important to the maintenance of their relationship they do, in fact, have little time for other people. Most Emotionals need a significant relationship in their lives before anything else, and consequently they give this the priority it demands.

Communication between the Emotional couple

The most important communication between the Emotional couple is oblique. Even when they are a chatty, articulate couple, what they say to each other is less important than what they don't say. Or, rather, the words are less relevant than what they are made to feel, and are often simply a useful method for triggering the important emotions in the relationship.

Emotionals don't find that talking about feelings has much of an impact on them. Even when they do, indeed, feel a need to talk about them it doesn't have quite the same effect that it does for other couples. For what happens when two Emotionals talk about a problem or a difficulty between them is that they reinforce what each other is feeling. They feel just as unhappy, or even angrier, or more gloomy than ever. Emotions are heightened by their interactions, verbal or not, rather than calmed. Neither believes in the power of 'solutions' or changes in behaviour, because emotions can't be 'solved', they just 'are'.

This is natural to them anyway — but because their relationship depends on the particular feelings it raises in them, good or bad, they are unconsciously committed to keeping them constant. Even when these feelings are bitter or angry, therefore, and even when they vow that they would feel better if they could change them or become more happy if something was done about them, they resist the opportunity.

Ms Emotional talks to her mother or her female friends about how unhappy she is. She finds fault with whatever they suggest, however. She brushes aside everything they say, and tells them that what they suggest is impossible. It might be as clear as day to them what should be done about her problem with Mr Emotional, but they can't get through to her. Indeed, she feels miserably misunderstood by them.

Embattled Emotional couples can sometimes seek help from a counsellor because they feel despairing. But I have heard stories from counsellors about how resistant these same couples are to the counselling process. Often what they are really seeking is an arbiter – or someone who will be on their side, and punish their partner for them. Couples like this often give up counselling quite quickly when they discover that they will not get this sort of 'help'. Those that stay the course for a while become visibly distressed by efforts to make them participate in communication that threatens to sort out their problems, or to tackle the power issues in their relationship. Indeed, sometimes when the counselling is a 'success' and one or both of them changes, the central point and uniting element of their relationship goes, and they split up. This can sometimes be for the best. The changes allow them to make different and better relationships with other people – often with someone of a different Sexual Style, with whom they can work more successfully on consolidating what they have learnt. Occasionally they can go on to make a healthier relationship with another Emotional whose needs are similarly healthy.

But a deeply-bonded Emotional couple usually prefer matters to continue as they always have and are motivated merely to refine their emotional communication skills to intensify the atmosphere of their relationship.

How this can work was brilliantly portrayed by Edward Albee in his play *Who's Afraid of Virginia Woolf?* The central characters, Martha and George, have been married for 23 years. All the action takes place late one night, after a party, in the company of a much younger couple, Nick and Honey, whom Martha has invited to join them for drinks. Not much happens except the continuing revelations of their painful but intense partnership, as all of them proceed to become very drunk. Martha has invited Nick and Honey so that she can use their presence to torment and humiliate George. The side-effect is that Nick and Honey, too, become drawn into the unpleasant atmosphere, and their relationship is rocked in consequence. This is clearly something that happens often around Martha and George. At one point, indeed, George, alone with Nick, notices that he is becoming increasingly irritated. 'So you're testy,' George says. 'Naturally. Don't ... worry about it. Anybody who comes here ends up getting ... testy. It's expected ... don't be upset.'

A telling exchange between George and Martha occurs when he is becoming more and more demented by her needling:

GEORGE: '[*barely contained anger now*] You can sit there in that chair of yours, you can sit there with the gin running out of your mouth, and you can humiliate me, you can tear me apart ... ALL NIGHT ... and that's perfectly all right ... that's OK ...'

MARTHA: 'YOU CAN STAND IT!'

GEORGE: 'I CANNOT STAND IT!'

MARTHA: 'YOU CAN STAND IT! YOU MARRIED ME FOR IT!!'

Towards the end of the evening, Martha is alone with Nick. She tells him that only one man in her life has ever made her happy, and she asks him to guess who this could be. He mentions an early lover she had told him about, but Martha says that he is wrong. It is George. 'George who is good to me, and whom I revile; who understands me, and whom I push off; who can make me laugh, and I choke it back in my throat; who can hold me, at night, so that it's warm, and whom I will bite so there's blood; who keeps learning the games we play as quickly as I can change the rules; who can make me happy and I do not wish to be happy. George and Martha: sad, sad, sad.' Albee displays the fundamental truth about couples of this kind: they don't want to change, even when they are as clever and knowing about their interaction as George and Martha are.

It *is* possible, of course, for the Emotional couple to change the way that they communicate, and still stay together. But it is extremely hard for them, and they need to want to very much.

I heard from a sex therapist about one couple who managed this. Nancy and Trevor were like Clara and Simon whom I described earlier — in that they too kept the hostile world at bay by having a close and exclusive relationship, with no friends, or even any involvement with family, apart from their beloved son. Their relationship was very peaceful on the surface. They needed each other so much that they were frightened to disagree about anything. This exclusion zone became threatened by a friendship that Trevor made with a woman at work — there was nothing sexual in it, but they were working together on a project that fascinated them both. Nancy felt a deep and terrible panic, which affected their sex life: she could not bear Trevor to touch her, but she didn't understand why. In fact, sex therapy revealed that she had never enjoyed sex much, but was satisfied because it expressed their closeness. Now that she thought they were not close, indeed, sex repulsed her. More terrified of losing Trevor than she was of the therapy, Nancy painfully learnt to tell Trevor what kind of touching she didn't like, and what she could accept. It was a revelation to her to discover that Trevor was not terribly interested in sex, either. He, too, liked the closeness and wasn't sure how else to express his feelings. They learnt that both of them needed hugs and cuddles more than they needed sex. Nevertheless, there were differences in their outlooks that needed to be managed, and with the therapist's help they talked these through. The unexpected effect of these conversations was that they realised that the differences didn't affect their closeness. Indeed, in being able to express them they felt less fearful and more intimate. Nancy learnt that Trevor's friendship needn't have an adverse impact on their relationship, and came to terms with it. What this couple discovered, and other Emotionals can too, is that it can be possible to keep the emotional content of their relationship as close as they want it, but also make it more pleasant.

Sex in the Emotional partnership

In common with Sensuals, Emotionals can continue to find their partners desirable throughout their relationship. They are not concerned with the superficialities of looks, only with the depth of feeling between them. Indeed, while Sensuals also care about the quality of love-making (particularly Ms Sensual), Mr and Ms Emotional think sex is about more than the mechanics. Sex is very intimate; it is a sharing that is wasted or devalued when there is not strong feeling between the couple. They find it difficult to understand the easy, carefree sexual relationships made by other people. When their emotional interaction is healthy and happy, indeed, they have the kind of sexual relationship to which many people aspire. One woman wrote anonymously to me after filling in a sex survey I devised for *Family Circle* magazine. 'I have been married almost 25 years now and still find my husband extremely attractive — I'm fortunate that I know this feeling is reciprocated,' she wrote. 'Although passion is not as intense as it was in our young years, it is still there and I believe always will be. Apart from other emotions, we have tremendous respect for each other, which for us is important. We had a short engagement and waited till marriage before sleeping together, though we certainly wanted to do "it". I am not against sex outside marriage, but I am against sex outside a caring and loving relationship. I believe today's youngsters get into deep emotional territory before knowing and understanding each other — or even having any real perspective on what they need and want from a relationship. Personally, I still see sexual intercourse as the ultimate giving of oneself — inhibitions to the wind with someone you can totally trust. I got lots of lusty feelings with men before meeting my husband, but there had to be a lot more "knowing" before I could be totally "giving".'

This woman's sentiments about what sex 'should' be like are shared by many. But when it comes to it, representatives of other Sexual Styles make compromises and behave differently from the ideal. My correspondent went on to write briefly about her past. She had been 'sexually and verbally abused' as a child. This, she said, meant, 'I grew up desperately wanting to be liked and loved by important people in my life – always being the "good little girl" and always willing to help anyone. "Miss Sunshine" they called me!' As her letter continues it becomes clear that, in common with other Emotionals, this imprinting has stayed with her. 'I still get a great kick from helping others – it gives me a buzz.' And, as is usually the case with Emotionals, she finds it hard to see beyond her own experience, and believes that other people would be happier if they were like her. 'It amazes me how selfish some people are – always thinking of their own needs first. We should be encouraging standards back into our lives – guidelines to help our young folk have sincere values again. Teaching them about kindness, understanding and consideration for others, about loyalty and respect.' Most people would agree with what she says – relationships would be better if these values were widespread. But the passion evident in her letter says more about her personally. She shows that she is still striving to be 'Miss Sunshine': 'I have experienced great hurt, yet bitterness does not bring you joy. I could be bitter because of things that were done and said to me (often I wish I had had a "normal" childhood) but there's no point.' She has daughters of her own, and worries about the sexual climate in which they are growing up: 'Casual sexual encounters are now commonplace entertainment on TV – it's no wonder youngsters emulate such behaviour – they are bound to think it's normal when they see it so often. My daughters' magazines horrify me at times with what they get up to at such young ages. No wonder they often look unhappy – so much on their young shoulders – totally confused by "what is love"? They think love is sex – how wrong they are.' Her advice is that the values of love and respect should be taught first; then: 'Learning about sex should come after all these basics. Although a natural and wonderful pastime it most certainly is one that is being much *abused* and misused in these days.' I chose to italicise the word 'abused'. Much of her sensitive thinking comes from her unhappy experience of sexual abuse as a child, and it colours her attitude to all sexual matters. She would find it impossible to understand, for instance, the Imaginative's carefree, unemotional approach to sex, or the Sensual's instinctive view that love indeed *can* be sex.

This woman is a fortunate Emotional, in that she has used her painful past to construct a healthy and happy present, which not all Emotionals are capable of doing. She ended her letter with a heart-warming sentence with which many Emotionals could identify: 'Perhaps if we loved more "choosily" real love would last much longer than it seems to do with so many couples today. Long live sex – but *long, long* live love.'

Many Emotionals are less able to break free from the effects of difficult experiences in the past. Instead, their sex lives continue to reflect them. Abused Emotionals, indeed, often find to their own horror that abusive sex continues to be the most potent and erotic for them, and sometimes the very unhappiness of a power struggle within their relationship keeps the sexual side alive and flourishing.

Love-making that does not grow out of strong feelings of one sort or another can appear futile. When the intensely loving feelings go, therefore, desire sometimes has to be stimulated in other ways. Emotionals who habitually row and then make up in bed need the adrenalin-rush of anger, the hot pulse in their blood, for their erotic feelings to manifest. Or the cold, despairing feeling of loneliness, which is then dispelled by the intimate contact of love-making. When these feelings are necessary for a continuing sex life, they will find ways to provoke each other in their daily life to achieve the result they need.

On the other hand, the 'wrong' feelings can switch off the libido, even in a highly-sexed Emotional. It was clear that the Emotional woman who wrote to me, for instance, would be turned off by anger, pain or fear. She needed, as she said, respect – and she made it obvious that her own self-respect was bound up with being 'unselfish', caring, joyful and unbitter. It is not too hard to see that her sexual feelings – the ultimate 'giving of oneself', as she put it – would naturally extend from caring, selfless tenderness towards her husband.

Sex is by no means important in all Emotional partnerships. There is very little middle ground here. Either it is powerfully uniting, happily or not, or it is almost irrelevant. When sex means little to the couple their closeness will be unaffected by a relationship that has almost no sexual contact. Quite the reverse, in fact. Sublimated erotic feelings can flow out into other areas of their relationship, increasing the bond. Sometimes there is a tacit agreement between Mr and Ms Emotional that sex is not necessary. With other Emotional couples there is more tension about it. They fight because one of them refuses the other sex, and this fighting invigorates them. Usually, however, the fight is somewhat stage-managed, in the unconscious Emotional manner. The one demanding sex does not really want it, but relies on the other to stop it for both of them. Similarly there is sometimes a sexual 'problem' which, in reality, is satisfying for them. A number of sex therapists have told me of couples presenting with vaginismus (where the woman's vaginal muscles seize up so that sex is impossible) or erectile problems (where the man can't achieve or maintain an erection), in which the couple become anxious when progress is made. One couple worked so successfully on the woman's vaginismus that intercourse became possible. Although it was what her husband had apparently been longing for, he then found he could no longer get an erection. Another couple came because he could not sustain an erection. When the sensate focus programme started to pay off, and he was getting strong and enduring erections, his wife said that the programme was 'boring' and they dropped out. Usually these kind of couples are perturbed by a problem because, from the outside, it looks 'abnormal'. In actual fact, they come to realise that it suits them profoundly.

Whether the couple have sex or not, or whether the sex is loving or hostile, or whether it involves an unusual interaction or is quite straightforward, it is usually an exact mirror of the rest of their relationship — more so than is the case with couples of other Sexual Style combinations. Even when they fight about it there is satisfaction, whether they recognise it or not — for two strongly bonded Emotionals have chosen each other instinctively because of their matching needs.

Long-term prospects

Usually, as has been seen, this couple make an exceptionally strong, close and enduring relationship. But this is not always the case. Two very damaged and angry Emotionals can find their interaction so powerfully unpleasant that they break up — indeed, they will often ricochet through life making a series of these cataclysmic relationships, never able to stay the course with one person. Most Emotionals, however, although they might have more than one important relationship in their lives, will tend towards staying with their partners for many years — and when their partners are Emotionals too, the union can be life-long.

It must be clear by now that Emotional partnerships can't be classified by the usual criteria. An unhappy or embattled couple are, in fact, 'happy' in their own way. At the very least, they feel that they are living out their destiny. Emotionals, like everyone else, have clear if unconscious expectations of life, and what it will bring them in terms of happiness or pain. While

Imaginatives, Romantics and Sensuals will all, to a degree, try to shape their lives to change the more negative aspects of what they have come to expect, Emotionals are helplessly driven to make their expectations come true. With another Emotional it is inevitable that they will succeed. So even when this leads to misery or despair there is a perverse satisfaction in knowing that they were right all along. Indeed, Emotionals who expect difficulties can be rendered unbearably anxious by periods of happiness and tranquillity: they know the axe is going to fall, and rather than have to wait for it, they hasten its descent.

This sounds negative, but for them it is normal. And of course, there are Emotionals with much happier expectations of life, much better childhood experiences, and therefore much happier and healthier outcomes. Two Emotionals like this will make the happiest and most intimate relationship of any combination. Their years together will increase their happiness, and they will know love more deeply and satisfyingly than anyone else.

The Romantic and The Sensual

'I slept and dreamed that life was beauty
I woke and found that life was duty.'

Ellen Sturgis Hooper

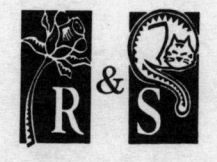

The Romantic and The Sensual

There could hardly be two people less alike than the Romantic and the Sensual. But despite this — and often because of it — there can be a strong mutual attraction. It's perhaps understandable that the mainly Sensual person is beguiled by the delightful person who is more Romantic than anything else. Most people *are* attracted to Romantics — after all, they tend to be fun, flirtatious and extremely desirable to be around. But the Romantic is also fascinated by the Sensual. When the Romantic woman sees a Sensual man, she sees 'man' writ large. This is the 'tower of strength'; this is the man who puts up shelves; this is the man who is masterful in bed; this is the man who will take care of all the practical things in life and let her take care of the good bits. The Romantic man who is drawn to the Sensual woman sees the potential dream wife. This is the woman who will love him in bed and out of it; this is the woman who will care for his future children; this is the woman who will soothe his fevered brow, be a practical helpmeet, look after the domestic details and leave him free to dream and soar.

Actually the Romantic will only find the better-looking and more stylish or talented Sensuals truly attractive, and the Sensual will be alert to the physical chemistry between them. But, all that being well, Romantics find the Sensual's qualities — so different from their own — somewhat exotic, and erotic. How do they manage to be so calm, so sensible? How do they understand the hieroglyphics on a bank statement? Needless to say, Sensuals also find the joyousness of Romantics and their attractive presentation of themselves extremely desirable. They bring a sense of excitement and drama into the routine of the Sensuals' lives.

This combination bodes well for an extremely intense and passionate affair. Romantics are at their most sexually responsive when they are first in love, and Sensuals can be almost romantic when they are swept up in the all-consuming passion of initial lust. Longer term there are likely to be problems but, even so, these people can complement each other well. If they can negotiate the inherent difficulties they can, as a couple, be more than the sum of their parts.

The beginning

The Romantic in love is a puppy dog. Whether there is any Sensual in his or her nature or not, he or she will be all over the beloved partner. The Romantic can't get too close, can't be too loving, can't do too much to demonstrate the deliriously excited extent of his or her loving feelings. Ms Romantic wants spontaneous and frequent love-making — it makes her feel so desirable and loved. Mr Romantic feels ardent and powerful, wants to ravish and conquer this wonderful woman — and her swooning submission to him makes him feel omnipotent and adored.

This couldn't be better for the Sensual, for whom love is best expressed physically, and especially sexually. The Sensual when first in love is a slightly demented creature. It's all a bit too much for the person who feels most content when jogging along in a pleasant, predictable routine. And the Sensual in love wants to own the beloved. For these reasons he or she can behave in uncharacteristically romantic ways to make sure that this new and adorable person will want to stay around. Mr Sensual will phone Ms Romantic constantly, remember to bring her flowers, take her out for good meals. Ms Sensual will be at her most concerned to look good, smell sweet, go along with all Mr Romantic's notions of fun in the interests of remaining as close as possible to him.

It's not surprising that they feel so *compatible*. They seem to want the same things, to show love in the same way. At its most intense they can't keep their hands off each other, and both, in their different ways, find this immensely gratifying.

Settling down

So they fall more deeply in love. Sometimes, of course, they do so without such a torrid start. For one reason or another there might have been very little love-making at the beginning. In either case, there is the deeper recognition of how each other's Sexual Style offers a missing component in their natures.

It is at this point, when they move in together, marry, or simply consolidate their relationship over a long period of months, that the cracks can start to show.

The fact is that Romantics want the passion to go on and on. If their sex drive is high, by passion they can also mean sex. The sex, however, must be special, thrilling, accompanied by loving displays and sweet nothings, between two people who continue to make the effort to look good for each other. But by passion they mean much more than sex. They want to keep the intensity turned up to maximum. They want to continue to be totally wrapped up in each other, for a current of excitement to run between them all the time. Their relationships must feel special, glamorous, even. They like to feel that their partners admire or revere them; they'd like to return that admiration at full blast.

This is not what the Sensual wants, or expects. Love is love, in the end, the Sensual would say. You feel it or you don't. It certainly shouldn't need to be stoked or nurtured. You show it through physical affection, by simply being there, by making love. Sensuals feel most comfortable in a relationship that has settled down.

Once Sensuals believe they have captured their prize, they want to get back to feeling normal: totally themselves. The Sensual woman wants to relax her vigilance over how she looks. She wants to be able to slop around, not wear make-up, carefully pack her sexy underwear away for use on birthdays and anniversaries. For the Romantic man, who has been beguiled by her gorgeous presentation, this can be extremely disappointing – almost alarming. The Sensual man, while remaining ready to bask in any attentions the Romantic woman showers on him, feels irritated if she expects him to go on saying how beautiful and wonderful she is. In fact, he has probably stopped noticing. Even when she has made a supreme effort to look her dazzling best for a special occasion she'll appear pretty much the same to him. If he's happy and generally contented with her it has ceased to matter much what she does look like.

These might seem superficial difficulties, but they do rankle. The Romantic whose Sensual partner has put on too much weight feels strangely uncared for. Doesn't the Sensual mind any more what the Romantic thinks? The Sensual who is aware of the Romantic's disapproval over external matters of appearance wonders what sort of love this is, or feels that there is something odd about the Romantic's need to look good all the time.

These can be the outward signs of a deeper discontent. For the Romantic love continues to flower when it is shown with ostentation. Ms Romantic positively needs to be told how much she is loved, and she wants the little gifts, the affectionate pet names, the continuing thoughtfulness, the surprise outings and the remembering of special anniversaries. The year is often littered with these for Romantic women – not just the obvious anniversaries and birthdays, but also the first kiss, the first love-making, the moment when love was declared and so on. None of this comes naturally to the Sensual man. Rooted in the here and now, anniversaries mean little to him; he's not greatly sentimental about the past, however exciting or loving it was. Romantic gestures seem somewhat bizarre and pointless, and he can be annoyed if they are expected of him. Alternatively, the Romantic woman needs to have continuing faith in the admirable, special qualities of her man – as a wonderful human being, great artist, brilliant businessman, or whatever. This can be a struggle when he is a Sensual man who leaves all that outside the front door and becomes, at home, something of a slob – clipping his toe-nails in front of the television, contentedly burping. Or even when he's the more refined Sensual, she wonders where all that brilliance goes as he potters around doing nothing very much at all, mindlessly and wordlessly happy.

Mr Romantic doesn't expect so much in the way of romantic gifts and mementos, but he does need to feel that his woman thinks he's quite perfect. The trouble is that Ms Sensual is too down-to-earth for this – she might think he's perfect, but that doesn't mean she's oblivious to his faults, and she won't think twice about mentioning them. She's being loving, but he sees it as quite the reverse. She can be more amused (or irritated) than admiring that he takes even longer to prepare to go out than she does: worrying about whether he needs a haircut; if those socks go with that tie; whether he's struck just the right note of casualness or elegance for the occasion. He wants her to be as glamorous, witty and enchanting at home as she was when they first fell in love. Instead she slops around, likes to have long stretches of comfortable peace and quiet, calls him to carry out a distasteful (for him) examination of a worrying mole she's discovered on her thigh.

The trouble is that Sensuals snuggle into domesticity with a sigh of relief. This is what all that unsettling excitement of intoxicating love was leading towards. If you love each other, you can just 'be'. Sensuals can be very deeply in love without needing to show it in any other way than gentle affectionate coddling, and sustained and pleasurable love-making. In contrast, for the Romantic, loving feelings start to diminish when not regularly topped up with outward displays of affection more tangible than a hug and a pat and a kiss and lots of sex.

Daily life

When there is plenty of love between the couple then these irritations ebb and flow, sometimes mattering more than at other times. If the Romantic has a strong dose of Sensual, and the Sensual also has some Romantic, then some of these differences can be smoothed out naturally, but not entirely.

It is daily irritations that often erode relationships far more than the big crises. The Romantic woman who discovers that her traditional Sensual man is expecting her to be the little housewife can feel like Cinderella, wondering where all the glamour and beauty of her life went. She might become defensively queenly, trying to make him see that she is above all that. Often what she wants to do is go out and buy something to cheer herself up — and she can think he is impossibly mean when he says they can't afford it. It's his *job* to make sure that they *can* afford it.

If Mr Sensual seems to switch off whenever they are alone together, or busies himself with tasks around the house, she can become flirtatiously coaxing, to make him see that she is more interesting than the humdrum chores. The Sensual man, who might have loved all this at the start, begins to find it irksome. Ms Romantic, feeling neglected and overlooked, looks for more powerful weapons in her armoury. She'll flirt with other men to make him jealous, or tell him about men who are after her. If she feels too ignored she'll pick a fight. She'd prefer him to show her that he loves her, but making him angry or upset will just have to do — at least when this happens she knows that his attention is being fixed on her. She's important; he's noticing.

The Romantic and The Sensual

Mr Sensual does not respond well to these tactics. He wants a quiet life, at least at home, and too much conflict can depress him. Too much lively interaction, even, is exasperating when he's tired or just doesn't want to have to think about anything much. He's hard to draw into a fight, and when he does get angry it's not a good sign. While the Romantic woman can work up a head of steam and then almost as quickly change her mood if things go right, the Sensual man will take longer to recover from his own rage. He'll tend to become warier, withdraw into silence — just the sort of behaviour that maddens Ms Romantic.

The Sensual woman whose Romantic man shows he much prefers the hubbub of life outside home to a cosy evening in can feel that what matters to her is not important to him. His attractive liveliness is all very well in its place, but she worries about how free he is with their money. He thinks that paying to have fun is just as essential as paying bills — sometimes even more so. He seems to treat money in his pocket as a windfall, and seems blithely convinced that another piece of luck will be along soon. It goes against the grain for Mr Romantic to use money for necessities: Ms Sensual wants to save to pay for the underpinning of the house; he wants to save for a holiday. For Ms Sensual, security is all-important, and if her partner has a rash attitude to cash she can be deeply disturbed.

Ms Sensual's belief that deep pleasure can be found in homely comforts can eventually bore Mr Romantic. He was instinctively drawn to this side of her nature, but he doesn't want his nose rubbed in it all the time. He can become fed up — literally — with her constant emphasis on serving delicious meals: there's only a degree of excitement and fun to be had in eating. Why does she expect him to be transported with pleasure over soft new bedsheets, a roaring fire, what's happening in the garden? In a way, all these things are beneath his notice and he finds her delight in them somewhat off-putting. Unlike Ms Romantic, the Romantic man is less likely to put effort into trying to provoke a different sort of response from his Sensual partner, or to change her. Instead he spends less and less time at home, and puts his energies into finding the drama and excitement he needs outside it. When the combination is this way round, indeed, there is a danger that the Sensual woman becomes more of a mother than a lover to her man, who turns into the recalcitrant little boy. Should this happen, however, he's also likely to lose desire for her. Then she is deprived of one her most compelling comforts: sex.

Communication between the Romantic and the Sensual

A lot of this is, not surprisingly, a communication problem. The Romantic and the Sensual have different ways of communicating about intimate matters. The Sensual, in fact, would rather not. He or she finds having to talk about relationships heavy work. It's not to do with whether Sensuals are intelligent or articulate — in other areas of their lives they can be the brightest sparks — but when it comes to love and sex they don't have much to say. If it all feels right that's fine — what's there to talk about? If it's uncomfortable and unsatisfying in any way, talking is not going to make much difference they feel. In either case, the Sensual wants to tackle the feelings in the way he or she understands best, by getting close. The happy Sensual wants to cuddle and make love. The unhappy Sensual thinks that things will get better if only they could cuddle and make love.

It's quite different for the Romantics. All their emotions are much nearer the surface and they tend to be quite open about what they feel. Indeed, they like to talk about themselves and what they are experiencing. If it's love, and they're happy, it's a favourite topic of conversation. They like all the lovey-dovey exchanges about how wonderful it all is and how lucky they both are. At these times the Romantic will hardly notice that the Sensual's main contribution is brief agreement and contented listening. When Romantics are discontented, however, they are more likely to complain and attack. The trouble is that when it is their Romantic expectations that are disappointed they never quite get to the root of the problem. They'll complain about the current petty aggravation in dramatic terms as if it were the worst thing that could possibly happen, because the real problem is virtually unsayable. How do you begin to explain — or even understand yourself — that what is missing is the grand, intoxicating excitement that welled up almost from nowhere and eventually disappeared like mist? This is one thing that Romantics share with Sensuals — they know that talking won't bring it back, but they ache with the knowledge that it is no longer there. The Romantic man can take it out on the Sensual woman, blaming her for letting herself go or for not keeping pace with him. The Romantic woman is more likely to question herself and her desirability. Both, however, can express these feelings in the same way — by having a melodramatic tantrum about something else, or picking a fight. The surge of adrenalin this creates floods them with the excited feelings they crave. It might be unhappy excitement, but it is better than nothing at all.

In other words, the Romantic confronts and the Sensual sulks. Neither of these methods help them tackle the real problem. When Sensuals are barraged with words they retreat into a mental bunker and wait for the explosions to die away. Deep down they fear that it might mean something is seriously wrong, but they'll wait and see. Sensuals who try their cure-all by taking hold of an angry partner, or making a sexual move will make the Romantic feel furious and violated. The Sensuals find that they have in their arms a physically rigid or temporarily violent person. Part of the trouble is that, in the early days when everything was lovely, these moves by the Sensual had the required result, and rage was replaced by melting love.

None of this is helped by the fact that both of them are equally clumsy when it comes to reading signals. If the

Romantic goes silent on the Sensual, he or she is blithely unaware that there might be a problem. Silence, after all, is often bliss. So long as the Romantic is *there* it must mean that everything is all right. Sensuals are quite capable of being completely oblivious to the implications even of a massive sulk. The Romantic, in turn, can fail to see that a prolonged campaign to educate and instruct the Sensual by complaints or exciting jealousy has resulted in a wounded and defensive partner. A frightened Sensual can appear to do all the things the Romantic wants, but it does not come from the heart.

Improvements can be made when the Romantic and the Sensual realise what's going on. Sensuals must understand that, while talking does nothing for them particularly, it is reassuring and helpful for the Romantic. Talking *will*, therefore, help in the end, because the Romantic will be happier and the relationship will feel better. Romantics must understand that some of the romance *can* be revived if they talk about their disappointments in the concrete terms that the Sensual understands rather than in generalised rhetoric or sniping. The Sensual needs to know, 'I loved it when you used to do [whatever it was] I'd be so happy if you did that again.' Sensuals must be prepared to *listen* to such specific requests, and act on them. It usually seems trivial from their point of view, so they can be truly amazed at how much difference it makes.

Romantics also have to recognise that the physical way that Sensuals show love really *is* love. It might be unglamorous, but it is steadfast. The Sensual who stops wanting to touch generally and to make love specifically is much more worrying. Telling your Sensual how you would like to be treated while you are embracing is much more likely to get the results you want. Even difficult things, such as 'I'd find you even more sexy if you lost a bit of weight' can be better 'heard' and accepted by the Sensual who is having a cuddle. Sensuals, for their part, must realise that they should never, never, *never* think sex will solve everything when their Romantic partner is seriously upset or angry. They will be rebuffed; Romantics will find it supremely unloving. Instead, the Sensual should make some effort to appeal to the Romantic's hurt feelings, be contrite, take interest. Romantics and Sensuals can both be warm-hearted, it's just that they need to understand each other's different needs and ways of showing love.

Sex in the Romantic and Sensual partnership

I once devised a questionnaire for *Family Circle* magazine, whose object was to find out about the sex lives of couples that had been married for a long time. Respondents were invited to write in with their comments if they wished. One heart-breaking anonymous letter came from a woman who had been married for nine years. It encapsulated the Romantic/Sensual dilemma. 'I am a romantic, unfortunately my husband is not,' she wrote. 'For many years it really got me that we seemed to be on different wavelengths. He thought romanticism was daft, and there was no point to it. He just sees sex as sex — not tied up with an atmosphere or image. We used to discuss it but no improvement ever came — and six months later we'd be having the same discussion. Eventually when he asked me what was wrong I'd say, "Nothing," because if I said, "You aren't romantic ..." or told him the real problem, he'd say, "Not this again." So whenever we have sex now I think of someone I like — currently a rock star. It makes sex bearable. My husband seems to think a quick grope down below will send me into multiple orgasms. If I say, "There's a problem between us, let's talk about it," he says, "I can't see a problem, Everything looks fine to me." He's always been complimentary about my body and says I've got a lovely figure. I do try with my appearance — day and night — and wear nice things to bed. But he makes no attempt to make himself look/smell nice. He comes to bed in his awful pyjamas he's had for 15 years. We've no one who can take the kids for a weekend so we can have a bit of space alone. He would see it as a total waste of money to go to a hotel anyway. I wonder whether I expect too much. I feel you're only young once, but he seems happy so long as the bills are paid. I often think and wonder if I will ever experience "real" love-making. Or is it just a fantastic dream that doesn't exist?'

There are no pat answers, especially when the Sensual man refuses to acknowledge that anything is wrong. In fact this woman didn't even ask for answers; she simply said, wistfully, 'I'll be interested to read your results to see if it is just me – or if many other women feel the same – caught up in the drudge of being taken for granted, bringing up kids, doing the washing, ironing, cooking every day.'

The trouble with the unawakened Sensual man is that he can derive just enough pleasure from unsensual sex to keep him satisfied. And because he's generally good at coping with disappointments in life, he finds it impossible to understand that these are much more devastating for his partner.

The anonymous writer was tackling the problem in the best way the Romantic woman knows – making herself alluring in the hope that it will effect a change in him. She tries to talk about what's going wrong, saying vaguely that she wants 'romance'. Eventually she is driven to say that 'nothing' is the matter, hoping he'll realise for himself. These strategies, unfortunately, are over the head of the Sensual man, however intelligent he might be. He's only dimly aware that she always looks nice. And when she complains he simply waits for her to stop – or as in the case of this Sensual husband, shrugs and says, 'I can't see a problem,' or, 'Not this again.' He only wakes up to the problem if she is strong enough to deny him sex altogether. That's something he *does* understand.

The Sensual man needs a much more direct appeal to his senses. If his Romantic woman introduces him to the pleasures of long, slow, intimate sex he can be delighted to find out what he has been missing. A few comments along the lines of 'I love it when you do that — don't stop' can also help. Buying him some new pyjamas, or some aftershave, or telling him that she finds him very sexy just after he's had a shower can also help in his re-education. Sadly, these strategies are difficult for the Romantic woman, who does not want to have to take the initiative or tell him what to do and finds it almost as unerotic to coax him as she does to have to put up with his caveman technique. She will be most willing to do so — and have most success — in the early days while they are still madly in love. If she waits too long — and having to fantasise about another man every time they make love probably *is* too long — then she will find it difficult to do more than yearn and nurse her resentment.

Often the issue of sex turns out not to be the main problem for Ms Romantic, just a focus for it. If the more aware Sensual man can learn to be more generally considerate and loving, she is less concerned about what they do sexually, and is more receptive. What she hates is to be treated as some kind of sexual receptacle whose feelings don't count. Her feelings about the relationship can radically alter if he makes her feel loved as well as desired, and is prepared to ignore the urgency of his sexual needs from time to time out of consideration for her.

There are similar problems when it is the man who is Romantic and the woman who is Sensual. She's certainly less concerned that he should look and smell nice, or behave romantically towards her, but she does need plenty of physical affection in and out of bed, and thoroughly enjoys prolonged love-making. The trouble is that once the romance goes out of the relationship for him he can't be bothered to waste much time over sex. He wants to make love when *he* wants to make love, and a woman who makes it clear that she wants more sex than he does, or at times when he doesn't, offends him. It feels like a criticism. And what can she expect? His Sensual lover has taken to going to bed in a musty tee-shirt and a pair of bed-socks and she expects him to be turned on! She has put on weight, only has her hair done for 'special occasions', yet thinks that he should be driven wild with desire! What's with this woman? Occasionally his body demands some sexual relief, and as she's there it might as well be with her, but he can't be expected to want to prolong the experience.

The Sensual woman in this situation is usually more motivated to change matters for the better than the Sensual man is – if only because sexual satisfaction for a woman is more complex than it is for a man, and she needs Mr Romantic's co-operation. She needs to meet him on his own terms: wooing him, making him feel special. She needs to vamp it up a bit, make sure she looks good, drape herself in the right clothes in the right light to bring out her best points and minimise her worst. He is more likely to feel desirous if there is a little more mystery and slightly less intimacy. He doesn't want to watch her preparing to look good, he prefers to be dazzled by the finished result. This is anathema, actually, to Ms Sensual, who wants to be natural and loved for herself. Similarly, she is not put off by a close physical relationship in which she is aware of all his bodily functions, crude or disgusting as they might be at times. When she loves him this doesn't make him a whit less sexy to her.

If she's not prepared to make the effort, however, or it hasn't occurred to her to try, he may eventually turn away from her sexually altogether. He might, indeed, look for sex elsewhere. The practical Sensual woman is often good at eventually sublimating her sexual drives, and looking for sensual gratification in other ways. If she can find this, her pragmatic approach to disappointment can mean that she does not feel quite so desperately frustrated as the Romantic woman who is not deriving the romance she needs from a relationship.

Long-term prospects

Some of the most successful Romantic/Sensual partnerships have a degree of practical difficulty about them. They can't see each other when they want – they might be having an affair, for instance, or one has to travel for work. This is particularly satisfying for Romantics, who often find that absence really does make the heart grow fonder, and romantic feelings return when they have to yearn a little for the presence of the beloved. It's not quite so comfortable for the Sensual, but it means that he or she focuses on the Romantic in the way the Romantic likes best when they are together, and this very focusing makes the Romantic most physically and sexually affectionate.

But more conventional relationships and marriages can work too, especially when each continues to value the differences that first attracted them. Romantics must realise that the very qualities that sometimes seem boring in the Sensual can also contribute to long-lasting love and fidelity. A faithful partner is essential to the Romantic of either sex. Sensuals need to realise that the unpredictability and volatility of the Romantic, which can be so exasperating at times, can bring a continuing lightness and excitement into their lives – something they are not very good at doing for themselves. If each can acknowledge the different strengths they bring to the union they can create a balance between stability and excitement that is very rewarding.

Marriages between Romantic women and Sensual men can suit them both well. It is the best way round for this pairing: he wants to be the man and she wants to be the woman – and if they can let each other do this in their own way they will both be happy. This is especially so when they put their various energies into creating a stylish and comfortable home and raising a family. The Romantic woman who has children gets in touch with the sensual (though non-sexual) elements in her nature. The primitive need to nurture and protect her offspring can deepen her need for stability and increase her appreciation of the simpler side of life. Mr Sensual can often be at his most romantic when his wife is the mother of tiny babies. He marvels at her femaleness and feels moist-eyed at the thought that she is nurturing the fruit of his loins – his investment in the future. He is likely to be at his most tender and considerate at this time. It does pass as the children grow up, but it can be extremely gratifying for Ms Romantic in the early, hectic days of motherhood.

The Sensual man who can also indulge his wife's need for glamour and image, and who can celebrate her femininity will keep her very happy. He might have to make notes to remind himself to acknowledge with little gifts and tender gestures the anniversaries that mean so much to her. She also needs to be taken out from time to time, and be given regular excuses for dressing up. When he does all this, she will blossom. In turn, she must recognise that he needs times that are simply quiet and comfortable, and prefers life in the house to out of it. He will feel more loved if she shows it rather than says it. Neglect these key issues and both of them will become very unhappy. It is in Mr Sensual's nature to still try to hang on to the relationship grimly, but, eventually Ms Romantic might find it unbearable and leave – particularly if they don't have children, and even if they do.

The Romantic man married to the Sensual woman can have a slightly more difficult time of it. As seen earlier, Mr Romantic can in this relationship become more of a boy than a man, and Ms Sensual can retreat into being more of a mother than a woman. When she does, in fact, become a mother, Mr Romantic can believe himself in competition for top place in her attention and affections, and he doesn't like it. Mr Romantic, indeed, is the man most likely to resent the commandeering of 'his' breasts for the purpose that nature intended. It's hard for him to continue to see Ms Sensual as a romantic figure when she is so evidently an earth mother. And because she is so talented at giving herself up to the experience of the moment, his importance for her can be as drastically reduced, for a while, as he fears.

Mr Romantic who can't find the romance he requires at home is much more cavalier about seeking it elsewhere – at work, or in the arms of another woman. This often happens because his romantic demands are less specific than the Romantic woman's and not so easily assuaged by attentive behaviour. But this combination can have a better chance of success in the long term than the reverse coupling. It suits Mr Romantic to have a base from which he can go out and find romance in whatever form he likes it, knowing that all the practical concerns are dealt with at home. He might, of course, leave if he falls in love, but not necessarily. Ms Sensual, for the sake of security, will forego a lot of the other things she needs in terms of sex and love, and is therefore prepared to tolerate a fairly empty marriage. She'll do more than put up with it if there are other compensations – children to love and fuss over and a relatively comfortable lifestyle.

It can be much, much better than this, however, so long as they can learn to find what they need in each other, rather than travelling along parallel lines. The Romantic man can be much more grounded and mature, and the Sensual woman can be much more fun and spontaneous if they learn to incorporate some of each other's excellent qualities in themselves.

The Emotional and The Imaginative

'It has been well said, that heart speaks to heart, whereas language only speaks to the ears.'

St Francis de Sales

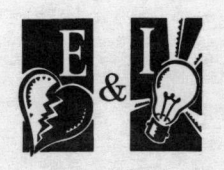

The Emotional and The Imaginative

The Emotional and the Imaginative are complete opposites. Emotionals trust their instincts, and what they feel: they don't have to have a 'reason' to respond or behave as they do. The motto of the Imaginatives could be 'I think therefore I am' — what can't be analysed or explained is disturbing to them. Emotionals experience the most important part of life deep in the recesses of their hearts, below the level of words; Imaginatives operate on the surface, through verbal communication. Emotionals thrive on intensity; Imaginatives are most comfortable in an emotional climate that is cool and allows for clear thinking.

Yet opposites, as the old saying goes, attract. The Emotional is fascinated by the quicksilver Imaginative, who seems to have something to say about everything, who is charming, articulate — and has the ability to be objective about life's vicissitudes. The Imaginative is intrigued by the deep waters of the Emotional. Here is a person who offers great potential for exploration. What you see is not necessarily what you get.

Ms Emotional watches in dazzled amazement as Mr Imaginative flies round the room talking to anyone and everyone. It's beyond her how he manages it — she finds chit-chat difficult, so caught up, as she is, in the undercurrents of what people really mean behind what they are saying. Mr Imaginative, flirting expertly with Ms Emotional, finds her intoxicatingly elusive. He can't get a handle on who she is and what she wants. He finds her more and more attractive.

Mr Emotional, treated to the full force of Ms Imaginative's personality, feels an immediate intimacy. She talks so openly about herself, and asks the most searching questions about him. Ms Imaginative sees in Mr Emotional a complex soul. What are his secrets? She *must* find out.

For this initial attraction to go any further, however, the Imaginative has to feel that the Emotional has an unusual mind, or an interesting sexual nature. The Emotional, in turn, will have to be drawn to something he or she perceives below the surface of the Imaginative's presentation, or something that touches — for good or ill — an important emotional chord: echoing, perhaps, a significant person in the Emotional's life who was equally bright and articulate, or similarly emotionally controlled and cool.

The beginning

Sometimes it is all over in a flash. The Imaginative who is a skilled sexual operator, and who can be so cavalier about sex, talks the Emotional into bed. A short while later, having mined the Emotional for all that is interesting, he or she is off looking for the next fascinating conquest. The Emotional, having mistaken the flurry of words for deeper communication, feels violated. Emotionals find casual relationships disturbing, even the men. Some Emotionals, however, seem to be drawn like iron filings to magnetic Imaginative heart-breakers who, as you might expect, break their hearts. They yearn to catch and keep one, but never seem to learn their lesson.

Often, however, this initial attraction is consolidated, and they fall in love. Both of them are pleasurably maddened by each other's very difference. The Imaginative finds the

Emotional's moods and passions mysterious. When, as sometimes happens, the Emotional is good at talking about everything but emotional matters, the Imaginative is tantalised by the knowledge that he or she is only seeing the tip of the iceberg in the beloved's nature. The Emotional's intense desire to possess the Imaginative can seem thrilling and unusual.

The Emotional envies and admires the Imaginative's ability to talk away difficulties, and finds he or she is lifted out of emotional chaos by the Imaginative's calm objectivity, or spell-binding stories.

Yet there seem to be great similarities too. Love by its very nature blurs the boundaries between people, especially in the early, heightened stage. Emotionals, newly in love, are going to be most open about their feelings, most willing to talk. Imaginatives will be at their most emotional, most focused on their partner, and less restless in their need to look for different experiences elsewhere. A clever or worldly Emotional, or one dedicated to a cause, can become a mentor for an Imaginative who has a thirst to learn. In this case, the Imaginative takes on the ideas and attitudes of the Emotional, at least for a time. This apparent sharing of what the Emotional cares for passionately can open the way to great love.

Settling down

'We're a couple now,' thinks the Imaginative. 'How can we make life even more interesting?' The Imaginative who needs a soulmate wants their partnership to develop in a stimulating, lively way – particularly Ms Imaginative. She wants their life together to be a continuing dialogue. She wants them to go out and about together and discuss what they think about what they've seen and done. What these Imaginatives, male or female, hope for from love is to have the ultimate best friend, so that they can say, in the words of William Cory, '... you and I/Had tired the sun with talking and sent him down the sky.'

The trouble is that none of this has the same allure for the Emotional. Yes, he or she might enjoy a certain amount of socialising and good conversation, but it's not what the Emotional is looking for from love. Indeed, some Emotionals find precisely the things that the Imaginative most enjoys superficial. Activities that are interesting but which don't engage them on a deeper level can even be irritating. An evening spent having dinner with a group of people that the Emotional doesn't particularly care about, and dissecting the interactions and the conversations afterwards, is not the Emotional's idea of fun either. Love might well include friendship, but it is certainly not dependent on it.

Emotionals need to bond. When they fall in love, they want the relationship to last. Some are almost chameleon-like in their ability to be what their partners need, so strong is their own need to hold on to them. The Emotional is perfectly capable of being the interesting, vital, sexually inventive partner the Imaginative wants in order to strengthen the commitment between them. As it happens, this kind of interaction is less important to the Emotional than what it produces: a profounder tie that makes separating less thinkable. Indeed, the Emotional is often unconsciously watching for the moment when the relationship has developed to this point, and he or she can drop the less natural Imaginative-type behaviour that has led to it.

When the Emotional no longer wants to play the Imaginative's games, as sometimes happens when the relationship has settled down over a period of months or years, and can no longer understand the Imaginative's need to continue the intense conversational dialogue between them, the relationship can become difficult for both of them.

The Imaginative reacts in the usual way: by looking for what he or she needs elsewhere. Imaginative is the Sexual Style that has least requirement to derive its needs from one other person. Feeling interested or intellectually engaged is far more important. This is the time that some Imaginatives take off for good. More usually, however, when they love their Emotional partners they will look to plug the gaps in their relationship instead. They will want to see other friends more often, go to the movies, to exhibitions, try all the new things that make them feel alive and happy — alone if necessary. They return to their partners refreshed and less demanding. Perhaps they chatter on about everything they've seen and done: the sound of their own voices obscuring the fact that they are getting back little of what they need from the Emotional in terms of response. In actual fact, although the Imaginative seems happy with this compromise, he or she is disturbed. Intimacy means sharing of thoughts and ideas. The Imaginative feels most loving and involved when having an exciting and open conversation.

The Emotional is disturbed too. And it is in the Emotional's nature to feel disturbance more deeply and painfully. The fact that the Imaginative is deriving so much satisfaction outside the partnership makes the Emotional insecure. If you love each other you shouldn't need other people and other activities to make you happy. The Imaginative's escapades make the Emotional feel unnecessary; unloved. These feelings are precisely the ones that make the Emotional close down in self-protection — in a way that is hurtful to the Imaginative. Or the Emotional becomes clingy and possessive, which makes the Imaginative feel suffocated. The Emotional doesn't want to hear about what the Imaginative did alone, and how exciting it was. The Emotional certainly doesn't want to discuss it.

It's hard for a loving Imaginative to curtail his or her enthusiasm for life outside the home in the interests of not hurting the Emotional's feelings. The Imaginative can't understand *why* it is hurtful. Imaginatives who no longer want to talk about their experiences or thoughts, indeed, are on the way to being very disaffected. Not talking about these matters feels unloving to them.

An example is a friend of mine I shall call Vera. She is an

Imaginative living with an Emotional, Denis. In an attempt to balance her life, she goes out regularly with a group of girlfriends to have fun. Vera, in the past, had many lovers, and sex without strings was extremely enjoyable for her. She loves Denis, and wouldn't dream of being unfaithful — not because it would matter to her, but because she knows it would devastate him. It is her habit, and her pleasure, to tell Denis every detail of her evenings out. Men often come up and flirt with her, which she enjoys without wanting to take it any further. She has always told Denis about these encounters too, because it's all part of the fun. If she had been a Romantic, her purpose in telling him would probably be to excite his jealousy, but it never occurred to Vera that it could — there was nothing to be jealous about. Once, in an excess of agony, Denis told her how much it hurt him to hear about these other men. Now Vera tries to remember not to include these details in her accounts, but she finds it hard. Not mentioning them feels like deceit. Telling all, when the Imaginative has nothing to hide, is an expression of love and commitment.

That's why the Imaginative can also feel anxious or even betrayed by the Emotional's very different view of these matters. Emotionals do not have the same need to talk through what they are doing, thinking or feeling. In fact it can be extremely hard for them to attach words to emotions — and seems unnecessary. They can also feel threatened by the Imaginative's belief that a rational explanation should be found for something as hard to describe as emotion — and feel alienated by the Imaginative's impatient dismissal of their unwilling and clumsy attempts to explain.

Vera has cited an example of this. For two weeks Denis was plunged into wordless gloom. She didn't know what she had done to cause it, but assumed it was her fault because she experienced his silence as hostility. Eventually, after much pushing he told her that he was depressed by the autumn schedule of television programmes. Their arrival meant that summer was over and winter would soon be starting. Vera was both exasperated and amused by this illogical explanation. Looked at from her point of view it *was* illogical. But Denis is a man who feels depressed during winter, and, as an Emotional, doesn't know how to be logical about this, or how to change his mood. Away from the arena of his emotional life, incidentally, Denis is a rational and articulate man, but he is unable to bring these skills to bear on this aspect of himself.

When the Emotional can't or won't talk about things, the Imaginative perceives it as secrecy, or as deliberate shutting out. The Imaginative needs to get inside a partner's head to feel truly bonded. 'I don't want to talk' sounds strangely like 'I don't love you enough' to the Imaginative. What is so important that it must be hidden? Both of them can find that the very qualities that drew them together so compellingly now seem to be driving them apart.

Daily life

The different pleasure-needs of the Imaginative and Emotional can be a source of tension. Even when they are happily in love there can be difficulties. An evening in, for instance, is not the Imaginative's favourite way of passing time, but if that's what they are going to do, at least they can talk. The Emotional can be supremely content to spend time alone with a loved partner, but doesn't believe they should have to entertain each other. Remember, the Imaginative finds talking intimate and emotionally satisfying; the Emotional can find talking *intellectually* stimulating but it has few emotional reverberations. The Imaginative whose attempts to start a conversation are rebuffed might retreat into a good book or television programme, and derive plenty of satisfaction from doing so – but he or she will feel distanced from the Emotional. The Emotional knows that something is wrong, but suffers because of it rather than trying to do something about it.

Or they go out. They do something that the Imaginative enjoys and the Emotional simply endures. Buzzing with the excitement, the Imaginative feels happy, while the Emotional – noting this – feels alienated because it is not the relationship that is causing this surge of happiness, but something outside it. The Imaginative, thinking it is just one of the Emotional's usual moods, is quite able to dismiss it as something merely irritating or unimportant.

When they are feeling less loving it is even harder. Ms Imaginative has had a bad day and is looking forward to talking it through with Mr Emotional – or doing something to take her mind off the problem. He hears her out, perhaps says 'poor you' and that is the end of the matter as far as he is concerned. In his experience talking doesn't achieve much, and certainly won't make you feel better. If he's very empathetic he can enter into Ms Imaginative's feelings too personally. 'How terrible,' he cries, becoming depressed himself. He's certainly no longer in the mood to do something frivolous and interesting which might make Ms Imaginative feel better. Her temporary gloom has pervaded them both.

If it's Mr Emotional who has had a bad day it is equally difficult. Ms Imaginative wants to make him feel better so she insists they talk about it. She comes up with some good ideas about how he should deal with the situation. Or she tells him something interesting to take his mind off it. All this makes him feel worse. He feels she is trivialising his experience by assuming it is so easily solved, and has no understanding of how he suffers. Under the volley of words he retreats deeper into himself and his feelings of misery deepen. In trying to make him feel better, Ms Imaginative is made to feel miserable herself, drawn into his uncomfortable world where her usual strategies don't work.

When the positions are reversed and the man is Imaginative and the woman Emotional, the problems are similar and sometimes more acute. Mr Imaginative arrives home to find Ms

Emotional in a state about something. He tries to be sympathetic and asks her to explain, but it all sounds so silly when she does. Typical female over-reaction, he thinks. After a few minutes trying to 'sort her out' he gives up. He doesn't want to be dragged down by her so he goes out or absents himself mentally by burying himself in some work, his computer, or a book. Now she feels lonely and unloved on top of everything else.

Mr Imaginative who is having a difficult time for one reason or another is less likely to look to his Emotional partner for support than Ms Imaginative is. Experience has taught him that Ms Emotional is unlikely to say anything useful, and has no talent for lifting his mood by suggesting interesting things to do or making him feel better by talking. No, she usually makes him feel worse, by catching his mood. He prefers to employ the tried-and-tested strategies of meeting up with friends, having a laugh, going out and doing something new, even flirting. Sometimes, if he's a sexually curious Imaginative with a high sex drive, he'll take the flirting further.

Imaginatives have feelings like everyone else, but they don't like being subject to their moods. They don't feel truly themselves when grappling with emotional undercurrents – they want to get back on an even keel. When united with an Emotional partner they are continually faced with intrusive emotions – their own and their partner's. Emotionals may not like their own moods but they respect the power of their emotions. An Imaginative partner appears to belittle what is fundamental to them. No wonder they both feel misunderstood or beleaguered at times.

Communication between the Emotional and the Imaginative

Of all the combinations, the Imaginative and the Emotional have most trouble communicating what is important to them. That is because their values and methods are so different.

Clear communication is considered the foundation-stone of a good relationship. Everything, it seems, is against the Emotional on this. Ideally, you work out what you feel and then express it simply, calmly and logically, in terms that the other person can understand. This is extremely difficult for an Emotional, who can't be calm when feeling strongly and who might *try* to be simple and logical about profound or disturbing emotions, but just hasn't the talent for it. Listening is an equally important part of communicating. But Emotionals don't listen with their ears, but with their hearts – or guts. It really doesn't matter what words are used – the Emotional hears the tone, or disregards the form of expression in favour of the content – what the Emotional believes is 'really' meant.

The Imaginative appears to hold all the cards in the communication game. No one could be better at calm, simple, logical expression. But the Imaginative is usually dealing with thoughts and reason, not feelings. Trying to tap into what he or she really feels, indeed, can be so difficult that the Imaginative often cheats – consciously or not – by coming up with something that sounds good but is not really authentic. The Imaginative also seems to excel at listening. He or she pays close attention to exactly what is said in the most literal way. But if it is inexact or woolly it seems incomprehensible. The Imaginative just doesn't have the knack of gauging what another person is feeling without being told in words.

To put it another way, the Emotional often 'hears' the anger behind the Imaginative's cool logic and reacts to that with reciprocal anger or misery. He or she doesn't necessarily care *why* or what it's about, the feelings are enough. The Imaginative hears precisely what the Emotional is saying, and takes it at face value. If it sounds inadequate or the Emotional can't explain, the Imaginative will dismiss it out of hand, hardly registering the significance of the underlying feelings. An example is Karen (Emotional) and Angus (Imaginative). They live in a cottage in the country, and after being made redundant, the only job Angus could find was in a faraway town. Commuting would have taken nearly six hours out of Angus's day, but Karen didn't want to move. Eventually Angus made the logical suggestion that he should get a small flat near work for weekdays, rejoining Karen at weekends. As an Imaginative he would not be bothered by these short separations, but Karen, as an Emotional, found the idea of them unbearable. He asked her to explain rationally what her objections were, or to come up with an acceptable compromise or suggestion herself. Instead, all she could talk about was how unhappy she would be and how lonely she would feel. Karen was not interested in Angus's logic. She 'heard' that he didn't mind not living with her for most of the week and she felt insecure. 'You don't care that we would hardly see each other!' she wailed. Angus 'heard' very well Karen's inadequate, emotional explanations but because they didn't address the practical issue of what was to be done he felt aggravated and dismissive. His feelings were just as Karen suggested: he didn't 'care' about the separations. But he knew he loved her, and anyway to him it wasn't relevant to the problem. Before Karen would be able to tackle the issue logically, Angus needed to spend time dealing with her feelings, and reassuring her how much she was loved.

And that's when they are trying to sort something out in a relatively civilised fashion. When the temperature is raised it's even harder. A cross or upset Imaginative will want to 'have it out'. The Emotional either refuses to be drawn or joins in the argument wildly, maybe incoherently. One is all reason, the other is all passion. No wonder they continue to 'miss' each other.

In these circumstances they can reach an impasse even when the Emotional is more articulate. Indra, an Imaginative woman I know, was involved with Seth, an Emotional man. Towards the end of their seven-year relationship they were having a lot of rows, which went nowhere. Indra hated this, as Imaginatives often do; Seth purported to hate it as well, but, for an Emotional, intensity good or bad can make the relationship seem more significant. Indra, in fact, was withdrawing emotionally — and Seth's acute emotional antennae sensed this. During their rows Indra would be calm and reasonable, saying the right sort of things, being logical about what was going wrong between them and how it could be put right. She wanted the rows to stop and the relationship to feel more comfortable. But this was maddening to Seth. He prolonged their arguments for hours — into the early hours of the morning. He kept asking her 'what she meant' when she 'looked like that'. He picked on her tone and expression as she said certain things. He could hear as plain as if she were shouting through a megaphone 'I don't really love you any more'. It was true — and he could hear it before she had even acknowledged it to herself.

The Imaginative can be well satisfied with less than happy relationships when matters are talked through, and decisions made. This is never enough for an Emotional. A counsellor once told me about Gary (Imaginative) and Melissa (Emotional). They came for counselling five years into their marriage, a second one for both of them, when they were in their 50s. They felt they were growing apart. Over a short period of counselling they grew much closer. The counsellor helped them talk to each other and they felt much better about their relationship. Gary, particularly, who had never talked much about intimate matters found it exciting and a revelation, as well as helpful.

Three months later, however, Melissa was back on her own. They were continuing to talk as they had been taught, and Gary felt completely at ease in their more 'intimate' relationship. Melissa was still unhappy, however, and wasn't sure why. Guided through the maze of her feelings by the counsellor's skills, Melissa was eventually able to identify that there was something chilly about all this talking for her. She wanted, she realised in the end, 'hugs and laughs' — she needed to *feel* warm, safe and loved — being told she was just didn't have the same effect. In some ways, she discovered, she was still the angry and resentful child she had been when she was younger. She wanted love as a child understands it — not this analytical grown-up stuff. Over a period of counselling sessions on her own she reported that she was able to convey this to Gary in the way he understood — in clear, logical language. And Gary responded to her requests in the way she needed. For them, a good marriage required a constant vigilance about balancing his need to talk and hers to experience their love in more basic ways through an emotional atmosphere.

The story of Gary and Melissa holds the key to communication — and happiness — for the Imaginative/Emotional couple. For the Imaginative intimacy is talking; for the Emotional intimacy is understanding and meeting emotional needs. If they can find ways to satisfy each other in these respects they both have the potential to develop further than they could alone — or even in a relationship with someone of a similar temperament. Imaginatives need to learn to be comfortable with, and respect, their own emotions, difficult and illogical though they might be at times. When they can do this they can also empathise more sincerely with other people. Emotionals need to be able to develop the ability to understand their emotions with their intellect so that they can express them in a way that means they are able to get what they need from others.

It's not easy, and each couple has to find the way to do it for themselves. One way for the Imaginative to help the Emotional, especially in the early, loving days, is not to demand explanations of feelings. Instead, the Imaginative should use his or her greater clarity to put suggested words to how the Emotional feels — not to analyse or explain, but simply to describe. The Imaginative also needs to know when to stop. Not to labour the issue, or go on too much once the Emotional has indicated that the right words have been found. This in itself is useless if the Imaginative does not then follow through by responding to the Emotional's feelings — not with words necessarily, but with appropriate actions, or silent compassion and concern. When the Emotional experiences the deep gratification of being accepted and understood in this way, he or she is more likely to want to learn to do this defining and describing of emotions that the Imaginative has started.

In return, the Emotional can help by recognising that the Imaginative feels most loved when he or she is talked to. Emotionals should make the effort as a gift of love. Imaginatives have the potential to reach an understanding of their own emotions if they are allowed to talk them through enough. The Emotional can help by prompting, 'How does that make you feel?' The Imaginative will often respond with what it makes him or her 'think', but patient digging can often result in a breakthrough. Similarly an Imaginative can be helped when saying, 'I know it sounds mad, but ...' or, 'I don't know why I should be feeling like this.' The emotionally sophisticated Emotional can reassure that there's nothing mad about it, or that he or she understands anyway, or that it doesn't matter *why*: the feelings are valid in themselves. This works best, of course, if the Emotional does not empathise so completely that he or she takes over the Imaginative's emotions and suffers for both of them.

These ways of communicating are unnatural to these Sexual Styles. But love will certainly increase and consolidate when they both make the effort.

Sex in the Emotional and Imaginative partnership

Sex is often an important element in the relationship between the Imaginative and the Emotional especially in the early days, as it is for most people. Lust often goes hand in hand with falling in love. Any Sexual Style can have a high sex drive, and these two are no different. A good sexual rapport at the start of the relationship can, however, obscure the fact that these two bring as different attitudes to sex as they do to communication.

Imaginatives, with a high sex drive or not, find sex delightful for what it is, but are physically moved by it rather than emotionally. Sex by itself neither makes them suffer nor makes them fall in love. Or rather, they are able to disengage emotionally from sex and put it, as they would say, 'in proportion'. This is the direct opposite of the Emotionals' attitude. For many, sex without love is at best an inferior experience and at worst deeply disturbing. Sex is intimately connected to love, and sometimes inextricably woven into feelings that are not so pleasant as love but equally powerful.

It can take time for these differences to show when lust is stronger than anything else. But when those initial feelings have died down another element of the Imaginative's approach to sex starts to surface: sex needs to be *interesting*. Imaginatives want to explore the sexual possibilities with their partners in order to keep love-making fresh and exciting. Or, if they are more cerebral Imaginatives they might not find it interesting at all, and not know what all the fuss is about. Emotionals have far less need for variety, but they need their emotions to be touched, and sometimes they need very specific and habitual sexual acts, games or positions to arouse their erotic feelings.

The Imaginative is often extremely willing to go along with the Emotional in this respect at the start. But if there's too much of the same, the Imaginative becomes bored. Equally, although the Imaginative is prepared to try anything once, if a sexual activity proves distasteful, he or she will be unlikely to want to do it too often.

The Emotional, who was happy to experiment sexually initially, begins to find an emphasis on sexual variety alienating. It stops feeling intimate and begins to feel contrived — as if it is outside the relationship and not dependent on the feelings within it. This can be extremely off-putting.

All this becomes most apparent when one has a higher sex drive than the other. When it is the Imaginative, the Emotional will feel harried into what seems like unloving sex for the sake of sex, and may well lose all desire for the Imaginative partner.

When it is the Emotional who needs more sex, the Imaginative starts to feel suffocated by the demands and the intensity, and wants to break away from the sexual pressure, which can begin to seem disgusting.

These differences are extremely difficult to resolve. The sexually-keen Imaginative needs to realise that to increase the Emotional's responsiveness attention must be paid to creating the atmosphere that the Emotional finds most erotic. This varies from Emotional to Emotional. For one it can be loving and tender, while for another it might need to be more angry, even abusive. These are the extremes, and there are many possibilities in between. Touch the right chord in the Emotional, however, and the way is more likely to open for the frequency – and the variety and experimentation – the Imaginative prefers.

When the Emotional is the more sexually eager, the approach is somewhat different. Knowing that the Imaginative finds talking loving, and can find mental preparation very erotic, the Emotional often has to prepare the ground for sex quite patiently. Conversational foreplay can be the most potent of all for the Imaginative, who then becomes more willing to agree to the Emotional's specific demands. Actually, both of them can sometimes find common ground through fantasy. Tentative exploration into what they both can tolerate and, preferably, enjoy, in the realm of verbal sex, can make whatever they do physically rewarding for them both.

Over time, however, neither of them believes sex to be the most important aspect of a relationship, even when they desire it frequently. Sometimes indeed, it can be quite peripheral. Imaginatives aren't necessarily interested in sex, and even when they have been in the past they often get to a point where their curiosity has been satisfied and they don't feel the same pressing need to make love. What's more important to them is for the rest of the relationship to be vital, interesting and full of engaging conversation.

Similarly, some Emotionals have never rated sex that highly, and others find their own sexual needs discomfiting. Either way, and even if sex is important to them, they can still feel passionately committed to a relationship in which, for one reason or another, sex has been sidelined, or is non-existent. So long as they feel profoundly moved by their partners, even if sometimes in an uncomfortable way, they will feel that their most important needs are being met.

Long-term prospects

These couples can make enduring relationships, although there are likely to be storms along the way. The Emotionals, in their tenacious drive to ensure their own emotional security, can hold on to the more flighty and emotionally independent Imaginatives until they have made themselves indispensable. Imaginatives, whose impulse is to move on to pastures new when they are not getting the stimulation and interest they need, find that being anchored to a relationship can be gratifying, and as long as they are not too smothered they can find their freedom within it.

Mr Imaginative and Ms Emotional are probably the best pairing, especially when they have children. Ms Emotional might continue to yearn for the kind of intimacy that she needs from her Imaginative husband, but finds it is much more obtainable — and controllable — from her children, particularly when they are young. But men tend to be less susceptible than women to emotional pressure, and Mr Imaginative is the least susceptible of all. He can brush off her demands — simply forget about them — as it suits him. Ms Emotional's need to feel that she has found a life-long partner will force her to tolerate the fact that he goes his own way, or buries himself in his own interests, even if it makes her unhappy. Mr Imaginative who does not get the sex he needs at home can make it his hobby to look for it elsewhere, but will rarely care enough about his lovers for it to affect his relationship with Ms Emotional. Similarly, if sex does not interest him, he can be willing to look for his intellectual interests outside the relationship if the Emotional woman does not come up to his exacting mental standards.

It can, luckily, be much better than this. Because the balance of power is often very important in Emotional relationships, Ms Emotional can even find Mr Imaginative's continuing mercurial elusiveness emotionally satisfying, even while it causes pain. Sometimes, indeed, she holds the balance of power. Her remarkable intuitive ability to sense others' feelings, and consequently their weak spots, can mean that she knows just the right buttons to press to keep her Imaginative man in thrall to her. Even when the power balance is not so obvious, they can 'divide up' the responsibilities of a relationship in a way that suits them both: she taking care of the emotional and perhaps spiritual aspects of life together, and he offering the practical logic and social skills that elude her.

Ms Imaginative and Mr Emotional often have a lot going for them as well, although this can be a more uncomfortable combination. It is harder for an Emotional man to tolerate his woman's needs for separateness and independence. When they have children, indeed, he will expect all that to stop. She dislikes domestic routine and, especially if she is confined to the home, will look to her Emotional man to provide the interesting elements that she misses from the world outside – particularly in terms of ideas and conversation. In this situation they can easily fall into the trap of condemning each other. She finds him suffocating and controlling; he finds her 'unfeminine' and demanding. Although she is less likely to be unfaithful than Mr Imaginative (or perhaps has less opportunity), Ms Imaginative who still retains a lively interest in sexual matters will add her disappointment over this to Mr Emotional's list of sins.

They, too, can manage their relationship much better if certain elements are right, or if they want to. Often having children opens up Ms Imaginative's emotional nature, and she naturally draws closer to him. Even if this is not so, Ms Imaginative can find herself the more powerful in the relationship, even though she rarely seeks to be so. In this case she may use this to coax her partner into giving her necessary latitude: 'space' — or taking it anyway. Sometimes Mr Emotional enjoys this at one level, while hating it at another — in other words, he enjoys hating it. But, just as she doesn't seek power in a relationship, Ms Imaginative also rebels against the wielding of it. If the Emotional man tries to restrict, constrict or control her, even in the name of love (and whether she has children or not) she will want to break away from him and may eventually do so.

It doesn't have to come to this, fortunately. The Emotional and the Imaginative have so much to offer each other, if they both want to take the opportunity. They will never be alike, but both can expand their horizons in their love for each other — and therefore also increase the richness of their lives.

The Imaginative and The Romantic

'Come live with me, and be my love,
And we will some new pleasures prove
Of golden sands, and crystal brooks,
With silken lines, and silver hooks.'

John Donne

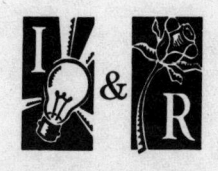

The Imaginative and The Romantic

The Imaginative and the Romantic find each other absolutely enchanting. Both in their own ways are expert at forging instant relationships, expert in the delightful dance of courtship and in investing encounters with thrills, excitement and charm. The Romantic is always eager to fall in love and re-experience the best and most intense feelings he or she has ever known. The slightly more cynical Imaginative is nevertheless open to all new people who promise the buzz of interest and the pleasure of connecting in a vibrant way.

Even when they don't fancy each other they'll have a delightful flirtation. A Romantic always likes the opportunity of testing that his or her powers of fascination are still intact; the Imaginative likes to dazzle or be dazzled by some energetic verbal interplay or wit.

When they *are* attracted to each other, however, stand back. The way they talk is the nearest thing to fully clothed sex. They don't even have to touch each other for the sexual electricity between them to be palpably obvious even to the casual onlooker. They both love this early, dynamic connection of erotic expectancy. The Romantic would like it to go on and on. Sex is more beautiful to the Romantic when it has been preceded by an almost agonising wait. The Imaginative is more impatient. He or she finds the anticipation exquisitely erotic, but is longing to see how the sexual reality matches up with the theory.

The movie *Four Weddings and a Funeral* perfectly illustrates the fascination that Imaginatives and Romantics have for each other. Carrie, as played by Andie MacDowell, is a pure Imaginative – most evident in the scene where she describes her lengthy list of lovers to the infatuated Charles, played by Hugh Grant. He is a Romantic, believing implicitly in the one and only true love, which he believes he has found in Carrie. Indeed, he fell in love with her at first sight. In Charles's own love-life, with its shorter list of conquests, he had never felt anything like it before. In typical Imaginative style, Carrie seizes the initiative, coolly taking Charles to bed on two occasions, despite being engaged to be married to the man she believes she loves. It's a romantic movie, and ends with them living happily ever after, in the unmarried bliss that suits the Imaginative best – unmarried there is always an escape route. In real life, however, when the violins stop playing the Romantic/Imaginative partnership is less smooth than the celluloid version.

The beginning

Talking is as important as sex to this couple, particularly at the start of the relationship. Romantics in love can't get close enough to their beloved. They want to know everything about them and what makes them tick. All their conversations seem to add to the heady, intoxicating aura. Romantics especially love to talk about 'us'. This emphasis on conversation suits Imaginatives beautifully. They love all the intense finding out as well, and although 'us' is only one interesting topic of conversation, so long as it doesn't become repetitious, they'll enjoy it too.

Sometimes what seemed to be an exceptionally promising relationship fizzles out soon after it starts. It's usually the Imaginative who backs away. The Romantic in love can be rather frightening to the Imaginative. There are few Romantics who don't fling themselves wholeheartedly into a new relationship when they fall in love. Even if they've been hurt; even if they swore they'd never do it again — when they fall 'madly' in love, the madness blinds them to any risk. Even if they are not swearing undying love they are usually showing the strength of their feelings in every possible way.

The Imaginative might be feeling very similar. The difference is that the Imaginative is more cautious about trusting the validity of these feelings, less convinced that they will last. Even while utterly bewitched and excited, the Imaginative will retain a modicum of detachment, a cool analytical portion of his or her brain that is ticking off the pros and cons of the relationship and the new partner. If the Romantic comes on too strong before the Imaginative has finished assessing the relative merits of this mental checklist, he or she can feel overwhelmed. This is particularly so if the Romantic becomes jealous, demanding or proprietorial. Imaginatives can't be 'owned', they have to give themselves freely. Too much love too early can seem like unbearable pressure, and the Imaginative reacts by taking flight. Of course, the Romantic is perfectly capable of losing interest too — and before the Imaginative. But when there are genuinely strong feelings on both sides it is the Imaginative who is most likely to cut and run in a seemingly inexplicable fashion.

All being well, however, the relationship continues, and the honeymoon extends. Imaginatives and Romantics have a lot in common and can bring out the best in each other, particularly while they are happy and in love.

Settling down

This is a lively, compatible partnership between two people who stimulate each other. Neither of them relishes routine, which they dismiss as boring, and so they act as a spur on each other to have a good time. Their relationship can continue to be sparky and lively long after other couples have settled into cosy domesticity. In their different ways both of them fight against anything that seems 'middle-aged' or predictable. No matter that their urges come from different needs, they dovetail beautifully.

The Romantic needs wonder, excitement, magic and fun in life to be happy and feel alive. The Imaginative thrives on variety of experience of all kinds, and a need to be interested and mentally engaged. They might have minor clashes about what they do – the Romantic prefers to go to a fashionable restaurant; the Imaginative wants to investigate a seedy dive – but they can usually compromise. The Imaginative's enthusiasm can often invest an adventure with the glamour that the Romantic needs even when it is, on the face of it, unglamorous. So long as they can continue to have an active and interesting life together they can usually be happy.

Once the besotted mutual fascination of first love has passed, however, some difficulties arise. The Imaginative doesn't mourn the passing of these feelings except momentarily, so long as the relationship has other interesting elements to it. The Romantic, as ever, takes it harder. Life is that much greyer. The Romantic always hopes that the intoxication will last, and begins to need more reassurance that he or she is still loved and adored. The perfect relationship is no longer perfect, and it is always a struggle for Romantics to adjust to this.

The Imaginative is rarely keen to indulge the Romantic's need to bring back the 'magic'. Imaginatives think it's boring to have to keep saying how much you love someone, or remembering to pass compliments or make the mundane special. Not *another* candlelit dinner, is their attitude. Even so, it's often fine while there is still a good deal of togetherness. Imaginatives who love and like their partners will enjoy talking to them endlessly, and Romantics love to be focused on in this way. It's harder when they are out in the world. At parties the Imaginative is off, talking with great excitement and intensity to other people. The Romantic experiences this as rejection. Ms Romantic feels humiliated that Mr Imaginative is not making it obvious that he 'belongs' to her. She infers that he is flirting, even when he's not, and she flirts herself — partly because it's in her nature, and partly out of revenge or to make him jealous. Gallingly, he doesn't even notice. He thinks she's doing what he's doing — simply enjoying the pleasure of meeting and talking to a lot of new people. Mr Romantic reacts similarly when his Imaginative partner circulates enthusiastically. His manhood feels threatened. He may flirt as Ms Romantic would, or he may hover menacingly behind Ms Imaginative, glowering at any man she talks to. Male or female, the Romantic is likely to give the Imaginative a hard time when they return home, or at least retreat into a mood that the Imaginative finds incomprehensible. A hurt Romantic is often too proud to explain what the matter is, and without an explanation the Imaginative is perplexed or dismissive.

It can be even more difficult when the Imaginative realises exactly what is going on in the Romantic's mind. Imaginatives hate to feel controlled. It is unbearably claustrophobic. Their impulse is to create more space for freedom, which makes the Romantic even more insecure. It's not too hard to imagine this happening to the Andie MacDowell and Hugh Grant characters from the movie. Carrie, used to doing what she wants, when she wants, and with whom she wants, doesn't seem to be the kind of woman who would change for the sake of Charles. He, already rather insecure, would find this increasingly hard to tolerate.

It is also somewhat shocking for the Romantic when the rose-tints fade and the admirable partner is revealed to have a catalogue of faults. If Mr Imaginative originally attracted Ms Romantic because he was excitingly dilettante, for instance, she can find herself eventually ruing the fact that he's not being more of a 'man': building a career, bringing home the bacon, giving her the lifestyle to which she wishes to become accustomed. Even the most successful Romantic woman yearns for a partner who exhibits what she sees as masculine traits. She doesn't want to wear the trousers; she wants to be cherished. His wit or his interesting conversation eventually palls if there is no solid follow-through.

Mr Romantic can't help wanting his partner to be something of a trophy to show off. Initially attracted by Ms Imaginative's ebullience, cleverness, and perhaps zaniness of outlook, he eventually finds himself wondering why she doesn't make more of an effort to look good when they go out. At home, he finds her intense interest in issues, the world, talking about other people, oddly impersonal. When is the subject going to come round to him and his preoccupations again? If their interests coincide, that's fine, but he's still sensitive to any hint that she is engrossed in matters that exclude him and their relationship.

When their interests don't coincide it is even more of a problem for Imaginatives. Sometimes they find their Romantic partner's concerns shallow. They don't understand the Romantic need for showy love. Romance seems somewhat superficial compared to their own interpretation of intimacy, which is mental, and to do with sharing thoughts and ideas. However intellectual the Romantic is, this kind of intimacy spells only interest, not love.

Problems are exacerbated when there turns out to be an intellectual disparity. Ms Imaginative can be in thrall forever to Mr Romantic if he is cleverer than she is, and this can be the best possible pairing. Her admiration suits his Romantic nature just fine. But even this can be difficult. The Romantic man doesn't have the same need to share his ideas in his intimate relationship, and she can feel shut out from the very aspect that she loves best in him. When she has fewer intellectual resources herself she needs more of the novelty and activity that also excites Imaginatives, and he may look down on her for it if what she wants to do doesn't meet his fastidious Romantic standards.

The other way round is even more difficult. Ms Imaginative who discovers that she is intellectually superior to her Romantic man can be bitterly disappointed. An Imaginative woman can be intrigued enough to fall in love with a man whose brain works very differently from her own — and this novelty can give mileage to an extremely unlikely relationship. But an Imaginative woman eventually feels very lonely if she can't share her thoughts and ideas with a responsive and understanding partner. Mr Imaginative can bear this better — he will often find the intellectual stimulation he needs outside the relationship — but Ms Imaginative has a greater need for it to be a feature of her intimate life. If there were ever to be a *Four Weddings and a Funeral Part Two*, the odds are that it would feature an extremely unhappy Carrie and Charles — if Carrie were even still around that is. Carrie, who initially found Charles's dithery British charm so compelling and exotic, was a decisive and clear-thinking woman. Years of putting up with Charles's woolly-minded thinking, difficulty in expressing himself, and chronic lateness would likely have taken their toll. Romantics will forgive a good-looking partner quite a lot; Imaginatives do not think that it makes up for other deficiencies.

Daily life

The happiest couples of this pairing have compelling enthusiasms and interests in common that they can pursue together, so that their off-duty lives are entwined satisfactorily. The Imaginative enjoys the feeling this gives of having a soulmate to share with, and the Romantic enjoys the feeling of being important in the partner's life. Paradoxically, this couple can be even happier with a relationship that involves some sort of enforced separation, so long as love and commitment is there — work keeps them apart for some time, or for one reason or another they have to live separately. This is perfectly comfortable for the Imaginative, who has built-in 'space' and whose commitment is refreshed by it. The Romantic may suffer more — but it is the kind of suffering he or she secretly enjoys — a yearning to be back together again, which is exciting in its own way. The reunions provide the romance that Romantics always require: they are delighted to see each other; they make time for each other; they want to catch up on the minutiae of each other's thoughts and activities; every moment is golden and special. A relationship like this can extend the honeymoon feelings indefinitely.

Whether they are apart a lot or together all the time, this couple is less good than average at looking at the deeper issues involved in a partnership. If what they are doing keeps them busy and excited they might rarely get round to tackling more fundamental aspects of life together. As both tend to be pleasure-seekers they'd rather ignore what is seamier and more disturbing. The Romantic wants to be happy, and pushes the issue away. The Imaginative doesn't want to drown in the murky waters of troubled emotions, so prefers to think of something else. When life becomes difficult, therefore, or a problem arises between them, they unconsciously collude to pretend it's not there. The trouble with this is that it can flourish unchecked, and in the future they are faced with something that has become too large to ignore and too big to handle.

This appears to be the case with Ralph and Candice, a couple who went to see a counsellor I once interviewed. They had been married for three years, supremely happily, so Candice said. 'Suddenly' it had gone wrong. Ralph had become distant and withdrawn, and wouldn't tell Candice why.

During counselling they talked about their life together. It had been 'ideal' Candice said, talking for them both. She listed all the things they did: everything that 'we' liked and didn't like. Ralph didn't contribute much at the first session, and said very little at the next. Towards the end of this hour, however, he suddenly put his head in his hands and started crying. He said he felt suffocated and controlled. Candice looked on, appalled. Ralph then pulled himself together, rose, and said, 'I've had enough of this – I'm leaving you!' He walked out of the counselling room and out of Candice's life.

Ralph's emotional reaction was typical of the way Imaginatives handle their feelings. Living, as they do, in their heads, they often don't know what their feelings are until they are suddenly overwhelmed by them, and then insight may come. To flee from such strong or unhappy feelings is also typical. The Imaginative doesn't want to go through the pain to a solution – he or she wants to be in a situation where the pain does not exist.

Candice continued counselling alone. Ralph's defection showed her clearly what had gone wrong between them. She, as a Romantic, had always wanted the 'ideal' relationship she thought she had with Ralph. When they were first in love they did so much together, and she always consulted his wishes. Later she forgot to do so. In pursuit of the ideal she slipped into dictating the terms of their relationship and their activities. Easy-going Ralph went along with it all, even when she started to groom him into greater perfection. She chose his clothes, sent him to the gym, vetoed certain friends. Ralph started to make small breaks for independence. She discovered he had started seeing again a friend she didn't like. He gave up the gym and took up archery. Then he became quiet and withdrawn. Candice knew something was wrong. She felt upset that he was no longer talking so much to her. What she didn't realise was that when Imaginatives come to the point of not wanting to talk to their partners it is a fatal sign of disaffection.

In daily life, to sum up, a balance has to be found between the Imaginative's need for a certain amount of freedom, and the Romantic's equally pressing need to feel that the connection between them is sufficiently significant to justify staying together.

Communication between the Imaginative and the Romantic

When they are happy and in love the Imaginative and the Romantic seem so similar. It's all that rushing around together doing exciting things, all that intensive 'relating' when they are alone. Both of them like 'communicating' – that is, talking together, and when they are mentally well-matched this can be an enduring source of pleasure to them. This can obscure the fact that emotionally they are very different.

It is the profounder sort of communication that creates problems for them – touching, as it does, on the emotional areas in which they are at odds.

The Romantic likes emotional intensity – he or she reaches for heightened emotion: great love; great bursts of anger; stormy tears. The Romantic, in effect, wants passion that explodes, not endures. The ache of long-term pain, gloom, despondency, and quiet empathy (all of which the Emotional understands so well) are foreign to the Romantic nature.

The Imaginative is altogether cooler. Imaginatives can have feelings as deep as anyone's, but they find them disturbing and distressing. They feel most themselves when their feelings are under control and they can be level-headed.

Actually, both of them have trouble connecting to their deepest feelings, and neither of them is aware of this. Romantics usually pride themselves on being in touch with their emotions. This mistake arises because they find it easy to express the feelings that well up in them, as they rage, or cry or throw themselves into their lover's arms. What they don't do is experience the more painful roots of sad or angry emotions. They know they felt furious, but they don't track the anger to its source, which could well be something that they don't want to look at – fear of rejection, or low self-esteem, say. They are like pressure cookers letting off steam, but the water is still boiling underneath.

Imaginatives also over-estimate their capacity to understand their emotions. They know they are not emotionally volatile, as are their Romantic partners, but they pride themselves on their mastery of such matters. They are good at analysing and coming up with rational explanations for what they think, oblivious to the fact that this is not the same as deciphering what they feel.

It is when things are going wrong between them that this discrepancy in the way they handle matters is exposed, and their difficulty in getting in touch with their true feelings begins to matter. Usually, what is at the bottom of it is what the psychologist Harriet Goldhor Lerner calls in her book of the same title 'the dance of intimacy'.

In a nutshell, the Romantic wants glorious togetherness and the Imaginative needs to feel that togetherness is a choice that is freely made.

The Romantic woman feels that the passion and intensity is going out of their relationship so she begins to turn up the temperature. She behaves to Mr Imaginative as she would like him to behave to her. She becomes even more feminine and alluring and she sets out to woo him. Unfortunately, Mr Imaginative is far more contented with the recent laid-back atmosphere of the relationship. They've done intensity and romance, and now it's time to get on with life. He can love her as much as ever, but he's tired of playing love-birds. He begins to find all her loving attention cloying, so he takes a step further back emotionally, and she feels rebuffed. He might try to get on with his own interests, see more people, build more activity into his life. He thinks she should do the same.

This behaviour makes Ms Romantic feel unloved; she simply can't believe that her Imaginative man loves her as much as ever or he'd want to be with her and *show* it. Perhaps if she explained at this stage how she was feeling and what she needed he'd be able to reassure her. But Ms Romantic is too proud. She doesn't want to have to *beg* for love, as she sees it. Instead, she goes in for more drastic tactics. She might try to make him jealous, or pick a row about something unrelated to her true feelings. At that moment she thinks they *are* her true feelings. Anyway, she quite likes rows, because they are personal and intense. Mr Imaginative often enjoys an intellectual tussle of wits, but he doesn't like emotional scenes. Neither does feeling jealous increase his interest (as it can do for the other Sexual Styles). He finds it very unpleasant. She is behaving in precisely the way guaranteed to alienate him.

It is similar when the woman is Imaginative and the man Romantic. Her independence and interest in things other than him makes him insecure. When he enjoys putting his woman on a pedestal, this apparent remoteness can increase his desire and his longing for her. He can become more adoring, which she perceives as craven; indeed she may despise him for it. Unable to empathise with his feelings she can even feel there is something slightly unhinged about his devotion. Ms Imaginative has a greater need for intimacy in a relationship than does the Imaginative man, but it is a different sort of intimacy from that required by her Romantic partner. It's about sharing ideas and feeling understood: adoration misses the point. When Mr Romantic treats her in these ways she becomes cold and retreats.

It is even harder when the Romantic man needs to know he is adored, as so many do. Ms Imaginative might well adore him, and pay him the rapt attention he craves. Equally, this might not be her style. Happy in her relationship, Ms Imaginative is just as likely to express this contentment by being more outgoing and ready to enjoy life generally. Mr Romantic is less prepared than the Romantic woman to try to get what he needs by guile. Instead he becomes autocratic and demanding. This results either in a crushed and resentful Imaginative woman, or one who breaks free once and for all.

When problems become entrenched, trying to sort them out

can be a nightmare. Whenever the Romantic's feelings run high the Imaginative is likely to look for an escape route. 'We'll talk about this when you are more reasonable,' is one of the milder Imaginative responses. It could just as easily be the distant bang of the front door. When the Imaginative is upset it is little better. The Romantic has become used to believing that he or she has the monopoly on emotion in their relationship and therefore underestimates the Imaginative's human capacity for hurt. As Imaginatives often struggle to be controlled and rational-seeming when distressed, the Romantic is misled into believing it's not too important. When the Imaginative explodes with rage or pain the Romantic believes it is similar to a Romantic flare-up – that it will pass without too much trace. In fact, it is much graver.

Learning to communicate these difficult emotions and issues more clearly in this partnership means careful emotional negotiation, and acting against type.

When the Romantic has what the Imaginative would call a tantrum it is a cry for attention, which needs to be taken seriously. Ignored Romantics shrivel inside – they don't 'come to their senses' as Imaginatives hope. The Imaginative should not walk away from the scene, but should use Imaginative powers of coolness and analysis to discover what the matter is – and not be too literal. It does not help for the Imaginative simply to respond to the immediate issue at hand in the interests of a quiet life. The Romantic might be raving about wet towels on the bathroom floor but is really feeling over-looked or unloved, for instance. Picking up the towels, or getting into a debate about them, or dismissing it all as over-reaction are unhelpful ways of handling the situation. On the other hand, Romantics always respond to reassurance that they are loved and valued. Imaginatives who 'pretend' to be Romantics, at least during these highly charged moments, and offer some openly loving comments, will find it pays off. Romantics should also be told, 'I'm really sorry that you're upset [or angry].' The Romantic who feels loved and cared for is less defensive, and more willing to get to the bottom of what the matter really is.

Romantics, for their part, need to watch for the subtle cues that their partners are distressed about something. They look for the blatant signs — the Imaginative is happy and involved with things outside their relationship — and misread them. They take it personally and believe that love is slipping away, which might not, in fact, be the case. It's more likely to be serious when the Imaginative raises an issue quietly, and has clearly given a lot of thought to it. It can be hard for the Romantic to hear out the Imaginative without getting worked up — but when the Romantic becomes emotional the Imaginative often switches off, or says it doesn't matter. Actually, it usually does. And it matters even more if the Imaginative stops raising these issues at all.

The Romantic, too, needs to use pretence — 'becoming' Imaginative for the time being. This means holding on to his or her own feelings, and simply asking questions to prompt. Imaginatives who feel understood from their own perspective are happier and more loving people.

What works well for this couple is not to leave these matters to chance, but to recognise that problems will arise and need to be sorted out. They should use the fact that they like talking together to make some regular time to do so about their relationship. This way they'll catch the problems small, and increase their intimacy while so doing. Waiting for problems to blow up makes it more difficult to use these loving strategies, and usually brings out counter-productive behaviour in them both.

Sex in the Imaginative and Romantic partnership

Sex can be great at the beginning of this relationship, but it can hit problems later. Imaginatives take sex less seriously than Romantics. They think sex is about sex, and Romantics think it is about love. When they are first in love their feelings seem to coincide. It is only after some time that they can realise they feel differently.

Sex is usually important to Romantics, even when they are not highly-sexed. This is partly because it is recognisably symbolic of love. Romantic women, therefore, rate virility high, even when sex is not particularly important to them — and especially when it is. But it is glamourised virility: strong and urgent, but gentle and infinitely tender. She must feel his desire is for her, and that he wants to please her, not that it's just a physical need. He must be in good shape and smell good, or she is too insistently reminded that sex is what animals do, which is not an especially erotic thought for her. Secretly, it's a version of the James Bond image that turns her on (although the sophisticated Romantic would never admit it): the bottle of champagne in one hand, the carelessly undone bow-tie, the sexual expertise combined with the thrilling sense of dangerous manhood.

Mr Imaginative can be content to play James Bond for a while, but he becomes bored. A sexually interested Imaginative man wants to sample all the different possibilities in sex. When he's in love he'll want to do so with his partner — and some of those possibilities will be crude, laughable, coarse or uncomfortable. Ms Romantic is prepared to go along with some of this in the name of love at the beginning, when simply being with him is erotic, but it doesn't suit her nature. The moment she suspects it is unloving, she is turned off. In some ways Ms Romantic is happier with the more aesthetic Imaginative man, with a lower sex drive, who is less interested in sex. Although he is not so likely to yearn for *outré* sexual practices, however, he is also unlikely to want to waste much time on sex, and it may be perfunctory and mechanical.

These differences call on all their powers of clear communication, and much of this falls on the shoulders of the Imaginative man. His Romantic partner doesn't like having to talk about sex or say what she likes. She wants it to be passionate and inevitable, and instinctively right for her. On the other hand, she's charmed to be asked, lovingly, whether she likes this or that, and whether he wants her to be gentler, stronger, stop what he's doing, or go on. Equally, when he makes her feel loved, and respects her wishes, she is more likely to enjoy experimenting sexually in ways that she might not have thought she liked.

Mr Romantic has an equally rose-tinted view of sex, and likes the woman he loves to live up to his specific high ideals. He sees the movies in which satin nightwear never creases, and a woman's hair and make-up is never messed up during sex or a night's sleep – and he can't help wanting real life to be the same. He can be delighted with an uninhibited, sexually fun-loving Imaginative woman at the start of the relationship, putting her response down to his sexual expertise. But if she later starts to demand more variety and experimentation he can become less keen. He feels criticised. He thinks there's something unfeminine and unloving about her attitude. He feels uncomfortable with the implication that he can't give her everything she needs, and he wonders if she'll stray. Indeed, he is often happier with the Imaginative woman who does not rate sex highly: the more cerebral type who does not include sex as one of her interests. It suits him best to have sex when he wants it, and not feel pressured at other times. He can also feel more virile with a slightly reluctant woman, so long as she doesn't actively dislike sex.

The sexually-keen Imaginative woman, therefore, has to be prepared to pander to his preferences. This can come easier to her than to other women, because she does not take sex so personally, and neither does it affect her deepest emotions. She can enjoy dressing up for him the way he wants, teasing out his fantasies, and acting on them. The trouble from her point of view is that too much of the same often kills her erotic feelings. Imaginatives need variety and novelty to stimulate desire. Nevertheless, if she becomes adept at making him think something was *his* idea, and at creating the atmosphere that best puts him in the mood for sex, then they both can be very happy.

Sex is not the be-all and end-all for either of them, however. They are perfectly capable of building a happy and fulfilling life together which includes very little love-making, so long as other elements in their relationship are enjoyable. But they should make efforts to construct a love-making pattern that suits them both while sex is important to either of them. A sexually-disappointed Imaginative is likely to go searching for it elsewhere, often casually. If one of these casual lovers turns out to be more 'interesting' than their partner, it could signal the end of their commitment. Amidst quantity, quality is sometimes to be found. A Romantic who is not sexually satisfied is even more dangerous. Romantics are more inclined to fall in love with sexual partners, and when in love they follow the dictates of their hearts.

Long-term prospects

Couples of this pairing who tackle the difficulties of emotional and sexual communication can make good and long-lasting relationships, especially when their interests coincide and they continue to 'play' and talk together. When this is the case, their lives remain stimulating and fun and they can seem much younger in their later years than some couples who have more natural staying-power. If they don't tackle the inherent difficulties, however, this can be an unstable union. Both of them, for their own reasons, value most highly the early days of a relationship. For the Romantic this is because it is the time of greatest intoxication, the most heightened feelings, when romance is naturally there, and doesn't have to be worked at or forced. The Imaginative is always most attracted to the new, and what is interesting — and however complex or fascinating the loved one, there comes a time, inevitably, when the Imaginative feels he or she knows all there is to know. The two- or three-year mark is usually critical for these couples, for it is the point at which they have to cope with knowing that something special for them has gone, and they have to make a conscious decision to continue. If, meanwhile, they have had children and built a home together, practical considerations can give them the impetus they need to make the relationship work over a longer period. But even when this is the case, Romantics and Imaginatives are equally likely to take the initiative to break up a relationship that has suffered a drastic loss of quality.

The Romantic woman and the Imaginative man have the greatest chance of success when he is successful and a good provider. If she can look up to him, and he can provide the kind of lifestyle she enjoys best, she is more able to forgive him for not being as romantic as she would wish. When they are a good mental match, and he is able to talk to her and respect her, he will, in turn, forgive what he sees as her emotional excesses.

If their daily lives diverge and they don't have too much in common apart from their family and domestic arrangements, however, the relationship can seem somewhat barren and bleak to them. Mr Imaginative will deal with this in his usual way – by seeking to compensate. He retreats into his own mental world; or throws himself into work; or places higher importance on his friendships or activities outside the home. This is guaranteed to make matters worse for Ms Romantic. To be ignored or disregarded is the most painful thing she knows. She reacts in the typical Romantic way: by trying to woo him into more togetherness; or with moods that are alternately frosty or demanding; or by a determined attempt to pique his interest by parading a troupe of admirers. These tactics, on both sides, only serve to drive them further apart.

Ms Imaginative and Mr Romantic can make the most stable union when their interests and ideas coincide and are more important to them than sex or shared domestic concerns. Ms Imaginative is not too interested in a beautiful home or a comfortable one, but she does need a stimulating lifestyle. If Mr Romantic pours his Romantic energies into work and outside relationships, nothing that he buys or does for her can compensate. This kind of Romantic man prefers a woman who exhibits traditional qualities – looking after the home and children (but looking beautiful while she does so), to free him to get on with living life the way he wants to. Ms Imaginative, who is so different from this type of woman, strikes him as unfeminine, and her dissatisfaction with what he offers is a serious blow to his Romantic pride.

The mundanity of real life and long-term relationships are always hardest for this combination to appreciate. Sometimes a series of failed relationships can give them a different perspective on life, however. When they find that what they most cherish has built-in obsolescence they can be more prepared to compromise in later life. Neither of them want relationships to be hard work, but even a modicum of effort on both sides can make a great difference. They have the ideal partner with whom to enjoy life and experience its diversity. They just have to recognise it, and act to keep up the quality in the relationship.

The Emotional and The Sensual

'Dumb swans, not chattering pies, do lovers prove;
They love indeed who quake to say they love.'

Sir Philip Sidney

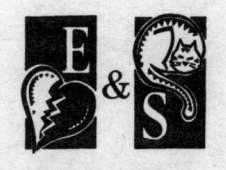

The Emotional and The Sensual

When this couple fall in love it can be for life. Both of them need steadfastness in relationships. In order to ensure it they are not so easily deterred by difficulties or even unhappiness as are the other two Sexual Styles, the Romantic and the Imaginative. They are only human, and they want the excitement, gaiety and thrilling passion of love, but they are also prepared to value a relationship that might miss some or all of these elements at times, and sometimes even when they are missing altogether.

Because of this, the relationships that they make also have the potential to be truly fulfilling, with the deep intimacy that can only come after many years and many experiences, good and bad, together. They can also discover, as only people in long-term partnerships do, that facing life together in this way offers much more than stolid endurance. Trust and deep contentment can lead to a renaissance of love in later life. When they cope as positively with their differences as they do their similarities, this couple have the capacity to be truly happy.

On meeting, of course, they don't know any of this. Both of them are instinctive people, however, and looking back they will often realise that their attraction for each other involved an unconscious recognition of a deeper compatibility. The Sensual, whose instincts are based in a physical reaction to the presence of another person, will be most aware of a sexual charge – pure lust. The Emotional, instead, gets strong feelings about another person — a gut reaction that might well include lust, but is usually a less definable sensation of being drawn towards this person. Somehow, they both know that something significant is happening, even if they are not sure what it is.

The beginning

At the start they are just in love, and like many lovers they don't stop to analyse why. They are the least analytical of the Sexual Styles anyway. It's just perfect, that's all; it feels so wonderful. The Sensual is probably the most shaken by what is happening. Heightened lust, good sex — the Sensual was expecting all this from the time they met — but not this whirlwind of excited emotion. The Sensual, like the Imaginative, is perfectly capable of separating sex from love, particularly Mr Sensual, and although Sensuals tend to feel fondness when they are sexually satisfied, it does not have to be anything stronger.

The Emotional is more ready for this intense burst of feeling. It is what he or she has been waiting for. Sex is never casual for Emotionals, and even if they have had so-called casual sex in the past it has always affected them — usually adversely, when no relationship has resulted. Emotionals can have strong sex drives that require satisfying, but until they fall in love this drive can be a mixed blessing — exciting in one way, but a millstone and a source of misery in another.

Whether they are both naturally highly-sexed or not, the beginning of the relationship will usually be physically passionate. Neither of them is particularly adept at expressing their love in other ways. They are often curiously shy about talking of their love, or simply not good at finding words that express the complexity and importance of it to them. In other areas of their life they might be exceedingly articulate and clear-headed, but not this one. The Sensual feels the love in every molecule of his or her body, and it is a short step from this to sexual desire. The Emotional is overwhelmed by feelings too grand and undefined to be categorised by mere words. Even sex is not quite enough to demonstrate these feelings, but it expresses the Emotional's overpowering urge to bond and merge.

One of the elements of this great attraction is their different emotional natures. Emotionals tend to be buffeted by life and moods. There is a strong pull towards the calmness and practicality of the Sensual, who, as they see it, has an amazing ability to cope whatever the circumstances. Sensuals make Emotionals feel safe from themselves. In turn, Sensuals are dazzled and perplexed by the way Emotionals are guided by their feelings above every other consideration. In a corner of their hearts they long to let go as well, but they don't know how, and are nervous about what would happen if they did. These mixed feelings translate into a compelling fascination, as mixed feelings often do.

Settling down

Unless the honeymoon period has revealed some basic incompatibilities between them, they both want the same thing: to settle down together for life. In their different ways they need the security of a relationship.

Sensuals need a base in life. Something that is safe, comfortable and predictable. These seemingly dull requirements are anything but boring to them. Harmony, stability and creature comforts reassure them. They need to be surrounded by what they know and like, so as to bring out their best side. They want to own what they love and like, as well — have it close and under control — and that includes people. Excitement and new love are all very well in their way, but there is an undercurrent of anxiety which is anything but comfortable.

Emotionals' needs are different, but have the same end result. They are at the mercy of their emotions, good or bad. So powerful is what goes on inside them that they can often feel misunderstood, cut adrift from other people. When they let someone into their hearts, which they don't do easily, they feel this person has become a part of them, and they don't want to let go. Breaking up with someone who has touched them deeply is always agony, and they feel compelled to cling on, sometimes even to relationships that are destructive. Whatever else they feel about the Sensual, Emotionals are deeply reassured by the instinctive knowledge that this person is not likely to skip off at the first opportunity – on the contrary, the Sensual will be there for them for a long time.

Mr Sensual and Ms Emotional settle down most readily together. It makes sense to them that he is the calm one who takes charge, and that she is the one who feels enough for both of them. Mr Sensual is particularly pleased when he is not feeling so madly in love. He wasn't sure it was real until now. Back to feeling more normal he can ask himself: 'Do I want to be here with her?' and if the answer is yes, he knows he truly loves her. Ms Emotional had no such doubts, but even if she misses the dramatically loving elements of their initial togetherness, the more even tenor of their life now is reassuring for her.

But when the combination is this way round – the man is Sensual and the woman Emotional – there is an inherent difficulty for them. It makes perfect sense to them both that he, as the man, should exhibit the steady, stable qualities of Sensuality, and she the more feminine, volatile, moody characteristics of the Emotional. Because of this they miss the precious opportunity to learn from each other and so develop into more rounded people by extending their emotional repertoire. Mr Sensual believes it behoves him to be controlled and sensible for them both; she gives her feelings full rein, knowing that in some strange way she is doing it for him as well. To be what each other needs therefore, they become entrenched in the less helpful aspects of their natures. Mr Sensual doesn't try to develop a better connection with his emotional nature. Instead, he becomes skilled – quite unconsciously – at pushing her emotional buttons when his own emotions threaten to surface. He's feeling angry,

The Emotional and The Sensual

so he makes her angry instead, and somehow feels better for it. Ms Emotional, for her part, never attempts to consider the appropriateness of showing what she feels. If she wants to get a hold on herself, therefore, she makes her anger or her misery even more obvious, secure in the knowledge that he will apply the brakes on her behalf. She doesn't know that she is doing it, or why. It is simply a habit that has developed.

Not surprisingly, this can lead to resentment on both sides. Mr Sensual, never learning to feel comfortable with his own emotional nature, feels bombarded by hers. Ms Emotional feels that he is cold and unfeeling, oblivious to the fact that she is pushing him into this sort of behaviour. Even so, the rightness of it for both of them maintains the bond, even when it is uncomfortable.

The partnership between Mr Emotional and Ms Sensual can be more stormy and appear less suitable, but for that very reason can also be more transformational for them both.

Despite being attracted to the Sensual woman for her calm practicality, Mr Emotional feels perturbed by her lack of emotional response. Like the Emotional woman, he can become more flamboyant in his emotional expression, but he is seeking to draw a similar response from her. With the Emotional's uncanny ability to read the emotional life of another person he may well find the way to open her up. Her anger flares, or she cries. Much as she wants to remain unflappable, she starts to experience more spontaneous emotions and begins the process of becoming more comfortable with them. Similarly, Ms Sensual can't help feeling that a man should be able to govern his emotions to a degree, and her Emotional man often secretly agrees with her. As she becomes more emotional he, paradoxically, can feel steadied. There is not the same need to go over the top to have his emotions 'heard': she has responded and it calms him.

As must be obvious, the Sensual/Emotional partnership is not always a bed of roses, but nevertheless it remains strong.

From the Emotional's point of view it is normal. Whatever relationship Emotionals find themselves in there is likely to be conflict, or at the very least strong feeling. Not so Sensuals, who prefer the quiet life. Even so, there is something stalwart about Sensuals. They are good at taking the rough when they know that there is the smooth to come. So long as there is stability and the kind of physical closeness they need, including regular sex, they can manage. It is also good for them to be close to someone who has more ready access to emotions. It shows them a side of life that is otherwise a mystery to them.

It is always hardest to categorise a relationship when one of the partners is Emotional. This is because Emotionals come in many guises, depending on which is their prevailing emotional state. A secure and deeply loving Emotional will have a quietly contented relationship with a Sensual partner. An insecure Emotional who has suffered many rejections will read betrayal into the Sensual's every action, and respond accordingly. Almost invariably, however, some kind of imbalance of power suits the Emotional nature. Even a loving need to be needed is a version of this, as the Emotional seeks to become so necessary to his or her partner that their union is assured. Sometimes the Emotional revels in being the needy one, in thrall to a more powerful partner. This is the reason some Emotional women seem incapable of leaving a violent or abusive partner, or leave only to make an identical relationship with someone else. Some Emotional men do the same. Indeed, when this is a facet of their personality these Emotionals feel impelled to act in ways to bring out this side of a partner's character – and succeed, even with the usually equable Sensual.

Sensuals like to be in control to feel that life is as they want it. Inevitably this includes controlling the people in their lives – partners, children, and so on. When this dovetails with the Emotional's need to be looked after or dominated, they both derive what they need from their relationship. When the Emotional needs to exert power, however, this couple can be very conflicted and unhappy. Mind you, the Emotional is infinitely more subtle than the Sensual, and is perfectly capable of manipulating and controlling so gently and skilfully that the Sensual doesn't even notice which of them is really in charge.

Despite the difficulties at times, Sensuals and Emotionals can draw great comfort from each other. So long as they continue to love each other their interaction can be very rewarding. Both, for their own reasons, like to be close. Sensuals enjoy showing and receiving physical affection — not always sexually. Loving and fond Sensuals want to sit next to their partners, cuddle them, hold their hands and so on. They show their love, rather than talking about it. The Emotional finds this gratifying, too. Emotionals don't need words of reassurance. Their instincts tell them what someone is feeling, and when the Sensual snuggles in they know they are loved. They too find actions speak louder than words and are just as likely to show love physically to the Sensual. Being embraced with kindness and affection is the way Sensuals experience love best — better than a passionate declaration. Indeed, when there is an absence of physical contact Sensuals cannot believe that they are truly loved, however much a partner tells them that they are. Similarly, when one of them is upset the other tends to offer physical comfort. The Sensual might not be good at talking the problem away, but he or she offers a steady shoulder to cry on. The Emotional might enter too deeply into a distressed partner's feelings, but he or she won't back away in alarm. This is one of the most powerfully uniting aspects of their relationship. It deepens intimacy, provides solace, and contributes to trust and staying power.

Daily life

Both of these people feel that their home life is important. Home is a haven, comfortable, and emotionally reassuring. Sensuals and Emotionals can become as deeply attached to where they live as they do to people. They only move when it is strictly necessary — because their family grows or because of financial constraints. They usually prefer to redecorate, improve or add-on, rather than to buy somewhere new. This shared love and need for a home-base is another uniting factor, and something that makes them think more than twice about breaking up a relationship, even one that has become unhappy.

This usually means that they value time spent at home, and often prefer it to going out. They are much more content than other couples with what can appear to be a fairly boring life. Time spent quietly together, particularly when there are plenty of good feelings between them, is deeply satisfying. They are particularly content when they have a family to raise, and are unlikely to feel that they are missing out if they have to forego outings and excitement. This can make them exceptionally good parents to younger children, but rather stultifying for adolescents who need to spread their wings. They can find it hard to understand why their children don't seem to share their delight in family life.

The fact that they draw most contentment from home life, however, works against them when they are less happy together. They are not so willing as other people to look for support or fresh pleasures outside — a practice that can sometimes bring a welcome perspective to relationship problems. In the absence of this outlet, bad feeling can fester. The Sensual and the Emotional are quite capable of carrying on silent feuds, sharing an enclosed space but acting is if the other did not exist. Neither is happy, but neither knows quite what to do about the situation.

It is hardest for a happier couple when there are enforced separations — particularly for the Emotional. The Sensual doesn't like it, but finds it perfectly easy to pick up where he or she left off, especially when reunions are marked by good sex and closeness. They 'remember' the good things with their bodies, by sex and hugging. Emotionals, on the other hand, need time to 'feel' themselves back into the relationship. They are not ready for sex until this has been re-established. One of the women who responded to the *Family Circle* magazine sex survey I devised, wrote about this problem. She, as an Emotional, was distressed by her husband's work in the navy serving on submarines. He was away a lot, and their only contact during these times was a weekly 'family gram' limited to 40 words. Her Sensual husband expected sex and attention immediately on his return; she, still feeling the pain of her loneliness needed time and more reassurance herself before she could feel sexual. It's hard for a Sensual in these circumstances to understand that a ten-minute cuddle doesn't recreate the necessary intimacy.

Usually, however, these couples try to work it so that they don't have to spend too much time apart. Both are in touch with what they need — the Sensual in terms of creature comforts, and the Emotional in terms of atmosphere. Often the pleasant routine of daily life, constructed around these needs, suits them well. The more busy they are with other commitments, the more they appreciate undemanding, quiet times together. They don't have to keep checking on the condition of their relationship, they know exactly where they are without words.

Communication between the Emotional and the Sensual

The strength of the instinctive communication between these two people is also a weakness. When you are happy words don't matter too much. As Gustave Flaubert said: 'Human speech is like a cracked kettle on which/we tap crude rhythms for bears to dance to, while we/long to make music that will melt the stars.' The Sensual and Emotional can, indeed, make such music without speech when everything is going well. When it is not, however, matters are different. Unhappiness needs to be understood before it can be sorted out. Neither of them respond too well to the concept of 'sorting out' problems; both of them are too ready to endure them in their own way.

When the problem is their life together, or their partner,

they both tend to be gloomily philosophical. This is a shame, because they miss the opportunity to improve matters. Coping with problems alone, especially when you have a partner, can be one of the loneliest experiences in life.

I know of a couple, Charlotte (Emotional) and Pete (Sensual), who show what can go wrong between two loving people of this style. They married young, and Pete, who felt he had never sowed all the wild oats he had meant to, had an affair within the year. Indeed, as a young Sensual man with a lot of maturing to do, he couldn't see that he had done anything particularly significant. He even told Charlotte about the affair, and that he was going to leave her for a while to live with this other woman, who had sexually enthralled him. It was soon obvious what a mess it was. His mistress told him that she was pregnant, and at this news he realised how little she mattered to him: he wanted her to have an abortion. A week later Charlotte announced that she was pregnant. That settled things for Pete. He knew which woman he loved and wanted to be with. He went home to Charlotte for good.

This incident was never once mentioned between them again. They got on with their lives. They had two more children. They were settled and, on the face of it, happy. But they were never intimate again. Charlotte accepted the pain of what happened and came to terms with it, but she became more secretive and focused on her children and her work. She never gave herself up to sex in the same way, and although their sex life was regular she made it clear that it was something she put up with for his sake. Sensuals derive most satisfaction from sex when they know that their partners are satisfied too, otherwise part of them feels rejected. Pete felt justified in having more affairs – clandestine ones this time; he had decided that he wanted to be with Charlotte for life, so he didn't want to rock the boat. Not that he thought there was a problem. Because Charlotte kept her sorrow private he was able to believe that it did not exist. Finding his most satisfying sex elsewhere deprived them of the best opportunity the Sensual and Emotional couple have to let down the barriers between them.

What this couple missed was the chance to draw closer after Pete's misguided first affair. Charlotte needed to let Pete know how badly she felt, and he needed to take her feelings into account and act accordingly. Emotionals can't necessarily be made to feel better by talking about the source of their emotions, but to be fully trusting they need to have it understood. It's not the emotional *interaction* that is so important to them (as it is, for instance, for the Romantic). It is the emotional *respect*. Strong feelings don't quickly fade, but the Emotional can process these better when the partner understands and values them. Charlotte, too, didn't want to rock the boat, because she loved and needed Pete. But by keeping her feelings to herself she prevented him from developing the responsiveness that can make the Sensual a better partner – and a more sensitive one.

Daniel (Emotional) and Gemma (Sensual) are a different example. They set up a business together which failed, leaving them deeply in debt. Daniel, as is common with Emotionals, had invested more than money in this venture. Emotionals rarely do anything without putting their whole hearts into it. Gemma was equally committed, and similarly devastated when they went bust, but as a pragmatic Sensual she did not give herself up to these feelings. He was plunged into a deep depression; she coped for both of them. Six months down the line, however, Daniel, who had spent time inwardly dealing with his feelings and allowing himself to 'go to pieces' was ready to put himself back together again, and was on the mend. Gemma, instead, who had endured the full blast of Daniel's feelings, and feared giving in to her own, was close to a nervous breakdown. Pushing her own feelings away had exacerbated them, and her disintegration was far harder for her to tolerate and manage than it had been for Daniel to contend with his own.

If the Emotional/Sensual couple can accept the message of these stories they can be much happier. They don't have to have endless dialogues about what they are feeling to make a difference, but they do need to have a few – and make them as honest as they can. That old saw 'a trouble shared is a trouble halved' is particularly true in their case. Both of them, in their own way, are realists who can take the bad news about a partner's feelings without backing off. The Emotional who makes the difficult transition from simply experiencing emotions to identifying and explaining them to the Sensual partner will usually find that the Sensual is motivated to make changes in the interest of more harmony between them. The Sensual always prefers peace to conflict, and can control their more selfish impulses to this end.

The Sensual, in turn, needs to be a little less good at coping, and very much better at noticing what he or she is feeling. For some, the route to this is an occasional emotional health-check of utmost simplicity: 'Do I feel sad, bad or glad?' When he or she is sure which, then a more complex analysis of what this feeling is and why it has occurred can follow. In the Emotional, the Sensual has the best partner in the world when it comes to empathising with feelings, difficult or beneficial. And if the Sensual can start the process of talking some of these feelings through with the Emotional partner, he or she will find that coping becomes easier. Controlled and restrained emotions have hidden dangers. Acknowledged and accepted emotions don't have the same disruptive power. Sensuals and Emotionals who learn to talk about their emotions when they are in love and happy, even if they don't do it very comprehensively and often, ensure a better future for themselves. If they wait until they are deadlocked and unhappy they will find it increasingly hard.

Sex in the Emotional and Sensual partnership

Although Emotionals and Sensuals bring different attitudes to sex, they share an important quality that also contributes to the long-term success of their relationship: sexual constancy. So long as their sex life suits them, they can continue to be sexually interested in a lover throughout their life together. Neither of them has a pressing need for novelty (as do Imaginatives), nor is physical shape or looks of paramount importance to them (as it is for Romantics). They can continue to feel desire for the right partner, which won't fade because of familiarity or changing physical appeal. It might diminish, it might change, but the erotic charge never disappears completely.

But the sex must suit them. For the Sensual this is a straightforward case of ensuring that love-making is physically satisfying. For the Sensual man, especially one who is not particularly sophisticated sexually, this is blissfully simple: intercourse when he wants it. The Sensual woman is less easily satisfied, as women's needs are more complex. She might need longer and slower love-making, with lots of the kind of caresses she needs to ensure that she reaches orgasm and is truly satisfied. A Sensual who has the right amount of sex, in the right way, is a happy person.

Sexual satisfaction is not such a simple matter for the Emotional. The right emotional atmosphere is equally important in sex as the actual love-making, or more so — at least for the Emotional to feel desire in the first place. According to the individual Emotional this can range from great tenderness to more complex and less seemingly happy feelings. Emotionals can also need quite specific turn-ons, in terms of scents, clothing, and sexual acts. In common with Sensuals, once Emotionals find out exactly what suits them sexually they like more of the same, and don't tire of it.

Sensuals with a high sex drive would do well to pay attention to the Emotional's sometimes strange-seeming needs, or they won't get the amount of sex they require. There has to be give and take on both sides. An Emotional man, particularly needs to understand his Sensual woman's physical needs as well as he understands his own emotional demands. If, by chance, he's into less straightforward sex, for instance, he must recognise that Ms

Sensual will only be happy to go along with this if she knows that he is also going to give her satisfaction in the way she likes.

In either combination, it is always that much harder when it is the woman who has the higher sex drive. An Emotional woman whose Sensual man does not need sex very often will find him quite stubborn and resistant to taking time to make love to her in the way she needs. It is even more delicate the other way round. An Emotional man with a lower sex drive than his Sensual woman can be turned off for quite a long time by her demands.

Emotionals, anyway, are most vulnerable to losing desire or potency when the emotional climate is wrong for them, or they are stressed or have any sort of worries. Sensuals are far less sensitive to these extraneous factors, and indeed can find sex works as a balm when there are other difficulties. There are no simple solutions for the Emotional when sexual appetite is dampened in this way.

A Sensual woman, also writing anonymously in response to my *Family Circle* survey, told her experience of this. Her opening lines express the positive side of long-term Emotional/Sensual partnerships. 'We are both in our mid-fifties and still content with each other after more than 30 years of marriage. Although I have always seemed to need sex more than my husband, for many years we had a reasonably satisfying relationship.' They had found a balance that suited them both, or, at least, for most of that time she was able to fit in with his preferences. 'He has always been reluctant to let me initiate sex and now that he's older he quite often is not moved by my approaches. As you can imagine, this causes me to feel resentment, frustration *and* unwanted! He's in a high-powered job, which involves long hours of work and a great deal of travel. In the past we used to have splendid sexy reunions. Now he's happy to cuddle me — but that's all. He has been concerned enough to buy (without telling me at first) a book on impotency, but couldn't find any relevance to himself in it

(I could: he's stressed and has been devastated when he hasn't been able to make love).'

This woman's love and concern led her to take the difficult route (for a Sensual) of discussing the problem. Like many Emotionals, her husband also found it difficult — talking never quite touches on the emotions, and neither does it relieve them. 'It was a painful conversation for him because he hates discussing his feelings. It was also painful for *me* — when he said he didn't like me kissing him! I certainly don't feel like giving up on sex yet, and I'm sure there are many wives in my position who would welcome advice on how to deal with their "proud" husband's diminishing virility. So please, please, *Family Circle*, can you help us young-at-heart women?' Actually, some of the solutions are hidden in her own question. An Emotional who is feeling stressed generally and sexually is going to find that his wife's sexual approaches, however loving, add to the pressure and turn him off further. At this stage of sensitivity even kisses can seem loaded with menacing demands. The best tactics at this stage are for her to back off completely, take the pressure off him while he is stressed and let him know that she is relaxed about the issue of resuming their love-life. This is, of course, one of the most difficult things for a sexually-interested Sensual woman to do, as she feels, in this woman's words, 'resentment, frustration *and* unwanted'.

An even more difficult problem occurs when Emotionals have developed distorted feelings about sex which take the happiness out of it. Bad relationships in the past or unpleasant sexual encounters in the Emotional's life can lead to love-hate mixed feelings about sex in which, eventually, the hate predominates.

This was the case with a couple called Helen and William, about whom I wrote in *The Relate Guide to Sex in Loving Relationships*, after I was told their story by a counsellor. Helen, the Emotional partner, had had a series of abusive and sexually violent relationships since she was 13. She had a great need for sex and climaxed easily, but she had disgusted herself with her promiscuity, and was deeply wounded by the fact that she never received love in return for sex. She met William, a kindly, reliable Sensual man when she was 28. By the time they came for counselling they had been married for 17 years and had three children. Helen had decided that she wanted no more sex. Despite the fact that William genuinely loved her and showed his love sexually, Helen was programmed to believe that sex was dirty and didn't bear any relation to love. She had needed frequent sex for most of their married life, but was quite specific about how she wanted it: William had to treat her like a prostitute, be rough, while she called out obscenities. She derived intense sexual pleasure from this, but felt disgusted afterwards. In the interests of getting the sex he needed, William went along with Helen's requirements, although he would have preferred more 'normal' sexual activity.

When Helen stopped wanting sex, William started to pester her. The counsellor suggested that he stop this, and that they agree a day and time for sex, so Helen would feel that she was making a free, unpressured choice. They said they'd try this, but they couldn't make it work. Helen would never agree on a time to have sex and William persisted in pestering her. Ultimately Helen said that they wouldn't be coming for counselling any more, and neither would she ever have sex again. She was prepared to give up something she enjoyed so intensely because it also made her feel so bad. Despite this, the counsellor had no doubt that they would stay together, even if they continued to fight about sex. This is exactly what I would expect of a Sensual and Emotional partnership. Deep commitment doesn't depend on happiness for them.

These are the sad stories. Most Emotionals have far healthier sexual requirements, and when they do they can be supremely compatible with their Sensual partners. For their continuing happiness as a couple it is even more important for them than it is for other Style combinations to get the sex right. They'll never become experts at verbal communication, but physical communion and harmony will ensure that they continue to show their deep love in a way that they can both understand.

Long-term prospects

As must be clear by now, the long-term prospects for this couple are extremely good – certainly in terms of staying together. Whether they live happily or unhappily ever after, however, depends on how well they manage their conflicts and how much effort they put into building on what is good between them.

Mr Sensual and Ms Emotional are the more comfortable pairing, in terms of how they naturally express themselves. Ms Emotional often finds motherhood answers her deepest emotional needs, so that even if she isn't obtaining quite the response she hopes for from her Sensual husband she can usually ensure she finds it in her children. Whether this is good or bad from their point of view depends on her own childhood experiences. All parents bring patterns from their past into the present with their children, but Ms Emotional is more deeply entrenched in these than other women. She is most likely to reproduce even the unlovely aspects of her own experience, however much she might determine to be different. Mr Sensual's ability to roll with the punches in life means that Ms Emotional doesn't have to be a constant support – she just needs to be there. This leaves her freer to concentrate on their children, and also on herself.

When the man is Emotional and the woman is Sensual there are similarities, but differences as well. As the steadier partner, Ms Sensual can find herself in the position of offering maternal care and love to her partner as well as her children. His capacity to be hurt, and difficulty in switching off his sensitivity in any area of his life, means that he will often find working and operating in the outside world rather draining. He needs much more succour from his partner than the Sensual man, and while he may love his children deeply he can sometimes feel that they are requisitioning the care and attention that is rightfully his.

These relationships can, of course, break down – although they will in general take much longer to do so than average. A common reason for relationship failure is the Sensual being driven beyond his or her limits of endurance. The Sensual's stoical qualities can be misinterpreted by the Emotional, who thinks that nothing much bothers or hurts the Sensual. The Sensual can become something of an emotional punchbag for the Emotional partner. There is only so much Sensuals can take, however, and when pushed too far they become rather a loose cannon emotionally. Not used to handling great anger or grief, or being too uncomfortably unhappy for too long, the Sensual can find it unbearable.

When the Emotional makes the break it is usually for different reasons. Emotionals can put up with almost anything but an absence of strong feeling. If they reach a point where they don't really care much what the Sensual says or does, the emotional vacuum is hard to tolerate. Emotionals also need a specific atmosphere that makes a relationship compelling for them. If this should change, then their feelings for their partner die. For instance, Emotionals who have a strong need to gain power through nurturing can find that if they do too good a job of it they can make themselves redundant. Such a one was Emma, of whom I heard from a counsellor. She fell for needy men – alcoholics, men with low self-esteem and so on. After a few years she always managed to rehabilitate these men, and as they became stronger she found she no longer loved them in the same way. She would move on to the next poor soul. Or there is her opposite, Clive, who was drawn to strong women, and then felt compelled to tear them down in some way. They usually left him.

Fortunately, Emotionals who are attracted to Sensuals are usually those who have a deep need for the kind of stability that this Style offers, That being so, they will be careful not to disturb the status quo if they can help it.

These two in combination can have a great love: not grand, but extremely special. Their natural preference for long-term relationships means they have all the time in the world to refine and deepen it. It's a chance that shouldn't be missed.

The Imaginative and The Sensual

'For God's sake hold your tongue, and let me love.'

John Donne

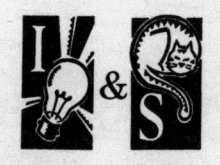

The Imaginative and The Sensual

Love often takes this couple by surprise. The Imaginative and the Sensual are perfectly capable of entering into a relationship fairly casually because they desire each other and want to go to bed together. They don't agonise too much about whether it will last, or what they have in common — mutual lust can be good enough. Mr Sensual and Mr Imaginative are particularly prone to make love first and ask questions later. Ms Imaginative and Ms Sensual may not be quite so carefree or careless, but unlike Emotional or Romantic women they have a robust attitude towards sex, and a philosophical perspective on relationships that turn out to be brief. When desire is strong, other concerns matter less.

Neither of these Sexual Styles quite trusts romantic love either. They fall in love of course, but they don't believe the feelings are reliable — at least, they don't when they are older and have experienced for themselves how deceptive they can be. But in some respects they are made for each other, and when they allow themselves to realise it a great love can grow from this initial attraction. In a way it is a quiet love — neither of them has a pressing need to be flamboyant about emotions, and both of them are happier when the emotional quality in their relationships is serene and not too intrusive.

That's one of the things that makes them compatible. But their love is also dependent on their differences. Sensuals are often captivated by the live-wires, who live life more spontaneously than they do. Ms Sensual is taken out of herself by the brilliance and energy of Mr Imaginative. Mr Sensual is thrilled by the quick-witted Ms Imaginative, who is so interested in him and so adept at understanding what he's saying, and casting a new light on his thoughts.

Imaginatives admire the steady strength of the Sensual. They like to be free and flexible, and they can be more themselves when they are partnered by someone who clears up their messes and sees to the practical side of life. Ms Imaginative feels empowered by Mr Sensual to develop herself without worrying about where she's heading. Mr Imaginative is liberated to concentrate on his intellectual considerations or pursue his interests because he knows that Ms Sensual won't let him starve or freeze to death. That said, however, the Imaginative needs to be interested in sex for the Sensual to fall in love and want the relationship to continue. And the Sensual needs to have a fine or interesting mind if the Imaginative is going to want to stay around. When these basic requirements are met, they are ready to forge a strong union.

The beginning

However intense and instant their coming together was they are likely to be cautious in every other way. They 'see how it goes'; they don't make plans too far ahead. Even when they are madly in love they don't necessarily consider it a sign of permanence, particularly when this isn't the first relationship for either of them.

The beginning of their relationship is usually characterised by plenty of highly-charged love-making. It is the way Sensuals express love best – even Sensuals who don't need a great amount of sex. Most Imaginatives find sexual exploration with a new partner exciting, and are as ready and willing as the Sensual to take every opportunity to make love. This enthusiasm and willingness, as much as anything else, is what changes the intoxication into love for the Sensuals. When a relationship feels this good, the Sensual's mind naturally turns to the future. He or she might be cautious about permanence, but permanence is precisely what the Sensual needs to be happy.

Sometimes, of course, this couple's cautious approach to the joys they are experiencing turns out to be justified. Sometimes it *is* just sexual. The Imaginative, as is his or her wont, becomes bored, and the Sensual finds that sex with this person is not as fulfilling as it could be. Neither is necessarily too hurt by this disappointment.

Often though, there is much more to it. From the Imaginative's point of view, even more exciting than good sex is the intellectual buzz of connecting mentally to the Sensual, and sharing new experiences. At this stage of the relationship the Sensual is most disposed to the kind of getting-to-know-you talking that the Imaginative values so highly. Stimulated by the Imaginative's eagerness and interest, indeed, the Sensual responds with a liveliness that can be out of character. The Sensual who wants to win the Imaginative will join in enthusiastically with the Imaginative's plans. Like any couple newly in love, time together is a happy blur of talking, love-making and activity. At this stage they are more alike than they will ever be, and they are entranced, unnerved and exhilarated by the strength of their intoxicated feelings for each other.

Settling down

Caution pays off, and they decide to live together, or marry. Usually the Sensual is the driving force in this. The Sensual knows what he or she wants, and is quite determined in the getting of it. The Imaginative is seduced into the delights of togetherness by the Sensual's ability to make it so comfortable. The Sensual woman seeps into Mr Imaginative's consciousness. He is charmed by the instinctive way she seems to know just what he needs before he knows it himself. She becomes indispensable to him.

Sexual Styles

George Bernard Shaw's couple, Eliza Doolittle (Sensual) and Professor Henry Higgins (Imaginative), are a telling caricature of this, particularly in the musical version, *My Fair Lady*. A dry, academic, confirmed bachelor, Higgins is intrigued by the cockney Eliza, who wants to learn to speak 'properly'. His intention is to teach her so well that she can pass as an upper-class lady. She moves into his house so that he can concentrate on her intensively. Eliza falls in love with him – and he with her, although he doesn't realise it until she leaves him. Then he finds he's uncomfortable without her; no one knows him quite so well, or understands his particular needs and creature comforts as she does. In the songs by Alan Jay Lerner and Frederick Loewe their different Styles are highlighted. Higgins sings 'A Hymn to Him' in which he wonders, 'Why can't a woman be more like a man?' bemoaning Eliza's irrational mind and nature – a typical Imaginative man's point of view. Eliza sings 'All I want is a room somewhere', expressing her delight in the Sensual pleasures of warmth, comfort, food, and 'someone's head resting on my knee'. In the musical there is the suggestion of a happy-ever-after ending. In Shaw's original, *Pygmalion*, the couple don't end up together, probably wisely. Eliza's education was a powerfully uniting interest. When it is over they have very little in common. Higgins didn't notice her womanly charms, and would continue to be exasperated by the intellectual disparity. Eliza would not find in him the man she craves: 'Warm and tender as he could be – who takes good care of me.'

Actually, when the woman is Sensual and the man is Imaginative, their partnership can sometimes work better than the other way around – and better than this fictional one, especially if the 'Eliza' is more interested generally in his concerns, and the 'Higgins' is less wrapped up in his own private world.

In the reverse combination – when the woman is Imaginative and the man is Sensual – she finds something seductive in his practical steadiness. She might not have had any plans to settle down, but there is something pleasurable – almost exotic – in the way that he always does what he says he'll do, turns up when he promises, constructs a lifestyle full of the agreeable details that she tends to overlook herself. She certainly wasn't searching for this kind of comfort, but now she has it she realises what she was missing before.

Ms Imaginative needs more intellectual satisfaction and congruence of interests from her Sensual partner, however, than Mr Imaginative needs from Ms Sensual. The Imaginative woman who commits herself is looking for intimacy in the way she understands it – a meeting of minds, and a friend to play with. The meeting of minds should be possible: Imaginative women often have quite a masculine cast of mind; certainly their thought-processes are less likely to be disturbed by their emotional state, and Mr Sensual often feels she is someone he can talk to, someone who will understand. The trouble is, he often doesn't feel like talking to her. Ms Imaginative can be unbearably frustrated by the fact that her intelligent, articulate Sensual partner seems to switch off as soon as he comes through his own front door – the same man who can be so witty and interesting at a dinner party. At home, he's content to lounge around and communicate in grunts. This is extremely wounding to Ms Imaginative, who, when she loves, needs to know her partner's thoughts as well as her own. When she says, 'How was your day?' She really wants to know – and in detail. She finds a one-word response, such as 'fine', or 'terrible' almost offensive.

This aspect is often less difficult for Mr Imaginative and Ms Sensual. Although some Imaginative men would also like to have a partner with whom they can share thoughts, it's not quite so central to them as it is to the Imaginative woman. They are better able to find other ways to satisfy this part of themselves – through work, other interests, and friends. This is fine for the Sensual woman who needs less stimulating interaction, and who can be content so long as he comes back to her happy and affectionate. It is harder for the Sensual woman if it means that he's rarely with her, or is isolated in his own world when he is. She doesn't need too much verbal interaction at home, but she does like cosy companionability, some affectionate touching, and, of course, a certain amount of sex.

This can be one of the stumbling blocks in the Imaginative and Sensual partnership. When Imaginative men or women feel mentally alienated from their partners they are not in the mood for physical affection. The Imaginative woman shut out of her Sensual man's thoughts is not going to be put in a favourable frame of mind by a hug, and the Imaginative man who does not find his wife interesting cannot spend a wordlessly happy time in her arms, although he might deign to have sex with her if he feels in the mood for it himself.

This is not a happy state of affairs for the Sensual, who needs affection to be shown physically in some form. This doesn't always mean sex, but without regular sexual contact there can seem to be a hollowness at the centre of the relationship. A sexually-interested Imaginative will understand why sex is important, but can find the Sensual emphasis on the physical in other ways rather incomprehensible. The Sensual's preoccupation with comfort in small things and in daily life can also seem unbearably trivial to the Imaginative. How can it matter so much?

This is related to the differences in their attitudes as to what constitutes fun. Fun, for the Imaginative, is doing lots of interesting things, getting out, meeting new people, exciting conversation and plenty of activity. From the Sensual's point of view, however, a little of this goes a very long way. Fun, for the Sensual is a small range of tried-and-tested pleasures, usually centred on the home. The occasional outing and party is quite delightful, but too much activity is unrestful and therefore irritating. New people are difficult, and certainly not so satisfying as old friends. Exciting conversation is all right in small doses, but can be wearing – and doesn't compare in satisfaction to the deep contentment of a harmonious, if quiet, evening spent with like-minded people. Indeed, to enjoy what the Imaginative enjoys, the Sensual needs plenty of relaxing calm in between. Too much stimulation will make the Sensual more resistant and mulish when out and about and in company.

Balancing these differences is important to the survival of the relationship. Actually, Sensuals need a partner like the Imaginative to get the most out of life. They are too quick to decide what they like and don't like, and to slide into a slothful, unvarying routine. The Imaginative can open doors to new pleasures for the conservative Sensual, and make the Sensual realise that life has much more to offer than he or she suspected. Similarly, it doesn't harm the Imaginative to slow down and reflect. Too much activity and a quest for novelty can inhibit them from truly appreciating what they do. With their eyes always fixed on the next pleasure, they don't derive the full satisfaction from the present one.

Indeed, some Sensual and Imaginative couples miss the opportunity to learn from each other. Instead, they go their separate ways: the Sensual at home, sometimes resentfully, the Imaginative out and about alone. This is most likely in the case of the Sensual woman and the Imaginative man. They might not be happy, but they can live for many years like this. When the Imaginative woman and the Sensual man don't try to integrate their different needs, however, the relationship is far more precarious. Mr Sensual won't be able to stand for too much independence from Ms Imaginative if he suspects she doesn't care enough for him, and if he tries to control her she may want to break free for good. In either case, too much separateness invites further dangers. The Imaginative of either sex who is too little connected to the Sensual has every chance of meeting someone new – someone more interesting. The Sensual, although not so inclined to look for someone new, might feel forced to do so if the relationship becomes lonely and barren. It's a shame if they let matters slide to this conclusion.

Equally, the relationship suffers if one of them is too dominant. A powerful Sensual who insists on life lived the way he or she prefers it will crush the Imaginative's spirit. A powerful Imaginative who drags the Sensual from pillar to post, will fill the Sensual with unbearable anxiety. It doesn't have to be like this. Fairly minor adjustments can make them very happy together – and happier in the long-term than a relationship with almost any other Sexual Style.

Daily life

The happiest couple of this combination are able to find a balance between their different needs. These needs are not so far apart as they might seem. The Sensual is not as resistant to the Imaginative's request for some stimulating conversation as he or she sometimes is to the similar-seeming Romantic's demands. Coded in the Romantic's proposals is emotional pressure to prove love, or to be the person the Romantic wants. The Imaginative, by contrast, is quite straightforward. The Sensual who is prepared to talk and open up is rewarded by the Imaginative's genuine delight. Nothing that is said is 'wrong', it must just be honest – and Sensuals are better at honesty than they are at courtliness or charm. When the Imaginative says, 'What are you thinking about?' he or she wants to know. When the Romantic asks the same question, he or she is secretly hoping that the answer is 'You!'. The bonus, from the Sensual's point of view is that the Imaginative who is interested and excited mentally, is also a more affectionate Imaginative. Indeed, for many men and women of this Style thrilling conversation is as erotic as foreplay, and increases their desire for their partners.

Similarly, the Sensual is more tolerant of the Imaginative's need for independence and interests outside the relationship than either the Romantic or the Emotional would be. The Sensual likes a happy partner, and doesn't feel threatened by a certain amount of absence so long as the Imaginative willingly returns to the family home, and is obviously still satisfied with the relationship. Being there is a good enough sign for the Sensual that love is still present.

Consequently, the Imaginative feels less threatened by the Sensual's need for a certain amount of boring togetherness at home. For the Sensual, this doesn't have to include a constant reaffirmation of love, neither does the Sensual need to feel powerfully important to the Imaginative. The physical presence of the person they love is quite enough to make Sensuals feel secure and content. The Imaginative is therefore free to read, work, or talk for hours on the telephone without feeling pressured into behaving out of character.

It helps the smooth running of their daily life that neither of them is particularly inclined to give the other a hard time. Both are happier without too much emotional tension or scenes. Sensuals might sulk a bit when things aren't going their way, and Imaginatives might do something to take their minds off it, but neither will make a big deal of matters going wrong unless they are extremely agitated or upset. In other words, they deal with it privately, and in their own way, which means that less important conflicts don't necessarily escalate out of control.

Communication between the Imaginative and the Sensual

Quite early on in the relationship the Imaginative might decide that they have a communication problem. This is when the Sensual can't seem to understand how important talking is to the Imaginative, and how intimacy for the Imaginative depends on it – particularly for Ms Imaginative. But, as has been seen, this problem can be resolved, so long as there is mental compatibility and mutuality of interests. Because the Sensual feels accepted by the Imaginative he or she is disposed to make more effort. Emotional pressure makes the Sensual retreat, genuine interest makes the Sensual bloom. When there is no such compatibility, however, there is little to be done about this difference of approach, and there will be far less happiness for them.

Actually, the *real* communication problem between them is less easy to solve, and is even more important to tackle. This is that neither of them is concerned to look particularly closely at emotional issues. Imaginatives are uncomfortable with strong feelings – their own and another person's. Sensuals are frightened that their coping abilities will suffer if they give in to their emotions. This means that unhappiness can isolate them from each other, and problems within their relationship are unlikely to be dealt with until they become severe.

What can happen – and how this can be resolved – is shown by the case of Jamie and Dawn, a couple I featured in one of my Relate books. Their relationship had lasted for many years in one of the typically unbalanced ways that can result when both partners in this combination act to type and don't adapt to each other. Dawn, the Sensual partner, was strong and steady for both of them She was a practical woman who made a lovely home, and mothered Jamie, as Sensual women tend to do. From this base, Jamie felt free to roam and indulge himself just as he wished – and what he wished for was to have plenty of exciting affairs. He enjoyed these, but they meant nothing to him. He wanted to stay with Dawn. And because the other women meant nothing, he made little attempt to cover his tracks. Dawn was always finding lipstick-stained handkerchiefs and hotel bills for two. She reacted in the Sensual way, by controlling her feelings and getting on with life. Controlling her feelings also meant controlling her tenderness. She was strict with Jamie, in her motherly way, and told him off about his affairs. Once 'punished' however, Jamie felt that the slate was wiped clean and he was free to sin again. Dawn seemed so strong. She was cross, yes – but Jamie had no idea how hurt she was. Until she left him, that is. Sensuals can put up with so much, but too much pain without an outlet is unbearable for them.

It was Jamie who dragged them both along for counselling.

He needed Dawn, and didn't want to lose her. The most important thing to emerge from the counselling was how little of their feelings they had ever shared. In the safety of the counselling room they were able to do so. Jamie had had a strict and domineering mother and had subconsciously deduced that closeness to a woman was uncomfortable. His affairs allowed him closeness that was not too close, and his behaviour had turned Dawn into a carbon-copy of his mother so that there was no real closeness there either. Imaginatives typically shield themselves from feeling too much by choosing or engineering a situation in which they don't have to. Dawn's Sensual stoicism had stopped her ever revealing how deeply hurt she was by Jamie's affairs. The turning point in the counselling came when Dawn broke down and wept on one occasion. Jamie was horrified to learn how much he had hurt her. It was a maturing moment for him to realise that his behaviour actually mattered to her — and that if he wanted to keep her he had to grow up and stop acting the little boy.

Dawn too had to realise something. When she started to weep, the counsellor had passed her a box of tissues. But she waved them away: she had brought her own. This led to a discussion about how Dawn had contributed to their difficult relationship by never showing any weakness and pretending to be strong. On a later occasion, when she cried again, she shrugged Jamie off when he tried to put his arm around her. She came to see that by hiding her vulnerability she made it easier for him to act irresponsibly.

Although facing these feelings was difficult for both of them it changed their relationship for the better. As matters improved, Dawn was able to show the tender side of her Sensual feelings, and Jamie discovered that being close to a woman could be rewarding and loving. He was confident that he would no longer need to have his casual affairs.

Sensuals and Imaginatives can learn a lesson from this couple. Sensuals can be too strong, and Imaginatives can be too flighty.

They draw closer by understanding each other better. And both have the ability to be understanding, if they try. Their emotional robustness means they are better able to tolerate what their partners tell them about their own feelings, without the over-reaction that typifies the Emotional or Romantic response. They both want serenity and happiness at home, and therefore are motivated to make changes to this end. The earlier they realise their own tendency to flee from emotions rather than facing them, and the earlier they try to fight against this tendency by talking to their partners about it, the more likely they are to develop a satisfying, long-term relationship.

Sex in the Imaginative and Sensual partnership

Sex means a lot to the Sensual, because it is important to his or her well-being and because it is a great pleasure. And, like the Imaginative, the Sensual can detach emotions from love-making. This similarity is a help when it comes to their sex life. An enthusiasm for sex on both sides can mean they have a perfectly good sexual relationship even if things aren't going too well between them. But there are important differences too. The Sensual's ability to remain emotionally detached is allied to a deep pleasure in love-making for itself — which means his or her need for sex remains fairly steady — a highly sexed Sensual will want a lot of sex, a Sensual with a lower sex drive will want it less often but fairly regularly. The Imaginative is more problematic when it comes to long-term relationships. Great sex at the beginning of the relationship doesn't necessarily mean that it will continue, sadly. The Sensual wants sex, great or not; the Imaginative is more inconsistent. The Sensual is happy to fall into a pleasing sexual routine, and will often be supremely content with a loved partner, even one who is no oil painting. For the Imaginative, on the other hand, sexual routine is anathema, and too much familiarity with a partner's sexual habits and physical appearance causes a drastic loss of desire.

The Imaginative and The Sensual

For the Imaginative to remain a willing partner therefore, there must be more variety for sex to remain interesting. A Sensual who wants to maintain the desired amount of sex in the relationship would do well to bear this in mind. Indeed, it sometimes suits them both for the Imaginative to take the initiative in what they do. The Sensual might not particularly care for some of the Imaginative's ideas on what *does* make sex interesting, but will often go along with it more equably than a Romantic or an Emotional would in the interest of keeping their sex life alive. Indeed, the Sensual who is often too quick to settle for something that feels nice, and do it over and over again, can be pleasantly surprised to find that some of the Imaginative's variations are even better.

When the man is Imaginative and the woman is Sensual it usually seems natural for him to take the lead in this way. The other way around it can be harder. Either Mr Sensual is more resistant or Ms Imaginative suffers in silence because she feels it is not her role to take charge. A sex therapist described to me a couple like this, both on their second marriage. The Imaginative woman was much more sexually experienced than her Sensual husband, but put up with his pedestrian love-making because she feared he would think her 'cheap' if she took the initiative and suggested things that she had done with other lovers. Sex therapy gave her 'permission' to expand their love-making activities, and her Sensual husband was delighted by the impact it had on their sex life. Sensuals enjoy anything that makes sex better, and for him it was a revelation.

It is harder if both of them are inexperienced, and the Imaginative woman has no idea what would make sex more exciting for her. One such woman wrote to me anonymously in response to a sex survey I devised for *Family Circle*. She had been married for 22 years to a 'wonderful, considerate and caring' Sensual. At the time of their marriage her husband was a virgin, and although she, at 24, had had a dozen previous lovers, she had never experimented much with them. Both husband and wife thought sex should always be in the 'missionary position' – anything else, she said, they thought was 'kinky'.

'When my children were young I would be very tired and because sex was a bit boring I wasn't terribly interested. We would make love maybe a couple of times a week but my husband was much keener than me.' Three years previously, however, she had met a young man. 'We became lovers and he opened up a whole new world for me. He was totally uninhibited and, with him, so was I. He introduced me to the delights of oral sex for me, and taught me lots of new positions.' Such an affair might well have put paid to the marriage for a woman of another Sexual Style, but Imaginatives are perfectly able to have sex with someone else and for their feelings to remain unaffected: 'I still loved my husband. He would have been suicidal if he had known of my affair and I never wanted to hurt him or even to be unfaithful – but that young man really enriched my life and stirred the glowing embers within me and set me alight, so I cannot feel guilty at all.' This young lover was a soldier, so they met very rarely. 'We would write letters and phone and he would tell me all the things he liked to do. Not wishing to appear ignorant I went out and bought *The Joy of Sex* – and I read some of those awful men's magazines. Part of me was really disgusted by the magazines and part of me was fascinated.'

As this experience opened up new possibilities for this woman, she shared them with her husband. 'My affair revolutionised my sex life with my husband. He just could not believe the change which had occurred in me – suddenly his wife had changed into this sex hungry woman who wanted sex every day and to try every new position she could think of. I felt, and still do feel, vibrantly alive and sexy.'

The difficulty for this woman, as with many Imaginatives, is that good sex with one person is never quite enough. She writes, 'I love my husband dearly – but in my heart I know I would like to have sex with other men to learn new things from them. He's a wonderful husband and I would want to stay married to him but I'd love to have other sexual adventures at the same time.' The affair with her young lover is over, but she has found an outlet that is almost as satisfying for the Imaginative: 'I like to hear other people's views on sex and to hear what they are doing with their partners – it gives me ideas of different things to try and I think that is good. I write to a lot of men and enjoy exchanging views about sex with them and hearing what they enjoy – that is helpful to both of us and there is safety in letters.'

Having affairs is not a recipe for contentment in this partnership, though some Imaginative men and women take this course. Sometimes they only desire sex with someone new and different, and however much they would like to feel sexual about their partners they can't. Sensuals feel fundamentally rejected if they find out that their partners have taken a lover – particulary Sensual men. Although both Mr and Ms Sensual for reasons of security might want the relationship to continue despite the infidelity, they will become unhappier, possibly depressed, and certainly withdrawn. When the withdrawal means talking and sharing even less with their partners, however, anything good that remains in the partnership is lost for both of them.

Sensuals too can have affairs that mean little to them, and might do so if their relationship is disappointing sexually. Mr Sensual can often put up with unsatisfying sex, so long as there is enough of it – but he is likely to show more interest in other women if this is the case. Ms Sensual needs sex to be more satisfying within her relationship. If she has a high sex drive as well, she will find being partnered with an Imaginative man who has less interest in sex hard to bear. On the whole, though, Sensuals much prefer to find what they need within their relationship, and can find the secrecy involved in being unfaithful very wearing and anxiety-provoking.

It's much better if they can possibly find ways of bringing back the excitement within their own relationship. Another counsellor told me about Fiona (Sensual) and Graham (Imaginative). Since the birth of their child 13 years previously their sex life had become infrequent and unsatisfying. Fiona, who came on her own for help, put it down to the fact that Graham had only wanted one child, and she felt that he was avoiding sex because of this. In fact, she wasn't seeking help about their sex life at all. As a stoical Sensual she was prepared to put up with little sex if she had to, even though she missed their love-making and knew she needed it. No, the problem, as she saw it was that Graham was a remote father. She felt her daughter was being emotionally damaged by this, and she wanted to know what to do about it. Graham had had a bad relationship with his father, which is why he was only prepared to have one child. He had handled his fear of parenthood in the typical Imaginative way — by not getting too close in case emotions were raised that he couldn't handle. Working through Fiona, however, the counsellor was able to suggest tactics that helped Graham become closer to his daughter.

While all this was going on, meanwhile, the counsellor learnt more about the couple's sex life. When it had been good, it was very good. They were married for five years before their daughter was born, and worked in tandem as travel reps, moving around the world with a holiday company, never staying anywhere longer than six months. Sex was very important to both of them at this time. Graham's Imaginative soul was stimulated by the travel, and their mutual interest in their work created an erotic charge for him. Since their child had been born they had settled in one place and rarely travelled at all. The counsellor suggested to Fiona that they should make efforts to reintroduce some of the adventurous excitement that had characterised the early part of their marriage. They started to take short holidays alone and this had a rejuvenating effect on Graham's libido and their sex life generally. Tellingly, Fiona once dropped in to say hello to the counsellor and reported that they had had a wonderfully passionate time on a walking holiday. 'You have to be resourceful and imaginative in a tent,' she explained happily.

A greater difficulty for this couple is when the Imaginative loses interest in sex altogether. This is always a possibility with Imaginatives, even those who were sexually enthusiastic earlier on in life. An Imaginative with little or no Sensual in his or her make-up, indeed, can find that sex becomes a bore once he or she has tried every sexual permutation that appeals. An Imaginative who finds sex dull is unprepared to try anything to revive interest. The Sensual may well put up with this because Sensuals, on the whole, dread breaking up a partnership, particularly one that has lasted a long time. But the relationship will suffer. However if the Imaginative is teamed with a Sensual who has a low sex drive it will matter far less. The Sensual will always look for compensatory sensual delights, where possible, and if the Imaginative also finds other elements in the relationship satisfactory, then both of them will have their own reasons for staying together.

Long-term prospects

Whenever one partner is a Sensual the relationship has a good chance of lasting. Imaginatives find it harder to make long-term relationships, because they are impelled towards the new and untried. Yet with a Sensual partner they can surprise themselves by feeling quite happy in the security of the relationship. Sensuals are possessive – but not in the suffocating way that Imaginatives perceive the Emotional or the Romantic. This is partly because they share a dislike of too much emotional relating and upheaval. With the Sensual, Imaginatives can live for long periods in the cooler emotional climate they prefer, while still receiving plenty of love. Neither needs to be powerfully in love, so they don't go in for too much introspective agonising if their relationship becomes more friendly and companionable than it is passionate.

An insecure Sensual, however, will suffer in a partnership with an Imaginative who appears to be emotionally independent. Billy and Marian are a couple like this. When they first married, Marian had become emotionally exhausted by her Imaginative lifestyle, and welcomed the steady security of her life with Billy, a wealthy, generous man. Both of them had children from previous relationships, and Marian nestled into life as Billy's wife, almost as a Sensual would do. When the children left home, however, Marian was ready to spread her wings. It wasn't much: she found a job, and started to contribute to the home. But Marian's pleasure in her job, and her new friends, unsettled Billy. He wanted her to give it up. He said he had plenty of money for their needs. What seemed like generosity now appeared suspiciously like controlling her through his money. The problem was that he didn't feel she needed him any more, and he feared she would leave him. Almost as a circumventing move, he formed a relationship with a woman who did need him, and told Marian he thought they had grown apart. Fortunately they went for counselling, and the process showed Billy that Marian loved him, even though she didn't need him in the way she once had. He finished with the other woman, and their relationship flourished satisfactorily.

Often, however, Mr Sensual is more secure and better able to tolerate Ms Imaginative's desire for some independence and separateness in their relationship. Her urge to break free, always lurking somewhere in the recesses of her heart, remains dormant because he lets her do what she must do to be happy. His desire for a relationship that is secure but not too invasive is similarly solved.

Ms Sensual and Mr Imaginative often make a more conventional pairing, and might try less to understand each other, or even to adapt to each other's needs. But this can suit very well their ideas about what a relationship should be. Where there is a genuine meeting of minds, as well as a satisfaction with the way they express their natures, however, they too can find they develop in ways that make them better individuals and more contented partners.

For, if they get it right, this can be one of the happiest, as well as one of the most enduring partnerships. The Sensual discovers more possibilities in a life that is brightened by a partner who will not allow him or her to become too entrenched. The Imaginative finds more contentment and deeper satisfaction with a partner who shows the extraordinary pleasure that can be hidden in the apparently mundane.

The Emotional and The Romantic

'Now laughing friends deride tears I cannot hide.'

Otto Harbach

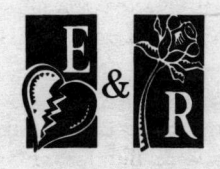

The Emotional and The Romantic

When the deep waters of the Emotional come into contact with the hurricane that is the Romantic you can expect tempests. This relationship is often the stuff of high drama: intensely passionate, full of feeling, thrills and everything but placid contentment.

The Romantic and the Emotional are both at the mercy of their emotions and both are attracted to people who understand the power of feelings to determine and change the course of life. They are drawn together by this similarity, and also, eventually, maddened and intrigued by their very differences when it comes to handling those emotions, and their dissimilar approach to life.

The Romantic is always attracted to the special. The Emotional who holds his or her attention must be good-looking, successful, talented – or dangerous and unobtainable. But the Emotional's specialness goes deeper than this – everything about the Emotional, indeed, is deep. Romantics love a challenge, and no human being is more challenging than the elusive Emotional.

Emotionals are drawn to the glittering exuberance of the Romantic. They, too, might be charmed by this person's looks, style and panache – but that's not the whole story. Emotionals are the least beguiled by appearance, even when they can appreciate the beauty of it. They are even more swayed by the Romantic's generous, happy radiance. Emotionals want some of that. Most of them are far better acquainted with the sadder more difficult side of life, and they long to taste joy – to have it as part of their experience. Perhaps, if they possessed the Romantic, they could possess the happiness too?

It is a combustible combination, and the first manifestation of this is grand and fiery love. Neither of them knows how to control overwhelming passions of any sort – and neither wants to. Both trust their instinctive attraction to other people and don't look closely at the nature of it. Love is destiny, they would say. You follow your heart where it leads – and your heart knows better than any other part of you what is right.

The beginning

Their relationship is very intense and passionate at the start. This passion might translate into great sex, but not necessarily immediately. Romantics and Emotionals who understand their own natures prefer, ideally, to wait before consummating their relationship. For Emotionals the best sex is an expression of commitment and strong feelings, and making love before they are sure can never be so satisfying to them. Romantics, too, prefer to feel that they are genuinely in love before they make love with a new partner – and although they are often sure quicker than the Emotional, they find the sex even more thrilling when they have had to wait before beginning. Indeed, Romantics and Emotionals who jump straight into bed with each other usually find that their early sexual encounters are less earth-moving than the later ones, when their feelings have developed and expanded.

Much more important and precious for both of them is the sensation that they are over-flowing with the strongest feelings they can know. Emotionals are at their happiest and freest at the beginning of a relationship when they are overwhelmed with the joy and excitement of new love. He or she *has* found the happiness that the relationship with the Romantic promised. It's hard, indeed, to tell at this stage which one *is* the Romantic. The Romantic, always in love with love, and in love with life when it is present, feels that he or she has truly found someone on the same wave-length. It all feels so wonderful and light-hearted, indeed, that neither suspects that it could be different.

Sometimes, after this glorious start, these two discover that there is a fundamental incompatibility between them. The more fun-loving Romantic finds that the particular intensity of the Emotional is of the wrong kind. An Emotional who is too gloomy or despondent can chase the Romantic off, as can a very angry or over-powerful Emotional. This kind of Romantic skips away with a sigh of relief into the waiting arms of an Imaginative, another Romantic, or even a Sensual. Or the Emotional is made too unbearably insecure by the Romantic's need to be shown love in the romantic way, or exasperated by the Romantic's inability to tolerate or understand the more complex and difficult aspects of the Emotional's nature. When their love consolidates and they stay together, therefore, it is because both are answering a deeper need in each other – and then their relationship can be very enduring.

Settling down

Some Romantics and Emotionals marry during the whirlwind excitement of new love before they have discovered whether there is a deeper compatibility. Sometimes these relationships last because of the sheer tenacity of the Emotional. Others quickly fail.

Those that go on to develop in a satisfactory way usually have a recognisable pattern, based on the Romantic's need for a relationship to involve admiration and adoration, united to the Emotional's need for a recognisable power balance, even one that is painful. Strong relationships that last for many years can be forged, in which the Romantic adores a powerful Emotional, or is adored by an Emotional who relinquishes all power to the Romantic. Because of this compelling interaction, there is great intensity, but often an absence of true closeness. This can contribute to holding the Romantic's interest because illusions remain intact – and illusion and image are important emotionally to the Romantic. Sometimes these relationships seem strange and uncomfortable, but they are deeply satisfying for the two people involved.

The best way to demonstrate this is by an example. In the following case the Romantic man's illusions seemed the reverse of romantic, but, nevertheless, that is what they were, as was clear when the relationship counsellor told me about it. Alan had come for counselling on his own, when his wife, Sadie, left him for another man. They had been married for 20 years and had a couple of children. Sadie was a deeply troubled Emotional, who suffered from crippling depressions, and early in their marriage had tried to kill herself. Alan was a Romantic who needed to adore: to feel that he was not worthy of his prize. The way he romanticised Sadie was to see her depression as a sign of deep sensitivity and fragility – quintessential femininity. He felt he had contributed to her depression by being a big, clumsy man who could not understand the depths of her suffering, and by making her pregnant and forcing her to become a mother. She had even had other affairs in the past, which had tortured Alan. But he put up with what other Romantic men would find unforgivable because it strengthened his conviction that she was the kind of woman every man would like to possess. By choosing to stay with him he was reflected in her glory.

Although the counsellor never met Sadie, it was clear from what Alan told her that Sadie enjoyed wielding power in the relationship and keeping Alan craven. She was contemptuous of him. She kept him at arm's length – which is often pleasurably maddening to Romantics, as it also means that they never have to get to know the 'real' person. Sadie had been in analysis for most of their marriage: another indicator of an Emotional. Although people of all Sexual Styles may choose analysis, the others tend to move on with it to a point at which they don't need it any more. Emotionals, however, are content not to move on — but to rehash over many years all their angst, keeping it fresh rather than learning from it and consequently changing.

Counselling forced Alan to confront his image of Sadie and to look at her more realistically. He realised that he had needed to see her as perfect, and it was uncomfortable for him to recognise that she wasn't.

Suddenly Sadie returned to Alan having broken up with the other man. The 'new' Alan said that he would only take her back if she joined in the counselling process, which she refused to do. He, in turn, refused to have her back. What would have happened if she had come for counselling is debatable. Alan's Romantic dreams were crushed; Sadie would no longer hold the same power over him. The compelling Emotional/Romantic tie that they had both contributed to keeping intact was unravelling, and it would have taken major work and commitment on both sides to keep the relationship going without it.

For relationships of this kind depend, as many of the Emotional/Emotional relationships do, on maintaining the particular tensions that keep it compelling. Romantics can tolerate discord, as Alan did, because it is a vivid and vital connection to the adored and admired partner. Romantics prefer happy and loving feelings, but they also thrive on anything that makes feelings run high.

It is these 'high' feelings that Romantics value most — excitement, love, anger, stormy sorrow — and they feel most alive when expressing them. The Romantic, indeed, mistakes these for deep feelings. But although the feelings that the Romantic is so good at letting out tend to be strong, the process of doing so leaves the emotional slate wiped clean — there's no long-term suffering involved. The deep feelings, which the Emotional knows so well, tend to be more enduring, less superficial, more painful and harder to handle and express, except in a wordless, depressive way. Because of this, indeed, the

Romantic often feels that he or she is the most emotional one in this relationship. Emoting is more dramatic and noticeable than suffering. The Romantic hates deeper feelings like this – will not tolerate them, and tries to avoid them.

So the Romantic feels invigorated and alive in a relationship that calls up these dramatic feelings, and an Emotional tests the strength of the bond by how deeply he or she feels about it. No wonder they can fit together so well. The Emotional is better than almost anyone at saying or doing things to keep a partner's feelings running high to the Romantic's satisfaction, and the Romantic's trigger-happy reactions and dramatic scenes churn up the deeper waters of the Emotional, which makes the relationship continue to seem so compelling.

Fortunately, there are also calmer Romantic/Emotional combinations than this, especially when there are grounds for genuine admiration, which can warm the core of the relationship. These are most enduring when it is the Romantic who admires the Emotional, or, best of all, when the feelings are mutual.

Daily life

The daily life of these two has the potential to be even more stormy than a pure Emotional partnership. I know one embattled couple who fight physically – or at least the Romantic wife does. She is always throwing things at her brooding Emotional husband, or hitting him – and she once pushed him down the stairs. His lack of reaction sends her demented – and although he knows this, what he needs is the fear this strikes in him, so he controls his reactions further.

In contrast, another couple of this combination I knew, who were married for many years, had a singularly peaceful life together – most of the time. The Emotional man worked quietly and very hard at home, and was subject to depression. She worked hard as well, and at home she tried to lighten the atmosphere by being charming and fun, and rarely allowing herself to become drawn into his moods. She was a Romantic who didn't like rows, and avoided them at all costs. But this controlled atmosphere is never compelling enough to hold the interest of either of these Sexual Styles. All the passion and tension of this couple's relationship was concentrated in, and provoked by, their social life.

The Emotional man purported to hate entertaining, or going to parties, or, indeed, meeting people at all. His Romantic wife loved it all. She was beautiful, vivacious and flirtatious. People loved her and were drawn to her, while her husband glowered in a corner, becoming more withdrawn and jealous by the minute. Their few rows always happened after these occasions. Both of them hated the rowing, but subconsciously sought it: it was when she knew how much he loved her and needed her; and he, as an Emotional, felt more committed when the intensity of his feelings were proved to him.

In one way or another, this pattern is often repeated in these pairings. The Romantic always needs more of a social life than the Emotional. The 'stage' of a relationship is never quite big enough for Romantics, who need other people to shine among and have fun with. Socialising is usually uncomfortable for an Emotional except on rare occasions, and on his or her terms. The Emotional, indeed, feels safest and most comfortable alone with the loved partner. The trouble is, at the beginning of the relationship Romantics feel the same; being together, alone, is all they want at this time. Unfortunately, this doesn't last, and sooner or later the Romantic will need more.

The Romantic will almost always activate the jealousy of an Emotional when they do see other people. It doesn't matter whether he or she is flirting or not — simply seeing the Romantic's sunny enthusiasm for something and someone that is not to do with their relationship causes the Emotional to suffer.

In the happiest Romantic/Emotional partnerships, the Emotional does more than tolerate the Romantic's need for this kind of fun, but recognises that it is essential for his or her happiness. Romantics who have a regular dose of glamour, excitement and fun will be at their most charming and loving to their partners – particularly while there are still plenty of good feelings between them. The more selfless Emotional is happy for the Romantic – and happier generally in consequence.

A powerful Emotional who manages to curtail their social life, in contrast, brings down the wrath of the bored and disappointed Romantic on his or her head. When there is too much stifling togetherness the Romantic seems impelled to generate the emotional fireworks that substitute for fun.

Communication between the Emotional and the Romantic

The Romantic is usually the live-wire in this partnership, and will often be the one who talks most – particularly Ms Romantic. Romantics prefer relationships which are lively, and in which there is much to say. But this is not quite so important to them as it is to the Imaginative. The Romantic needs *attention* more than interaction. He or she can put up with an Emotional partner who is less interested in conversation, so long as he or she doesn't feel ignored or over-looked. The Emotional needs to feel the compelling importance of the relationship. This is why, for both of them, good conversation can be replaced by rows when there is less harmony between them – at least the Romantic has attention, and the Emotional derives the required feeling that this is significant, if not happy.

Not surprisingly, therefore, 'communication' between them often misses the fundamental point. This couple has a lot invested in not burrowing too deep into the whys and wherefores of the relationship and sorting out any problems. It is often precisely the problems that hold the attention of both involved.

Sometimes, indeed, the relationship rests on the fact that

there is almost *no* communication. This tends to be the case when the man is Romantic and holds the power. Romantic men are more likely to look for what they need outside the relationship than are Romantic women, particularly when they are sure of the admiring, fearful love of their Emotional woman.

This was so in the case of Dan and Sally. She was an Emotional woman ready to be subservient and adoring. He was a good-looking charmer – and, when they met, he was also her boss. When Dan asked Sally to marry him, she couldn't believe her luck. Again, this story was told to me by a counsellor, who saw the couple about nine years into their marriage. Dan was having an affair, which Sally knew all about. He was tortured with guilt, and she was desperately unhappy so they came to seek help.

Sally looked years older than her age. She was very overweight. She had stopped working soon after their marriage, and stayed at home to bring up their children. This was lonely for her, and in common with other Emotionals she used food to comfort herself – since finding out about Dan's affair she had put on even more weight. Dan partly blamed Sally for his infidelity. Romantics find it hard to tolerate a partner who doesn't look good and he felt that she had given him the right to look elsewhere.

Rather unusually, the counsellor took the step of inviting the couple to see her separately – they seemed incapable of saying anything in front of each other. In actual fact she was reinforcing their usual pattern – of not really talking to each other about what was important. Dan's guilt, it transpired, had little to do with Sally, and more to do with his feelings about himself. Romantics are acutely concerned with image – their own, as well as other people's. In Dan's case, his self-image was of a fine, upright man, with magnificent self-control. Having an affair did not fit in with this image and, he admitted to the counsellor, it was not his first. Sally was pathetic and down-trodden when she spoke to the counsellor alone. She didn't know why Dan stayed with her. He was worth so much more. She also confessed to secret drinking, which, with her overeating, combined to keep her overweight, which was disgusting to Dan and disgusting to herself. He must never know; he'd despise her even more. Not surprisingly, the counsellor learnt much about this couple, but they learnt little about each other. Bound by confidentiality, she couldn't tell either of them what had been said in their absence. In the end Dan moved out to live with his mistress for a few months as a trial.

Sally was devastated. The only thing she felt that she could do was to make herself a better person to try to win him back. With obsessive Emotional tenacity, and without Dan around, Sally was able to institute and maintain a health and fitness programme to curb her eating, drinking and weight. Before the counsellor's eyes she became weekly younger, trimmer and more attractive. But having to live without Dan effected a greater change in her. The bond of humiliating dependency was inevitably weakened — and with that went her feelings of great love for Dan. He didn't seem so wonderful any more; she began to understand his subtle cruelty. Dan, for his part, on seeing the emergence of a newly glamorous and confident wife wanted to come back to her, but she wouldn't have him. The emotional point of the relationship was lost as far as she was concerned. The counsellor suspected that Dan would not have been happy with the less admiring Sally anyway: 'With Sally aware of Dan's imperfections, he would have had to confront the side of himself that he already despised.'

What makes communication difficult for this Sexual Style combination, is that neither really wants to understand emotional motivations. Indeed, the Emotional can often only do so once the motivation has gone (as in Sally's case). When they try to communicate these important matters, Emotionals don't want to find solutions to feelings, they just want them 'heard'. They want empathy and reinforcement. In contrast, the Romantic struggling with difficult feelings wants them to be magicked away — for everything to be made all right again. They both, therefore, approach each other's feelings in their own way, even when they are in love and want to help. The Emotional seeks to empathise with the Romantic — enters into strong feelings, and says how terrible they are — making the Romantic feel worse. Romantics try to jolly along the Emotional — laughing off the importance of strong and unhappy feelings. The Emotional feels misunderstood and lonely; the Romantic feels exasperated and dragged down. It's common, indeed, for such a couple to divide up the emotional life between them. The Romantic 'does' happiness, and perhaps all the volatile emotions of anger and sentiment, wilfully ignoring deeper unhappy feelings; the Emotional 'does' misery and gloom, making no attempt to lighten up or express feelings more openly.

But this couple can find that learning to understand and value each other's feelings, and coping with their own in a new way, has a revolutionising effect on their relationship. A couple I wrote about in *The Relate Guide to Better Relationships* demonstrate this. One of the interesting things about Beverley (Emotional) and Jack (Romantic) was that both of them had a similar problem which they dealt with completely differently according to the dictates of their Sexual Styles. Both had had childhood experiences that had caused them to feel lonely and excluded. Emotionals are often driven to maintain the feelings and atmosphere of these early experiences — it is what they have come to expect of life, and everything they do makes these expectations come true. Romantics, on the other hand, react to early painful experiences in the opposite way — by trying to behave in ways that make their lives happier, so that they won't have to suffer again.

Beverley was a quiet loner. In company her feelings of exclusion were amplified. She didn't try to talk to people or make friends, because she thought she would be rebuffed.

Jack was the opposite. He was a sociable creature, who made himself the life and soul of the party. Beverley initially came for counselling on her own because she was convinced that Jack was about to have an affair with the wife of a couple with whom they were friendly. This had happened once before. With both these couples Beverley had felt excluded from the merry interaction, and had sat lost in her own world while they all chatted.

Beverley talked with the counsellor about these lonely feelings, and began to see that she assumed people were leaving her out even when they weren't — often she left *herself* out by not joining in. She also told the counsellor about Jack's lonely and difficult childhood, and how left out he had been. She reported these conversations to Jack, who had never really thought about it before, but he agreed that, yes, he too had felt painfully excluded in the past. This was when he decided to join in the counselling.

This was a turning point for them, because they learnt that their different ways of handling these feelings was the sole cause of the problems between them. Jack's Romantic attempts to be happier and never feel lonely again made him gregarious in company. This made Beverley feel insecure about losing him, so she would put him down and tell him how stupid he appeared. She retreated further into her shell. This exacerbated Jack's behaviour. As a Romantic he was as much distressed by Beverley's contempt as he was by the possibility of being lonely. He became more manic, more concerned to make people like and admire him, and Beverley became gloomier and lonelier. Jack had, indeed, had one affair, but he had no intention of doing so again, nevertheless Beverley was convinced that he would do so — and exclude her again. Their clashing behaviour meant that they both felt lonely in their marriage. Beverley, in common with other Emotionals, particularly Emotional women, used food to give herself love and had become very overweight. Jack, feeling undervalued by Beverley, suspected that he was only good at making friends, and put no effort into his working life.

Sharing and understanding these feelings made a great difference. Armed with the knowledge of what they were doing to make matters worse, they started the slow process of changing how they behaved. Jack had to make every effort to include Beverley in the fun, and pay her attention when they were in company. In return she had agreed that she would not make him feel bad about being out-going, or put him down. This worked. They came for counselling for months, and the counsellor watched their happiness and confidence grow. Beverley lost weight. Jack was proud of the way she looked and how she blossomed in company – paying her attention had paid off. Jack, feeling better about himself, took a new job and became successful. Beverley's pride in him – and her admiration – meant that he was calmer and more self-contained in company. He didn't have to prove what an attractive and likable man he was any more. He knew it to be so.

Other Romantic/Emotional couples can learn from this. A compelling but unhappy interaction *can* become an attentive and loving one, so long as both want it to be so, and make the effort to understand each other and change.

Sex in the Emotional and Romantic partnership

This couple's sexual relationship is very rarely quiet, safe and predictable. Sometimes a battling relationship generates erotic tensions that make for a very steamy sex life. On the other hand, it can put one of them off – particularly the Romantic, who needs there to be something beautiful about sex to make it erotic.

A couple I know, whom I shall call Felicity and Carlos, exhibit one way in which the sexual tensions in a Romantic/Emotional partnership can manifest. They have been married for 15 stormy years. Felicity is the Romantic, and she fell in love with Carlos chiefly for his glamorous Latin looks, his exotic foreign personality and his rather effete style. He was highly intelligent and well-educated, but hadn't done much with his life by the time they met. In her Romantic way, she was convinced of his potential to be great and that one day he would look after her as his cherished wife.

Carlos came from a family dominated by powerful matriarchs, who ruled over their weak and work-shy husbands. He was attracted to Felicity for her beauty, her vivacity — and also the potential he sensed in her to be as powerful a woman as the ones in his family. At any rate, in his inimitable Emotional way, he set about turning her into such a woman. He was unreliable, rarely worked, never did what he said he would do. At first she was too in love with him to care, and she continued to think that he would change: he would become powerful, successful and rich. After their children were born, however, sheer self-preservation meant that she had to take control, work for the family, try to build a stable home life. She tried pleading with him, nagging him — and eventually bullying him into behaving more like a 'man'. This was just what Carlos subconsciously wanted, what his Emotional nature demanded, although he often appeared shell-shocked and unhappy. He certainly made no attempt to change for the better. Indeed, Carlos was obsessively in love with Felicity, and her bad treatment — so right for his Emotional expectations — only served to increase his love.

Initially their sex life had been very good. Carlos was a highly-sexed Emotional, and Felicity was a Romantic in love. While he was still her prince she desired sex as regularly as he did. He was an expert lover, with a lot of experience before he met Felicity, and he took infinite pains to make love to her so as to make it deeply physically satisfying. But, as Carlos failed to live up to Felicity's hopes and image of him, her desire for him went as well. She avoided sex as much as possible.

Eight years into their marriage, the inevitable happened:

Felicity fell madly in love with someone else, and, in the typical Romantic way, within weeks of meeting him she left home, work and Carlos, and took the children hundreds of miles to live with her new man. He was quite the opposite of Carlos. A steady, dependable widower with a well-paid job, he seemed the epitome of manliness after her feckless husband. Felicity burst like a hurricane into his life – almost unannounced. Sex with him, she confided, was 'wonderful'. But he was a poor lover, who was not very interested in sex. What made her swoon with lust was the feeling of his large body on top of her – it was so 'masterful' and she felt like a tiny, feminine woman.

In fact the relationship went wrong quite quickly. Felicity's lover's neat, ordered life was threatened by the liveliness – and mess – of her and her children. Within a few months she was back with Carlos: back working; back to being the domineering matriarch. The relationship is far from ideal, but the one thing that keeps it going for the Romantic Felicity is that Carlos does love her – deeply, unwaveringly, however she behaves. Sex is something she concedes to Carlos on occasion, but she is quite unmoved by it. His ardour, if anything, has been increased by the chain of events, and by the strict, whip-cracking wife he has turned Felicity into. She remains quietly hoping for another prince to appear and take her away from all this; perhaps when the children are grown up. It keeps her going.

As this story illustrates, for both the Romantic and the Emotional sex is as much about the atmosphere within the relationship as it is about physical pleasure. Felicity needs to feel admiring, womanly, that she has a man to take care of her. Without this no amount of careful and expert love-making can turn her on. Carlos finds cruel and domineering women erotic, and a more gentle and complaisant woman just wouldn't do.

It depends on the dynamic between the couple how their sex life works. I know another Romantic woman paired with an Emotional man, who, like Felicity, needs to feel that her man is masterful. She also needs to feel desired. The trouble is, this Emotional man, unlike Carlos uses the withdrawal of sex to punish her. When he is upset or angry, he will not touch her. He knows that this makes her feel unfeminine – which a Romantic woman finds unbearable.

The hardest thing about getting their sex life right is that the right feelings must be generated. With this couple, technique is only a minor factor in arousing desire. In other words, however good the physical sex, both will be unmoved if the atmosphere is not right. When it is, however, sex will be intensely moving and important to them. It varies in individuals and in different couples, but there are some broad similarities, at least among the Romantics. Ms Romantic must feel loved, needed and desirable. She likes to feel that her man is a man, but not too animal. Even when sex isn't that important to her, the adored Romantic woman can graciously concede sex to the worshipping Emotional – particularly if is he a bit of a hunk. Or in her adoration, she lets the powerful Emotional man do what he wants with her.

Mr Romantic needs his woman to look desirable, and to make him feel good about himself. He can adore a powerful and contemptuous Emotional woman, but he's unlikely to be able to make love to her. Neither is he able to feel good about himself if his Emotional woman makes it plain that she needs more sex than he does. Paradoxically, this can send him into the arms of another woman, simply to prove to himself that he is still a man.

Mr and Ms Emotional's needs are more complex and harder to classify. Sometimes more negative feelings can act as an aphrodisiac on them, depending on their experiences and the power of their libidos. Sex can be a great force in their lives, or be of minimal importance.

Actually, this is true of the Romantic as well. Some long and enduring partnerships of these Sexual Styles are virtually sexless, even while passions rage out of bed. Their sex life can be an exact mirror of these passions, or they can use up so much energy that love-making seems irrelevant.

Long-term prospects

As has been seen, there can be a vibrant, long-term connection between this couple that can keep the relationship alive and satisfying for both of them, even when it means there are upsets. The Emotional often acts as the anchor to the more volatile Romantic, and will do everything to keep the relationship going. This very need of the Emotional's, indeed, answers the Romantic's corresponding need to feel important and essential to one other person. Romantics are even prepared to renounce the loving happiness that they really crave when they are made to feel that their partner would be lost without them. I know of a number of long-lasting relationships of this kind, in which the Romantic is unhappy and not in love, but feels that the Emotional's life almost depends on the relationship continuing. There is a perverse satisfaction in this, touching as it does on the Romantic's belief in his or her unique specialness.

Mr Romantic and Ms Emotional often make the most comfortable and enduring relationship, particularly when she adores him. When they have children together, she can often often derive the deeper emotional gratification she needs from them. Mr Romantic often likes a firm base from which he can wander and adventure, and an adoring or forbearing Emotional wife makes him feel more secure about himself. Her jealousy or misery contributes to his good feelings about himself. They can also be very happy. The more secure the Romantic man feels, the less likely he is to want to make her jealous or miserable, and no one could be better at giving him the steadfast love he needs than a certain type of Emotional woman.

When Ms Emotional holds the power, however, this relationship can be less stable. The admiring Mr Romantic is ever-vigilant about the object of his adoration. Is she still so beautiful, so successful, so clever? If not, his devotion can waver. The most lasting relationships of this pairing, indeed, tend to be when the man romanticises wild unpredictability or emotional turmoil (as Alan, mentioned earlier, did). This aspect in her nature is likely to remain constant.

Ms Romantic and Mr Emotional can have a somewhat harder time of it. Ms Romantic needs more gratification from her central relationship than does the Romantic man, and she is less likely to try to meet her romantic needs outside the relationship. If she does so, indeed, she is also likely to leave her Emotional partner. While she can be very happy so long as he adores her, she also needs to be able to admire him in some way as well, even if it is mainly for his physique. An attractive, successful older woman, indeed, can fall for an adoring younger Emotional man, but the relationship won't last if adoration is all he has to offer. Romantic women paired with Emotional men, in fact, are more constant if they are the admirers. She can put up with his moods if he is brilliant and successful, and she will be less concerned about his physical attractiveness than would be a Romantic man. The Romantic woman in thrall to an Emotional man, however, often finds that her lighter and more frivolous side is thwarted. When he holds the power, he will dictate what they do or don't do, and usually that means less of the glamour and excitement she needs to be truly happy.

These relationships are rarely easy – but Romantics and Emotionals who are attracted to each other aren't looking for comfort. They are searching instead for the person who plays on them to activate their emotional life. With each other, the centre of their existence is rich and compelling – and, for good or bad, they know that they have to be together.